ALSO BY ELIZABETH SOMER

Age-Proof Your Body

Nutrition for a Healthy Pregnancy

Nutrition for Women

Food & Mood

The Origin Diet

The Essential Guide to Vitamins and Minerals

The Nutrition Desk Reference

The Food & Mood Cookbook

THE
Food & Mood
COOKBOOK

Recipes for Eating Well and Feeling Your Best

Elizabeth Somer, M.A., R.D., and
Jeanette Williams, R.N.

An Owl Book HENRY HOLT AND COMPANY | NEW YORK

The nutritional and health advice presented in this book is based on an in-depth
review of the current scientific literature. It is intended only as a resource
guide to help you make informed decisions; it is not meant to replace
the advice of a physician or to serve as a guide to self-treatment. Always seek
competent medical help for any health condition or if there is any question about
the appropriateness of a procedure or health recommendation.

Henry Holt and Company, LLC
Publishers since 1866
115 West 18th Street
New York, New York 10011

Henry Holt® is a registered trademark of
Henry Holt and Company, LLC.

LIBRARY OF CONGRESS CATALOGING-IN-PUBLICATION DATA

Somer, Elizabeth.
    The food & mood cookbook: recipes for eating well and
    feeling your best/Elizabeth Somer and Jeanette Williams.—
    1st ed.
        p. cm
    Includes index.
    ISBN 0-8050-7338-8
        1. Nutrition. 2. Mood (Psychology) 3. Nutritionally
    induced diseases. 4. Cookery. I. Williams, Jeanette. II. Title.
    RA784.S6468 2004   2003050825
    613.2—dc21

Henry Holt books are available for special promotions
and premiums. For details contact: Director, Special Markets.

First Edition 2004

Designed by Richard Oriolo

Printed in the United States of America

10 9 8 7 6 5 4 3

For Leah, my angel on earth and comrade in the kitchen,

and in memory of my heavenly angels, Amanda and Ben,

who especially loved the Lemon Cheesecake Piled High with Blueberries.

ELIZABETH

To my beloved father, Leo,

the Frenchman who inspired me with his

late-night creativity in the kitchen.

To my mother, Doris,

who through her love defined the true meaning

and significance of a table set for seven.

Gary, Alex, and Amy, you are my inspiration for life.

JEANETTE

▪ Contents ▪

Introduction   **xi**

Breakfasts and Breads: **Fatigue Fighters**   **1**
Why Breakfast? ▪ Smart and Happy ▪ Breakfast Eaters Are Leaner ▪
Breakfast Eaters Are Healthier ▪ Not Just When, But What ▪ Breakfast Rules ▪
Breakfast Recipes

Appetizers, Snacks, and Quick Fixes: **Eat to Relieve Stress and Improve Sleep** **29**
Stress, Hormones, and Weight Gain ▪ Stress = Nutrition Meltdown ▪
Eat to Cope and Sleep ▪ Snack When Stressed ▪ Appetizer and Snack Recipes

Lunchables and Sandwiches: **Midday Energy Boosters**   **57**
The Power Lunch ▪ Midday Fat: Don't Overdo It ▪ The Importance of Regular
Meals ▪ Ironing Out Fatigue ▪ Watch Out for the Midday Quick Fix ▪
Lunch Recipes

Soups and Stews: **Emotional Eating**   **85**
It's a Chemical Thing ▪ The Diet Connection ▪ Stuff It ▪ Check In ▪
Comfort Foods ▪ Caloric Density: The Case for Soups and Stews ▪ Soup and
Stew Recipes

Salads: **Overcoming Overeating with Truly Tasty Foods**   **113**
Flavor: A Matter of Taste and Aroma ▪ Taste, Memories, and Emotions ▪ Sifting
Fat from Flavor ▪ The Yum Factor ▪ The Golden Rules of Salads ▪ Salad Recipes

Entrées: **Taming Out-of-Control Appetites**　　　　**143**

Appetite versus Hunger ▪ Eat Less, Weigh More ▪ Simple Steps ▪ Live to Eat or Eat to Live? ▪ Entrée Recipes

Pasta, Rice, and Potato Dishes: **Carbs for PMS, SAD, and Depression**　　　**171**

Nerve Chemicals, Mood, and Cravings ▪ When a Craving Goes Bad ▪ The Common Thread in PMS, SAD, and Depression ▪ The Carb Solution ▪ Habit, Not Chemistry ▪ Pasta, Rice, and Potato Recipes

Vegetables: **Antiaging Mind Boosters**　　　　**201**

The Three Tenets of Brain Smarts ▪ Exercise Your Mind and Body ▪ Brain Food ▪ Avoid the Rust ▪ Why Your Brain Needs Antioxidants ▪ Vegetables and Fruits = Total Recall ▪ How Many Vegetables Do You Need? ▪ Vegetable Recipes

Desserts, Chocolate, and Other Sweets: **Curbing Sweet Cravings**　　　**229**

Your Sweet Origins ▪ Are You a Sugar Addict? ▪ Sugar Binge ▪ The 12-Step Program ▪ Dessert Recipes

Beverages: **Boost Energy**　　　　**259**

Why You Need Water ▪ What's Your Water Quota? ▪ Drink to Lose Weight ▪ Water versus Soda ▪ Am I Thirsty or Hungry? ▪ Have a Smoothie ▪ Beverage Recipes

Selected References　　　　**287**

Acknowledgments　　　　**301**

Index　　　　**303**

· Introduction ·

"**I NEVER KNEW** I could feel this good!" Those words continue to remind me how important what we eat is to how we feel. The woman who shared those words with me was in her mid-40s and already in good shape. She exercised, felt good, and thought she ate pretty well, but decided to make a few changes in her diet after reading my book *Food & Mood*. I met her a few weeks after she had adopted my Feeling Good Diet, and she was already enjoying even greater energy and sharper memory.

Ever since the first edition of *Food & Mood* was published in 1995, people have told me how much better they feel once they start eating in tune with their bodies' chemistry. They tell me they are sleeping better, have more energy, and feel less stressed. They are thinking more clearly and remembering more. Uncontrollable cravings for chips and chocolate no longer rule their lives. Symptoms of premenstrual syndrome (PMS), menopause, depression, and winter blues, for the first time, are manageable or have disappeared.

I'm not surprised at these reports. I've been reading the research on food and mood for about 25 years. Scientists continually report that what and when we eat has a profound effect on how we think, feel, and act. What we choose to eat affects whether or not we battle a sweet tooth, overeat, and struggle with our weight. It determines how well we cope with stress, sleep, and even whether we have the energy to get things done. Something as simple as spreading our food intake into little meals and snacks throughout the day might be all it takes to boost energy level, improve thinking, and even drop a few pounds! (One client of mine lost 30 pounds by following that one tip alone!) What's rewarding is that the research can be applied to people's lives in such simple, easy steps and still have remarkable and consistent results!

The *Food & Mood* Promise

You wouldn't dream of putting sawdust into the gas tank of your car and then expect it to run right. Yet, most Americans are eating the nutritional equivalent of sawdust, grabbing highly processed foods, skipping meals, and eating way too much fat and sugar. They wonder why they can't think straight, feel tired all the time, gain weight, and are frequently stressed out. The connection is simple. Live on chips, fast food, and soft drinks, and you function on fumes, living and enjoying only a fraction of the life you could have. Eat well and in tune with your body's chemistry, and you will be amazed at your energy level, how much quicker you think and how much more you remember, how good you feel, how well you sleep, and how little you are controlled by food cravings and insatiable appetites. Not only will you feel better, you will look your best. I promise. I've seen it over and over again during the almost ten years since *Food & Mood* was first published. I've seen it in men and women of all ages, teenagers, children, seniors, athletes, pregnant women, stressed-out workaholics, you name it.

Why a *Food & Mood Cookbook*?

People are always asking me to suggest a cookbook that reflects the guidelines of the Feeling Good Diet outlined in *Food & Mood*. I was at a loss as to what to recommend. That's why I asked Jeanette Williams to join forces with me to create a cookbook that put know-how into practice with the best mood-boosting recipes for every meal and snack, every occasion, and every craving. The recipes had to

- address all the aspects of the Feeling Good Diet,
- be simple and easy to prepare,
- taste great, and
- be incredibly satisfying, while low in calories, sugar, and saturated fat.

In other words, the recipes had to boost mood, rev energy, improve thinking, satisfy taste buds, and fill you up without filling you out. The cookbook also had to include an overview of each aspect of food and mood, not only for those who had not read *Food & Mood*, but for those who had and wanted more information.

Enjoy the Foods That Make You Feel Great

This cookbook gives you hands-on recipes and cooking tips to feel and think your best. It combines Mother Nature's super-mood foods with the best that modern food technology has to offer to cut calories without sacrificing taste. In short, the recipes that follow allow you to have your cake and eat it, too, both literally (wait until you try some of the delicious desserts!) and in terms of mood and energy levels.

But it's much more than that. We believe that food should look good, taste good, smell heavenly, as well as be good for you. The recipes in this cookbook will convince even the most stubborn skeptic that eating well doesn't mean feasting on groats and drinking wheat grass smoothies. It doesn't mean cardboard meals and hard-to-chew foods. It doesn't even have to take much time. In fact, all of the more than 200 recipes in this book will convince your taste buds that they have never had it so good! As Jeanette says, "This is jazzy-flavor fusion in action!"

The American palate is changing. Salsa now outsells ketchup, Italian food is no longer considered "ethnic," and Asian, Cuban, Latin American, and regional Mexican dishes are on many menus across the United States. What sounds adventuresome today will be mainstream recipes tomorrow. We took advantage of the wealth of new foods on the market that add zest, pizzazz, fun, and exciting and rich flavors, as well as creamy to crunchy textures to foods. We've paired interesting flavors—from fresh mint and ginger, chipotle peppers, and toasted sesame oil to garlic, cumin, curry, and more—to create feeling-great foods that taste delicious, smell yummy, and look festive. The result: You will thoroughly enjoy the foods that make you feel great!

Time: A Little Goes a Long Way

Jeanette and I are both working moms. We typically arrive home at night with only 20 minutes to create a pleasing meal for our families. We are well aware of the time crunch that many people face, which leads them to order takeout or grab a frozen entrée instead of making a home-cooked meal. It wouldn't make sense to create a cookbook designed to improve mood that only added more stress to your life with demanding, complicated, time-consuming recipes! That's why most of the recipes are quick, easy, and require a handful of ingredients that are stocked in the Food & Mood kitchen.

On the other hand, taking a little time to create a festive, feeling-good meal for you and your family should be fun. Jeanette's eyes light up when she talks about food: "My favorite childhood memories are laced with the smells of home-cooked meals and the table set for dinner." The research bears this out and shows that children from families that sit down together for a daily meal perform the best in school and are more apt to slide through those childhood years free from major emotional problems. The kitchen has always been the center of the home, a sanctuary, a gathering place. To bring that serenity into the heart of your home when preparing meals is as important an aspect of feeling good as the recipes themselves. You'll find that cooking attracts people, like moths to a flame. So put on some soothing music and relish this time, even if it's only a few minutes, to create foods that will nourish you and your family's health and mood today and in the future.

The Four Categories: Comfort, Quick, Adventurous, and Special

The *Food & Mood Cookbook* offers a wide variety of recipes for both the novice and the experienced cook. All the recipes use the freshest ingredients whenever possible, such as fresh herbs and vine-ripened tomatoes. Some recipes are classic comfort foods (you can't have a cookbook about mood without comfort foods!) that have been given a low-fat face-lift. Many recipes are quick-fix items for those days when you have only a few minutes to fuel your mood. Most of the comfort foods and quick fixes are also kid-friendly recipes. Other recipes are adventurous; they take average culinary skills to the next level with some interesting ways to pair flavors and experiment with new ethnic dishes. Finally, we've included recipes for special occasions in each category, from breakfasts, beverages, grains, and snacks to lunches, soups, salads, dinners, and desserts. These are the gourmet foods that have an added tinge of romance or elegance not typical of everyday fare.

To help you find the right recipe for your needs, we've assigned each recipe in this cookbook to one or more of these four categories, designated by capital letters that follow the recipe names.

C —COMFORT FOODS: These recipes are old favorites as you've never had them before, such as Frothy 'n' Rich Hot Chocolate; Chunky Chicken Noodle Soup; Grilled Turkey Reuben on Dark Rye;

Individual Meat Loaves with Fresh Thyme; Old-Fashioned (Low-Fat) Macaroni and Cheese; and the Ultimate Bittersweet Chocolate Pudding.

Q —QUICK FIXES: Easy-to-prepare time savers pack a mood and taste punch, such as Wake Up and Smell the Mocha Cooler; Quick Oatmeal with Bananas and Maple Syrup; Mexican Five-Layered Spread; Beans, Greens, and Roasted Garlic Soup; 1-2-3 Sloppy Joes; Shrimp Curry in a Hurry; and Busy-Day Brownies.

A —ADVENTUROUS FOODS: These innovative recipes offer a powerhouse of flavor, so you are satisfied without feeling stuffed. They include Ginger-Pumpkin Muffins; Toasted Crostini with Brie, Spicy Shrimp, and Peach Chutney; Smoky Sweet Potato 'n' Corn Chowder; Sesame Salmon and Spinach Salad with Asian Vinaigrette; Fish Fajitas with Creamy Chipotle Coleslaw; and Pan-Seared Asparagus with Gingered Onions.

S —SPECIAL OCCASIONS: The recipes in this category provide a little extra flare and are great for company or when you are looking for elegance, romance, or just a cut above the norm. The festive recipes include Peach Blush Bellinis; Bay Shrimp Omelet with Sautéed Spinach and Gruyère Cheese; Chili-Spiced Shrimp Spring Rolls; Build-Your-Own Fish Tacos; Grilled Asian Flank Steak with Wasabi Cream Sauce; Zucchini-Tomato Lasagna with Fresh Thyme and Caramelized Onions; and Low-Fat Panna Cotta with Fresh Raspberry Sauce.

Where Art Meets Science

The *Food & Mood Cookbook* presents the latest research on how eating well can help you feel your best. That's always been my forte. I love research. Call me the "Food Police" if you will, the nutrition junkie who is always concerned with healthy eating. Every recipe in this cookbook had to meet high nutritional standards to get my approval.

While I'm the Food Police, Jeanette is the "Mood Master." She continually reminds me that cooking is as much an art as a science. You learn about food and flavors by experimenting, becoming inspired by and delighted with a dish, then adding your own special touch. We both agree that you must trust your palate and feel free to change any of the recipes in this book to better suit your preferences by adding a favorite herb or spice, tinkering with the ingredients, or exchanging one vegetable for another. In short, food is as much passion as it is nutrition.

It is the blending of those two worlds—science and art—that makes this cookbook unique. May the following recipes bring you and your family and friends joy, health, good memories, and boundless energy.

Elizabeth Somer, M.A., R.D.

The Food & Mood Cookbook

Breakfasts and Breads

Fatigue Fighters

IS YOUR HOUSE a zoo in the morning? Do you scramble to get up, get coffee, get showered, get dressed, and get going? Wait a minute. Something is missing, and that something could make or break your energy, mood, and thinking all day long. It could even influence whether or not you battle a weight problem. It's breakfast.

Why Breakfast?

You probably heard the old adage: Breakfast is the most important meal of the day. Well, it's true. "Anyone, from kids to adults, who wants to function well in the morning should eat breakfast," says Barry Popkin, Ph.D., a professor of nutrition at the University of North Carolina, Chapel Hill.

The brain is fueled by glucose, which is supplied regularly throughout the day in grains, fruits, milk, and legumes. Eight to 12 hours elapse between dinner and breakfast, during which time the body uses most of its easy-to-burn glucose just keeping you alive. By morning, your brain is on red alert for a glucose fix to restock depleted fuel stores.

In an effort to persuade you to eat something, your brain releases a nerve chemical or neurotransmitter called neuropeptide Y (NPY), which triggers preferences for the best source of glucose: grains. It's no wonder that our favorite breakfast foods are toast, cereal, oatmeal, pancakes, waffles, and doughnuts! Eat a healthful breakfast, and not only do you satisfy NPY, you restock your fuel stores to maximize energy throughout the morning hours.

If you are a breakfast skipper, you're not alone. As many as 4 out of every 10 Americans skip this meal. Fifty percent of Americans eat breakfast sporadically. Granted, breakfast skippers probably begin the day with ample energy, if only because they are well rested. Just below the surface, however, they are functioning on fumes, which will take its toll by catapulting the body into metabolic stress later in the day.

Smart and Happy

Breakfast eaters reap a world of benefits. They have the best memory, thinking ability, recall, and problem-solving skills. Breakfast influences how well you learn new information and remember that information, how easily you grasp complex concepts, and how quickly you react to new stimuli. Compared with breakfast skippers, breakfast eaters score higher on intelligence tests, are more creative, have more sustained energy throughout the day, are more cheerful, and are less likely to battle fatigue. They are also calmer and less stressed. These benefits are most apparent in children and seniors, but people of other ages would profit from a morning meal as well. "Every child should eat breakfast," says David Schlundt, Ph.D., an associate professor in the Department of Psychology at Vanderbilt University in Nashville and an expert on breakfast.

Breakfast Eaters Are Leaner

People trying to lose weight skip breakfast more often than any other meal. Big mistake. Skipping breakfast is likely to add extra pounds, not help you squeeze into last year's jeans. According to the National Weight Control Registry (an ongoing study that has tracked more than 3,000 people who have successfully lost weight and kept it off for long periods of time), eating breakfast is a habit shared by people who have conquered the diet game.

How could adding an extra meal to the day's quota lead to weight loss? The 95 percent of dieters who mistakenly avoid food in the morning, thinking it will save calories, actually stack the deck in favor of eating more food, and often less healthy choices, later in the day. They gobble more fat and calories from lunchtime to bedtime than breakfast eaters consume all day long.

Skipping the morning meal upsets your appetite chemistry. NPY levels, which normally drop after breakfast, remain elevated into the afternoon hours, when they are joined by other chemicals such as serotonin. This arsenal of chemicals wages an all-out attack on your willpower, encouraging not just a snack but a binge on chips, cookies, ice cream, and other junk food. "The normal meal pattern with three meals and perhaps a snack evenly distributed throughout the day is very important for weight management. Without that consistency, irregular eating patterns develop that can lead to weight gain," says Dr. Popkin. It's not surprising that a study from Vanderbilt University found that people who ate breakfast lost more weight than did breakfast skippers.

Breakfast Eaters Are Healthier

Taking a few moments in the morning to eat breakfast makes it easier to meet your daily quota for all fatigue-fighting nutrients. A study from Cardiff University in Wales found that people who ate high-fiber breakfasts were more energized throughout the day and were less likely to battle emotional and memory problems. For one thing, breakfast eaters consume more

- folic acid (aids in memory and mood),

- vitamin A (improves concentration and mood swings),

- vitamin C (helps fight fatigue, depression, stress, and memory loss),

- vitamin E (important for mental function and memory),

- calcium (helps curb symptoms of premenstrual syndrome),

- B vitamins (essential for optimal thinking and good mood), and

- iron (combats fatigue and poor concentration).

According to several studies, if you skip breakfast, you never make up the difference in lost nutrients later in the day. In fact, it's downright impossible to meet your needs for fiber, vitamins, and minerals without eating at least three meals each day.

Not Just When, But What

What you eat is just as important as *when* you eat. In fact, if you are not careful, you can pack in an entire day's allotment of fat, saturated fat, cholesterol, and sodium

12 QUICK-FIX BREAKFASTS AND BREADS

1. **THE NEW YORK SPECIAL:** Toast a sesame bagel and fill it with smoked salmon, fat-free cream cheese, and slices of red onion, tomato, and green pepper. Serve with orange juice.

2. **THE ONE-MINUTE PANCAKE:** Freeze extra whole grain pancakes, reheat in the microwave, and top with fruit. Serve with low-fat milk.

3. **BLUEBERRY WAFFLES:** Toast frozen whole grain waffles and top with fat-free sour cream or yogurt and blueberries. Serve with calcium-fortified soymilk or nonfat milk.

4. **BREAKFAST PARFAIT:** Layer fruit, low-fat yogurt, and low-fat granola in a parfait glass.

5. **CANTALOUPE CUPS:** Fill half a cantaloupe with lemon yogurt and top with whole grain cereal.

6. **PEANUT BUTTER WRAPS:** Spread peanut butter on a slice of whole wheat toast, wrap around a banana, and serve with yogurt or milk.

7. **TOAST AND CREAM CHEESE:** Top a slice of whole grain raisin toast with fat-free cream cheese and apple slices. Serve with low-fat or nonfat milk.

8. **THE COMFORT BREAKFAST:** Cook oatmeal in nonfat milk and top with dried cranberries, chopped walnuts, and brown sugar. Serve with orange or grapefruit juice.

9. **POCKET BREAKFAST:** Stuff half a whole wheat pita with fat-free cottage cheese and sliced peaches or pears. Serve with orange juice.

10. **CEREAL TWIST:** Don't like whole grain cereal? Try mixing equal parts of your favorite sugar-coated cereal with a whole grain variety (such as whole wheat raisin bran, Grapenuts, shredded wheat, Kashi, or NutriGrain). Serve with fruit.

11. **PEANUT BUTTER KRISPIES:** Microwave 2 tablespoons reduced-fat peanut butter just until it starts to get runny. Pour peanut butter over 1 cup fiber-rich cereal topped with slices of banana.

12. **A BRITISH MCMUFFIN:** Top a whole grain English muffin with 1 ounce low-fat cheddar cheese and 2 thick slices of tomato. Broil until cheese melts and tomato is hot. Serve with orange juice.

before lunch. "It is a lot easier to get a healthy breakfast if you stay away from many of the typical breakfast items, such as sausage, bacon, doughnuts, and other processed foods," says Dr. Schlundt. The old-fashioned breakfast of eggs, sausage, bacon, and pancakes provides two days' worth of cholesterol, almost 50 grams of fat, and more than 1,000 calories. Even a Belgian waffle with butter and syrup can tally more fat than two Quarter Pounders.

There is also the issue of sugar. Most people wouldn't eat a candy bar for breakfast. Yet some pastries, such as an almond croissant, have more fat, sugar, and calories than two candy bars! Commercial cinnamon rolls, doughnuts, scones, and the like are basically breakfast cakes. Cereal bars and toaster pastries are more like cookies than breakfast foods.

BREAKFAST SUPERSTARS

Breakfast is a great time to load up on some diet superstars like antioxidants and polyphenols, substances in foods that protect your brain and body from damage and premature aging.

- TEA: Drink a cup of tea in the morning (green or black tea) for a dose of polyphenols.

- SOY: Soy contains compounds called isoflavones that help prevent memory loss. Drink a glass of calcium-fortified soymilk, add soymilk to pancake or waffle batter, or toss some tofu into your scrambled eggs.

- BERRIES AND DRIED PLUMS: These fruits are some of nature's best sources of antioxidants. Top waffles with blueberries, add strawberries to morning smoothies, or top cereal with chopped dried plums.

- SALMON: For breakfast? Yep. Salmon is one of the best sources of omega-3 fats that protect your brain from damage and memory loss. Add smoked salmon to a poached egg on a toasted English muffin for a healthy alternative to eggs Benedict.

- OATMEAL: The soluble fibers in oats lower heart-disease risk and help fill you up without filling you out. Cook in nonfat milk or soymilk and top with chunks of apple, maple syrup, and pecans to make a crunchy, flavor-packed, and nutrient-dense breakfast.

A quarter of your daily nutrients should come from breakfast. It's possible to build a great meal for only 400 to 500 calories, one that provides hefty doses of all the vitamins and minerals needed to boost your energy, mood, and mental ability. In fact, the best breakfast combines whole grains, low-fat or nonfat milk or yogurt, and fruit. "One of the best and healthiest breakfasts is a bowl of whole grain cereal with skim milk and fruit," recommends Dr. Popkin. No other breakfast offers so much fiber, vitamins, and minerals for so few calories and so little fat. This fiber-rich breakfast helps maintain an even blood sugar level and keeps you feeling satisfied and full throughout the morning hours. You'll stay more alert, energetic, and happier, and will be less likely to overeat as a result.

When selecting a cereal, look for varieties that supply at least 3 grams of fiber and no more than 3 grams of fat per serving. Avoid cereals that list hydrogenated fats in their ingredients list, since these fats contain *trans* fatty acids that damage arteries and contribute to heart disease. On the other hand, a type of fat called the omega-3 fats is good for both your arteries and your mood, lowering the risk for depression, memory loss, and irritability. Boost your intake of these fats by trying the Salmon Hash with Dill Cream (page 22) or by sprinkling flaxseed meal on your cereal or adding it to pancake batters.

Keep breakfast low-fat, since the benefits to energy level, mental function, weight management, and mood are noted with low-fat fare. Replace high-fat spreads like cream cheese and butter with fat-free cream cheese and all-fruit jam. Also, pay attention to portions. A serving of grain is a little less than 2 ounces, not the 4 to 5 ounces in many commercial muffins, bagels, scones, and other pastries.

Breakfast Rules

There are three simple rules for creating an energizing breakfast.

Rule 1: Combine high-quality carbohydrates with a little protein. The carbs provide the fuel your brain needs to function and the protein helps you feel full and energized longer. A rule of thumb is to include:

- two fruits or vegetables like a glass of orange juice and a banana;

- one protein like a glass of milk or a cup of yogurt, a slice of low-fat cheese, 2 ounces of turkey ham, or an egg; and

- one to three carbohydrate-rich foods like whole grain cereal, toast, or waffles.

Some examples of these combinations are:

- Pocket Breakfast: Scramble eggs with a little low-fat grated cheddar cheese, and salt and pepper to taste. Fill a whole wheat pita bread with egg mixture. Serve with orange juice.

- Pancake Wrap: Make extra pancakes on the weekend and freeze a few for during the week. Heat one of these pancakes in the microwave for two minutes, fill with a sliced banana, roll up, and top with apricot sauce or preserves and put a dollop of light whipped cream on top. Serve with low-fat milk.

- Super-Simple Breakfast: Cinnamon-raisin toast dunked in low-fat cinnamon-apple yogurt and served with 100 percent fruit juice.

Rule 2: Avoid high-sugar and high-fat breakfasts.

Rule 3: Be time savvy. Time is no excuse to skip breakfast. It only takes five minutes to prepare a good breakfast.

The recipes in this chapter fit rules 1 and 2. All are easy to fix, and some even take five minutes or less to prepare. Enjoy!

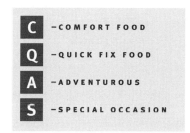

C —COMFORT FOOD

Q —QUICK FIX FOOD

A —ADVENTUROUS

S —SPECIAL OCCASION

Spinach and Ham Quiche Cups

Serve these yummy quiche cups with a slice of whole wheat toast and a glass of orange juice for an energizing, quick-fix breakfast. Freeze leftovers and briefly reheat in the microwave for instant breakfasts later in the week.

---

cooking spray

4 ounces turkey ham, minced

⅓ cup onion, minced

1 clove garlic, minced

1½ cups baby spinach, chopped

5 eggs (or use the equivalent in egg substitute)

salt (optional)

pepper

1 cup low-fat cheddar cheese, grated

baby spinach

Preheat oven to 350°. Coat 6 cups in large muffin pan with cooking spray. Spray non-stick skillet with cooking spray.

1   Sauté turkey ham, onion, and garlic until onion is translucent. Add the chopped spinach and toss until wilted, about 2 minutes. Remove from heat and divide spinach mixture among the muffin cups.

2   Whip eggs. Add salt and pepper to taste (turkey ham is salty, so go easy on added salt) and cheese. Mix until thoroughly blended.

3   Pour egg-cheese mixture over spinach mixture in cups until nearly full.

4   Bake for approximately 15 minutes or until eggs have set. Allow to stand for 2 minutes before removing from muffin cups (you might need to gently separate egg cups from pan with a knife). Place on bed of baby spinach and serve with melon or other fresh fruit.

MAKES 6 EGG CUPS

NUTRITIONAL ANALYSIS PER EGG CUP **126 calories** ▪ **47 percent fat (total fat 6.52 g, saturated fat 2.5 g)** ▪ **8 percent carbohydrate (0.5 g fiber)** ▪ **45 percent protein.**

Q

Cranberry-Orange Bread

While other fruit breads supply 160 to 200 calories a slice and up to 9 g of fat, this tasty, festive bread is 30 percent lower in calories and contains a third of the fat. It's a great gift bread, an addition to a buffet table, an appetizer for a holiday party, or a breakfast bread. Top with sugar-free marmalade or marmalade mixed with fat-free cream cheese, and serve with a glass of nonfat milk or cup of Frothy 'n' Rich Hot Chocolate (page 272).

(page 272)

MOOD TIP

Wheat germ is an excellent source of vitamin E, a nutrient that helps lower the risk for dementia and Alzheimer's disease.

cooking spray

1¾ cups all-purpose flour

⅓ cup toasted wheat germ

⅔ cup sugar

2 teaspoons baking powder

¼ teaspoon baking soda

1 tablespoon orange zest

1 teaspoon lemon zest

½ cup plus 2 tablespoons dried cranberries

1 generous cup apple butter

¼ cup canola oil

¼ cup liquid egg substitute (equivalent to 1 whole egg)

2 teaspoons vanilla extract

Heat oven to 350°. Coat bread pan with cooking spray.

1   In a large bowl, blend flour, wheat germ, sugar, baking powder, baking soda, and fruit zests with a wire whisk until thoroughly mixed. Stir in cranberries and set aside.

2   In a medium bowl, thoroughly blend apple butter, oil, egg substitute, and vanilla.

3   Add apple butter mixture to flour mixture and blend only until dry ingredients are wet.

4   Pour into bread pan. Bake for 50 minutes or until wooden toothpick inserted into center comes out clean.

5   Cool on wire rack for 10 minutes, remove from pan, and continue to cool to room temperature. Slice and serve.

MAKES 18 SLICES

NUTRITIONAL ANALYSIS PER SLICE: **158 calories** ▪ **20 percent fat (total fat 3.5 g,** saturated fat < 0.5 g) ▪ 74 percent carbohydrate (1 g fiber) ▪ 6 percent protein.

C

Very Berry Lemon Pancakes with Blueberry Sauce

To cut back on sugar, use Splenda or other sugar substitute. (This will cut 28 calories per pancake or 15 percent of the calories.) Cool extra pancakes on a cookie rack and freeze for future breakfasts. Wheat germ loads these yummy pancakes with nutrients, from vitamin E and zinc to the B vitamins. The sauce is also great on fat-free vanilla frozen yogurt.

MOOD TIP

A study from Tufts University found that blueberries (as well as strawberries and spinach) reversed age-related memory problems, including dementia. People who eat up to two cups of blueberries a day show improved short-term memory, too!

PANCAKES

cooking spray

1½ cups all-purpose flour

⅓ cup toasted wheat germ

½ teaspoon salt

3 tablespoons sugar

1¾ teaspoons double-acting baking powder

2 eggs, separated

2 tablespoons canola oil

1¼ cups nonfat milk

½ cup plain nonfat yogurt

2 teaspoons lemon extract

1½ cups blueberries (fresh or partly frozen)

fat-free sour cream (optional)

SAUCE

⅔ cup water

2 teaspoons lemon zest (grated lemon peel)

4 cups blueberries (fresh or partly frozen)

4 tablespoons sugar

⅔ cup water

2 tablespoons cornstarch

Preheat pancake griddle to approximately 380°. Coat with cooking spray.

1   With a whisk and using a large bowl, thoroughly blend flour, wheat germ, salt, sugar, and baking powder. Set aside.

2   In a medium bowl, thoroughly blend egg yolks, oil, milk, yogurt, and lemon extract. Add dry ingredients and stir until wet. (Don't over stir.) Gently blend in blueberries.

3   Beat whites until firm but not dry. Fold into pancake batter. Batter should be slightly thin.

4   Pour ½ cup of batter onto griddle for each pancake. Turn when bubbles on top begin to break.

5   To make the sauce: Heat ⅔ cup water and lemon zest in saucepan over high heat. Once the mixture reaches a boil, cook for 3 minutes to soften peel. Add blueberries

and sugar and heat through, approximately 3 minutes. Blend thoroughly ⅔ cup water and cornstarch and add to blueberries. Stir until sauce turns clear. Remove from heat.

6   Top each pancake with ¼ cup sauce and a dollop of sour cream (optional). Serve with orange juice.

MAKES 12 (5-INCH) PANCAKES AND 3 CUPS SAUCE

NUTRITIONAL ANALYSIS PER PANCAKE WITH ¼ CUP SAUCE **189 calories** ▪
18 percent fat (total fat 3.9 g, saturated fat 0.6 g) ▪ **70 percent carbohydrate (2.4 g fiber)** ▪
12 percent protein.

C

Oat 'n' Dried Plum Muffins

These multigrain muffins supply a hefty dose of antioxidants, B vitamins, calcium, iron, and magnesium and are a sweet, but nutritious, addition to breakfast or a midmorning snack. You also get a half serving of fruit in each muffin! Top with peanut butter or apricot jam and serve with a glass of nonfat milk.

MOOD TIP

In a study from Tufts University in Boston, researchers found dried plums had twice the antioxidant activity of any other fruit or vegetable studied. An antioxidant-rich diet helps prevent memory loss.

cooking spray

1¼ cups all-purpose flour

½ cup old-fashioned rolled oats

¼ cup sugar

¼ cup Splenda

¼ cup cornmeal

¼ cup toasted wheat germ

1½ teaspoons baking powder

½ teaspoon baking soda

1 teaspoon ground cinnamon

pinch of salt

1 cup packed pitted lemon-essence dried plums, chopped (approximately 30 plums)

1 cup nonfat plain yogurt

¼ cup canola oil

¼ cup liquid egg substitute (equivalent to 1 whole egg)

Heat oven to 400°. Coat a 12-muffin pan with cooking spray and set aside.

1   In a large bowl, whisk together until completely blended: flour, oats, sugar, Splenda, cornmeal, wheat germ, baking powder, baking soda, cinnamon, and salt. Set aside.

2   In a medium bowl, blend dried plums, yogurt, oil, and egg substitute. (An alternative method is to place ⅓ cup plums and rest of ingredients in blender and whip until smooth. Mix rest of chopped plums into this liquid and proceed to step 3.)

3   Make a hole in the middle of the flour mixture, pour the plum mixture into the hole and stir until dry ingredients are barely moistened.

4   Spoon batter evenly into 12 muffin cups. Bake for 15 to 18 minutes or until a toothpick inserted into middle of muffin comes out clean. Set on rack to cool.

MAKES 12 MUFFINS

NUTRITIONAL ANALYSIS PER MUFFIN **203 calories** ▪ **23 percent fat (total fat 5.2 g, saturated fat ‹ 0.5 g)** ▪ **67 percent carbohydrate (2.8 g fiber)** ▪ **10 percent protein.**

C

Baked Apple–Cinnamon Pancake

A meal in one, this pancake combines the three basic elements of a healthful breakfast: grain, low-fat milk, and fruit. It is so light, sweet, and delicate, you'll feel almost sinful, yet it is low in fat, sugar, and calories. Serve with juice or fresh fruit and a hot cup of tea, cocoa, or cider.

MOOD TIP

While apples don't hold a candle to oranges as a source of vitamin C, one study found that the phytochemical content in apples Is so high that one apple has the antioxidant equivalent of 1,000 milligrams of vitamin C.

2 tablespoons butter

3 large tart apples, peeled, cored, and thinly sliced

cooking spray

1 cup nonfat milk

1 cup liquid egg substitute (equivalent to 4 whole eggs)

3 tablespoons sugar

1 teaspoon vanilla extract

¼ teaspoon ground cinnamon

salt, to taste

⅔ cup all-purpose flour

3 tablespoons brown sugar

powdered sugar

Heat oven to 425°.

1   Place butter in 9-by-13-inch pan and place in oven until butter melts, approximately 5 minutes. Remove from oven and line bottom of pan with sliced apples, overlapping them tightly to distribute evenly. Coat with cooking spray and bake for 10 minutes or until apples are slightly tender.

2   While apples are baking, combine milk, egg substitute, sugar, vanilla, cinnamon, and salt in a medium bowl. Add flour and blend until smooth.

3   Pour milk-flour mixture over apples. Sprinkle with brown sugar and bake for 20 minutes or until sides pull away from edges and top is puffed and golden brown.

4   Let cool slightly, sprinkle with powdered sugar, and serve warm.

MAKES 4 SERVINGS

NUTRITIONAL ANALYSIS PER SERVING **339 calories** ▪ **22 percent fat (total fat 8.3 g, 4 g saturated fat)** ▪ **64 percent carbohydrate (3.1 g fiber)** ▪ **14 percent protein.**

C

Ginger-Pumpkin Muffins

A great breakfast or snack for the holidays, these muffins are also worthy of attention year-round. Serve with peanut butter or applesauce and a cup of warm milk flavored with almond extract.

cooking spray

4 plus 2 tablespoons candied ginger bits

½ cup dried cherries (or use cherry-essence dried plums, cut into bits)

2 tablespoons dark rum or 5 teaspoons water and 1 teaspoon rum extract

2 cups all-purpose flour

1 tablespoon ground ginger

2 teaspoons pumpkin spice

1½ teaspoons baking soda

pinch of salt

2 large egg whites

¼ cup liquid egg substitute (equivalent to 1 whole egg)

¾ cup canned pumpkin

½ cup low-fat buttermilk

1 teaspoon vanilla extract

¾ cup plus 1 tablespoon brown sugar

¼ cup apple butter

¼ cup canola oil

Heat oven to 375°. Coat a 12-muffin tin with cooking spray and set aside.

1   Place 4 tablespoons of the ginger bits, the dried cherries, and rum in small bowl. Blend and set aside.

2   In large bowl, mix with a wire whisk flour, ground ginger, pumpkin spice, baking soda, and salt. Set aside.

3   In small bowl, whip egg whites until frothy, but not stiff. Add egg substitute and blend. Set aside.

4   In medium bowl, blend pumpkin, buttermilk, vanilla, ¾ cup brown sugar, apple butter, and oil. Add egg mixture and blend. Fold the mixture of ginger bits, dried cherries, and rum into the batter.

5   Pour pumpkin-egg mixture into flour mixture and mix until dry ingredients are wet. (Don't overmix, since this will result in flat, tough muffins.) Divide batter evenly among 12 muffin cups.

6   Mix remaining 2 tablespoons ginger bits and 1 tablespoon brown sugar and sprinkle over tops of muffins before placing in oven. Bake for 25 minutes or until a toothpick inserted into muffin comes out clean.

MAKES 12 MUFFINS

NUTRITIONAL ANALYSIS PER MUFFIN **213 calories** ▪ **21 percent fat** (total fat 4.9 g, saturated fat ‹ 0.5 g) ▪ **69 percent carbohydrate** (1.4 g fiber) ▪ **8 percent protein**.

A

Strawberry Yogurt Pancakes with Coconut

Light, fluffy, and easy to make, these pancakes can be served for breakfast during the week or for a special weekend brunch. They are especially good when topped with fresh sliced strawberries and a dollop of reduced-fat whipped cream.

---

cooking spray

2 cups prepared/complete low-fat pancake mix (buttermilk pancake mix works best)

1⅓ cups water

1 (6-ounce) container nonfat strawberry yogurt

3 tablespoons Angel-flake coconut, sweetened

Coat griddle with cooking spray and preheat to 375°.

1 In a large bowl, combine pancake mix and water. Stir with a wire whisk. (Batter will be lumpy; do not overmix.)

2 Add yogurt and coconut. Mix to blend.

3 Pour about ¼ cup batter per pancake onto preheated griddle.

4 Cook pancakes 1 minute per side or until golden brown.

MAKES 14 4-INCH PANCAKES

NUTRITIONAL ANALYSIS PER PANCAKE (WITHOUT TOPPINGS) 45 calories ▪ 10 percent fat (total fat < 0.5 g, saturated fat 0 g) ▪ 77 percent carbohydrate (0.5 g fiber) ▪ 13 percent protein.

Whole Wheat Banana French Toast

It's well worth the effort to stop by your favorite bakery to pick up a loaf of fresh whole wheat bread for this simple wholesome breakfast. Additional sliced bananas piled on top provides a flavorful touch.

½ cup liquid egg substitute (equivalent to 2 whole eggs)

¼ cup low-fat buttermilk or fat-free half-and-half

1 teaspoon vanilla extract

½ teaspoon ground cinnamon

1 teaspoon Splenda

2 bananas, peeled and cut into 1-inch chunks

1 loaf honey wheat bread (round unsliced works best)

cooking spray

light maple syrup

1   In a shallow bowl, combine egg substitute, buttermilk, vanilla, cinnamon, and Splenda. Mix well.

2   Place bananas in a blender or food processor and blend until smooth. Pour into egg mixture. Mix well.

3   Slice bread into 8 thick slices (approximately 2 inches thick). Save remaining bread for sandwiches.

4   Heat a nonstick griddle or pan on medium high. Coat well with cooking spray.

5   Submerge each slice of bread in batter. Turn to coat each side.

6   Cook on hot grill for 3 to 5 minutes per side or until crispy brown. (The bread may stick, so spray pan again before turning over the slices). Serve hot with light maple syrup.

MAKES 8 SERVINGS

NUTRITIONAL ANALYSIS PER SERVING **132 calories** ▪ **14 percent fat (total fat 2.1 g, saturated fat < 0.5 g)** ▪ **69 percent carbohydrate (3 g fiber)** ▪ **17 percent protein.**

Ham, Cheese, and Spinach Frittata

You can add your favorite vegetables to this recipe. For example, replace the tomatoes with diced red pepper or sun-dried tomatoes, or replace the spinach with an equal amount of frozen chopped broccoli. Further cut cholesterol (from 125 to 9 milligrams) by replacing whole eggs with an equal amount of egg substitute. Serve with whole wheat toast and a glass of orange juice for breakfast, or Crusty French Bread (page 18) and a salad for lunch or dinner.

FOOD TIP

The difference between an omelet and a frittata is that you mix, rather than fold, the filling into a frittata. Frittatas can be served at room temperature, making them perfect for brunches or large groups.

cooking spray

½ cup yellow onion, diced

4 whole eggs, whipped

1 cup liquid egg substitute (equivalent to 4 eggs)

½ cup low-fat (1 percent) milk

salt and pepper, to taste

1 cup tomatoes, chopped

1 (10-ounce) package frozen chopped spinach, thawed and thoroughly drained

⅔ cup low-fat sharp cheddar cheese, grated

⅔ cup turkey ham, diced

Heat oven to 400°. Spray a 9-inch square baking dish or deep-dish pie pan with cooking spray.

1 Spray a medium, nonstick pan and place over medium heat. Add onion and sauté until transparent, approximately 5 minutes. Set aside.

2 In a medium bowl, blend eggs, egg substitute, milk, salt, and pepper. Add remaining ingredients and blend thoroughly.

3 Pour mixture into greased pan. Bake for 40 minutes or until frittata puffs and turns golden brown.

MAKES 8 SERVINGS

NUTRITIONAL ANALYSIS PER SERVING **144 calories** ▪ **39 percent fat (total fat 6.2 g, saturated fat 2 g)** ▪ **13 percent carbohydrate (1.2 g fiber)** ▪ **48 percent protein.**

Crusty French Bread

Spraying the oven with water during baking gives this classic bread an extra-crusty crust (just make sure not to squirt the oven light!). French bread goes well with any soup or salad. It is best eaten right out of the oven but also makes great sandwiches the next day. Use two-day-old leftovers for French toast or croutons.

FOOD TIP
A loaf of French bread is also called a baguette because of the traditional elongated shape of the loaf.

1 package dry yeast

1 cup warm water

2 tablespoons sugar

2⅔ cups plus ⅓ cup all-purpose flour

1 teaspoon salt

cooking spray

1 small egg white, lightly beaten

1 teaspoon water

1   In a large bowl, dissolve yeast in water. Stir in sugar and let stand for 5 minutes.

2   In a medium bowl, thoroughly blend 2⅔ cups flour and salt.

3   Slowly add flour mixture to yeast, first stirring with whisk (for first 1 cup of flour), then mixing with wooden spoon. Finish kneading dough until dough is smooth and slightly sticky. Sprinkle remaining ⅓ cup flour on clean surface, transfer dough to floured surface, and knead until all flour is incorporated and dough is smooth.

4   Coat large bowl with cooking spray, place dough in bowl, and spray top of dough. Cover with a clean towel and let rise in a warm place, free from drafts, for about 45 minutes or until dough has doubled in size. (I place the bowl on a heating pad to ensure adequate warmth in the wintertime.)

5   Punch down dough, knead four or five times to evenly distribute temperature, and shape into long, thin loaf (approximately 14 inches by 4 inches). Place on cookie sheet sprayed with cooking spray. Cover and let rise for 30 minutes or until double in size. (Again, I use a heating pad as the warmer in the winter.)

6   Preheat oven to 400°. Blend egg white and water. Set aside.

7   Uncover dough and make 4 diagonal cuts ¼-inch deep across top of loaf. Brush with egg-water mixture.

8   Bake for 20 minutes or until loaf sounds hollow when tapped. Spray sides of oven two or three times during baking with water (steam helps form crust on bread).

MAKES 15 SLICES

NUTRITIONAL ANALYSIS PER SLICE **99 calories** ▪ **2 percent fat (total fat < 0.5 g, saturated fat 0 g)** ▪ **86 percent carbohydrate (0.8 g fiber)** ▪ **12 percent protein.**

C

Breakfast Oat Scone Cake

To save time in the morning, prepare this cake the day before. Just reheat a slice or two in the microwave or toaster oven! For the best mix of carbohydrate and protein, slice scones in half like a sandwich and spread with peanut butter or low-fat cheese. Serve with mango or papaya slices and a cup of Frothy 'n' Rich Hot Chocolate (page 272).

cooking spray

½ cup plus 2 tablespoons cake flour

1 cup quick-cooking oats

⅓ cup brown sugar

2½ teaspoons baking powder

½ teaspoon salt

¼ cup butter-oil replacement*

1 large whole egg

¼ cup nonfat milk

2 tablespoons orange marmalade

1 teaspoon vanilla extract

¼ cup currants

½ cup fresh raspberries

1 teaspoon powdered sugar

Heat oven to 375°. Coat a 9-inch cake pan with cooking spray.

1   In a food processor, add cake flour, oats, brown sugar, baking powder, and salt. Pulse off and on for 30 seconds.

2   Add butter-oil replacement. Pulse off and on until mixture starts to form into a crumble.

3   In a medium bowl, mix together egg, milk, orange marmalade, vanilla, and currants. Add crumbled mixture, stir well to combine.

4   Pour into prepared cake pan. Bake for 30 minutes or until top is brown and center springs back when touched.

5   Cool in pan for 10 minutes. Place on flat plate. Cut into 8 wedges. Sprinkle with fresh raspberries and powdered sugar.

MAKES 8 SERVINGS

NUTRITIONAL ANALYSIS PER SERVING **145 calories** ▪ **14 percent fat (total fat 2.3 g, saturated fat < 1 g)** ▪ **76 percent carbohydrate (2.2 g fiber)** ▪ **10 percent protein.**

*Butter-oil replacement is a nonfat product made of dried fruit puree (water, dried plums, and apples). You can find it in the baking section of your grocery store. You also can use baby food prunes.

Quick Oatmeal with Bananas and Maple Syrup

Toasted wheat germ in this recipe adds a nutty taste and lots of brain-boosting nutrients! You can replace the bananas with your favorite fruit or berry.

3 cups nonfat milk

½ teaspoon ground cinnamon

⅛ teaspoon ground nutmeg

¼ teaspoon salt

1½ cups quick-cooking oats

¼ cup toasted wheat germ

4 tablespoons light maple syrup

1 banana, peeled and chopped

fat-free half-and-half (optional)

chopped walnuts or pecans (optional)

brown sugar (optional)

1   In a medium saucepan, add milk, cinnamon, nutmeg, and salt. Bring to a boil. Add oats and wheat germ to boiling milk and stir constantly for 3 minutes, until thick and creamy.

2   Remove from heat. Stir in maple syrup. Divide mixture evenly in four bowls and sprinkle with chopped bananas. If desired, serve with half-and-half, nuts, and/or brown sugar.

MAKES 5 SERVINGS OF APPROXIMATELY 1 CUP EACH

NUTRITIONAL ANALYSIS PER SERVING **286 calories** ▪ **10 percent fat (total fat 3.1 g, saturated fat ‹ 1 g)** ▪ **72 percent carbohydrate (4.6 g fiber)** ▪ **18 percent protein.**

Denver Egg 'n' Cheese Muffins

Satisfying and nutritious, these breakfast sandwiches take only 10 minutes to prepare. They are also a great snack or a quick lunch. Add salsa for a spicy variation. Serve with orange juice or fruit. The following makes one sandwich, so multiply ingredients according to how many sandwiches you need.

cooking spray

2 tablespoons onion, diced

2 tablespoons red bell pepper, diced

⅓ cup liquid egg substitute (equivalent to 1½ whole eggs)

pinch of dry mustard

salt and pepper, to taste

drop of Tabasco (optional)

1 whole wheat English muffin, lightly toasted

1 ounce low-fat cheddar cheese

Heat broiler.

1   In a medium nonstick skillet sprayed with cooking spray, sauté onion and pepper over medium-high heat, stirring constantly, until onion is transparent, approximately 2 minutes.

2   Lower heat to medium and add egg substitute, mustard, salt, pepper, and Tabasco if desired. Mix with onion and pepper and cook, stirring occasionally, until egg is cooked through, about 1 minute. Remove from heat.

3   Spoon egg mixture on half of toasted English muffin, spread evenly, and press down. Top with cheese.

4   Place on a cookie sheet under broiler for 1 minute or until cheese melts and just begins to bubble. Remove.

5   Top with other half of English muffin.

MAKES 1 SANDWICH

NUTRITIONAL ANALYSIS PER SANDWICH **240 calories** ▪ **22 percent fat (total fat 5.8 g, saturated fat 2 g)** ▪ **42 percent carbohydrate (4.2 g fiber)** ▪ **36 percent protein.**

Q

Salmon Hash with Dill Cream

Easy, yet rich in flavor and packed with omega-3 fats (each serving has 2 grams), this recipe is a great way to use leftover salmon, a great brunch selection, and a delightful switch from typical breakfast fare. If you're not using leftovers, the salmon can be grilled, baked, or poached, as long as you make it simple.

MOOD TIP

When researchers monitor eating habits across countries, they find that as fish consumption goes up, depression rates go down. In fact, there is a sixtyfold difference in depression rates across countries from the highest to the lowest intake of the omega-3 fats found in fish.

DILL CREAM

1 cup fat-free sour cream

2 teaspoons dried dill

1 teaspoon fresh lemon juice

pinch of salt

HASH

cooking spray

1 tablespoon canola oil

1 (28-ounce) bag frozen O'Brien Potatoes (mix of cubed potatoes and chopped onions and peppers)

1 teaspoon Dijon mustard

salt and pepper, to taste

1 pound salmon fillet, cooked

¼ cup green onions, finely chopped

1 teaspoon dried dill

1 In a medium bowl, blend all ingredients for Dill Cream. Set aside.

2 Spray a large nonstick skillet, add oil, and place over medium heat. Add potatoes once skillet is hot. Break any clumps into individual pieces and cover. Cook for 8 minutes, stirring occasionally, or until potatoes are hot. Remove cover and increase heat to medium-high. Pat down potatoes with a spatula and cook for 5 minutes, turning occasionally until potatoes are brown and beginning to crisp.

3 Mix in mustard, salt, pepper, salmon, green onions, and dill. Toss to coat thoroughly, but not to break up potatoes. Cook until heated through, approximately 2 minutes. Serve immediately and top each serving with Dill Cream. Serve remaining cream at table.

MAKES 4 SERVINGS

NUTRITIONAL ANALYSIS PER SERVING **404 calories** ▪ **34 percent fat (total fat 15 g, saturated fat 3 g)** ▪ **35 percent carbohydrate (21 g fiber)** ▪ **31 percent protein.**

Hot Polenta Cereal with Honey

Polenta, also known as corn grits, is high in fiber, and when cooked in milk, it blends carbs with protein for the perfect 5-minute breakfast.

½ teaspoon salt	2 tablespoons honey	honey to drizzle over hot cereal
3 cups nonfat milk	1 cup dry polenta	1 cup fat-free half-and-half

1   In a medium saucepan over medium-high heat, bring milk and salt to a gentle boil.

2   Whisk in polenta, reduce heat to medium-low, cover, and cook for 5 minutes. Whisk frequently, until thick and creamy.

3   Remove from heat, stir in 2 tablespoons honey.

4   Divide evenly among 4 bowls. Drizzle with honey. Top each bowl with about ¼ cup half-and-half. Serve immediately.

MAKES 4 SERVINGS OF APPROXIMATELY 1 CUP EACH

NUTRITIONAL ANALYSIS PER SERVING **246 calories** ▪ **5 percent fat (total fat 1.4 g, saturated fat 0 g)** ▪ **77 percent carbohydrate (3.4 g fiber)** ▪ **18 percent protein.**

Fresh Fruit Parfaits with Strawberry Coulis

This parfait is especially good with Ham, Cheese, and Spinach Frittata (page 17), or serve it as a dessert.

STRAWBERRY COULIS

1 cup strawberries, fresh or frozen

juice of 1 orange (add enough water to make ⅓ cup)

1 tablespoon honey

1 teaspoon Splenda

½ teaspoon almond or vanilla extract

PARFAITS

3 (6-ounce) fat-free lemon chiffon yogurts

zest of 1 medium orange

1 cup blueberries, fresh or frozen

½ cup of fresh or frozen strawberries, sliced

1 medium orange, peeled, separated into segments, and diced

1 banana, peeled and diced

⅓ cup low-fat granola of choice (maple works well)

⅓ cup fat-free whipped cream

2 teaspoons low-fat granola

1 In a blender or food processor, place all ingredients for Strawberry Coulis. Puree until smooth. Add additional orange juice or water if too thick. Cover, place in refrigerator until ready to use. (Will keep in an airtight container for up to 24 hours.)

2 In a medium bowl, mix thoroughly lemon yogurt and orange zest.

3 Add equal amounts of yogurt mixture to bottom of 4 parfait glasses, about ⅓ cup each. Layer with equal amounts of fruit, Strawberry Coulis, and granola. Continue layering until all ingredients are used. Be creative; it doesn't matter which ingredient ends up on top. Dollop with fat-free whipped cream. Garnish with a sprinkle of granola.

MAKES 4 PARFAITS

NUTRITIONAL ANALYSIS PER PARFAIT **259 calories** ▪ **8 percent fat (total fat 2.3 g, saturated fat 1.5 g)** ▪ **79 percent carbohydrate (4 g fiber)** ▪ **13 percent protein.**

S

Overnight Crunchy French Toast

Serve with fresh, sliced strawberries and low-fat maple syrup. If you can't find the recommended cereal, use cornflakes.

cooking spray

1 cup liquid egg substitute (equivalent to 4 whole eggs)

1 cup low-fat buttermilk

2 teaspoons Splenda

1 teaspoon vanilla extract

½ teaspoon ground cinnamon

¼ teaspoon salt

4 cups Crunchy Rice and Wheat Flakes with Strawberries cereal, crushed

1 loaf Ciabata bread or French bread, sliced diagonally into thick 2-inch slices (about 8 slices)

light maple syrup

fresh strawberries

Spray a flat cookie sheet or baking pan with cooking spray. Set aside.

1. In a shallow bowl, combine egg substitute, buttermilk, Splenda, vanilla, cinnamon, and salt. Mix well. Set aside.

2. Place crushed cereal in a shallow bowl.

3. Dip each slice of bread in egg mixture, turn to coat each side. Allow time for each side to absorb egg mixture. Dip bread into crushed cereal, coating both sides. Place on cookie sheet. Cover. Freeze until ready to use. (May place in Ziploc plastic bags after 1 hour of freezing time or leave French toast on cookie sheet if baking the next day.)

4. Preheat oven to 425°. Place cookie sheet with frozen French toast in oven for 25 minutes or until golden brown, turning once. Serve hot with light maple syrup and fresh strawberries.

MAKES 8 SERVINGS

NUTRITIONAL ANALYSIS PER SERVING 185 calories ▪ 12 percent fat (total fat 2.4 g, saturated fat < 1 g) ▪ 68 percent carbohydrate (1.6 g fiber) ▪ 20 percent protein.

S

Egg and Sausage Enchiladas

Low in fat and high in taste, this hearty breakfast uses turkey sausage, which has half the fat and saturated fat of pork sausage. Serve with fresh fruit slices and a Wake Up and Smell the Mocha Cooler (page 271).

---

cooking spray

½ pound turkey sausage links (cut into small 1-inch slices)

2¼ cups liquid egg substitute (equivalent to 9 whole eggs)

½ cup nonfat milk

1 (4-ounce) can diced green chilies, drained

1 (1-pound, 3-ounce) can red enchilada sauce

10 (8-inch) whole wheat tortillas

1 cup reduced-fat cheddar or Monterey Jack cheese, shredded

1 cup commercial salsa

Preheat oven to 350°. Coat a shallow 11-by-7-inch baking dish with cooking spray.

1   In a medium nonstick skillet over medium heat, brown turkey sausage until no longer pink in center, approximately 7 minutes. Stir frequently to prevent sticking. Remove sausage from pan, transfer to a plate lined with a paper towel. Wipe excess fat from pan and set aside.

2   In a medium bowl, whisk together egg substitute, milk, and green chilies. Reheat skillet used for sausage over medium-high heat. Add egg mixture and sausage and scramble until eggs set, but are still soft, stirring frequently. Set aside.

3   Pour enchilada sauce into a shallow, large bowl. Dip each tortilla in enchilada sauce to moisten and coat both sides. Place one tortilla at a time on a flat plate and spoon about ⅓ cup of egg-sausage mixture on the edge of each tortilla. Sprinkle with 1 tablespoon cheese. Roll tortilla and place seam-side down in baking dish. Repeat this process until all tortillas are filled and placed in baking dish. You will have leftover enchilada sauce.

4   Add salsa to remaining enchilada sauce and mix well. Pour evenly over enchiladas. Cover with foil and bake for 40 minutes or until enchiladas are hot and bubbly. Serve immediately.

MAKES 10 ENCHILADAS

NUTRITIONAL ANALYSIS PER ENCHILADA **288 calories** ▪ **45 percent fat (total fat 14.4 g, saturated fat 7 g)** ▪ **31 percent carbohydrate (2.6 g fiber)** ▪ **24 percent protein.**

A

Low-Fat Eggs Benedict Florentine

Hungry for a morning feast? Thinking of something creamy, rich, perhaps with a sauce? This classic breakfast dish is just for you! Serve with fresh fruit.

SAUCE

1 tablespoon reduced-fat margarine (Brummel & Brown spread made with yogurt works well)

1 tablespoon all-purpose flour

¾ cup fat-free half-and-half

¼ cup liquid egg substitute (equivalent to 1 whole egg)

2 teaspoons lemon juice

zest of 1 lemon

1 teaspoon Dijon mustard

⅛ teaspoon nutmeg

¼ teaspoon salt

¼ teaspoon pepper

EGGS BENEDICT

4 whole eggs

2 whole wheat English muffins or bagels, split and toasted

4 slices thick red tomato

2 cups cooked spinach, drained

paprika for garnish

1   Melt margarine in a small saucepan over medium heat. Blend in flour, mix well. Add half-and-half, stir continuously until mixture starts to boil. Continue to cook for 1 minute. Remove from heat. In a small bowl blend a small amount of hot mixture into egg substitute. Pour egg substitute mixture back into same saucepan, mix well. Cook and stir until mixture starts to simmer. Remove from heat, stir in lemon juice, zest of lemon, Dijon mustard, nutmeg, salt, and pepper. Keep warm until ready to use.

2   Poach eggs. In a medium saucepan or skillet add enough water to cover eggs. Bring water to a boil; then reduce to a simmer. Break each egg into a small bowl or saucer. Carefully slip egg into water. Cook about 5 minutes or until whites are firm and yolks are firm but not hard. Remove with a slotted spoon and drain off excess water.

3   To serve, place a half toasted muffin or bagel on each plate. Add 1 slice tomato, spread ¼ cup spinach evenly on tomato slice. Top with a poached egg, pour sauce over top. Garnish with a pinch of paprika. Serve immediately.

MAKES 4 SERVINGS

NUTRITIONAL ANALYSIS PER SERVING **201 calories** ▪ **26 percent fat** (total fat 5.8 g, saturated fat 1.6 g) ▪ **45 percent carbohydrate** (4.4 g fiber) ▪ **29 percent protein.**

Bay Shrimp Omelet with Sautéed Spinach and Gruyère Cheese

Crabmeat would also taste great in this omelet. Another alternative would be to replace the Gruyère cheese with several slices of fresh avocado. Serve with Fresh Fruit Parfaits with Strawberry Coulis (page 24).

---

1 teaspoon reduced-fat margarine

2 cups fresh spinach, chopped

¼ teaspoon salt

¼ teaspoon pepper

½ cup cooked salad shrimp, cleaned and patted dry

1 cup liquid egg substitute (equivalent to 4 whole eggs)

1 teaspoon cooking sherry

¼ teaspoon ground nutmeg

cooking spray

¼ cup Gruyère cheese, grated

1   Melt margarine in a nonstick large skillet over medium-high heat. Add spinach, salt, and pepper. Sauté spinach until wilted. Add shrimp and gently mix into spinach. Remove from heat. Spoon spinach-shrimp mixture into a small bowl. Keep warm.

2   In a medium bowl, whisk together egg substitute, cooking sherry, and nutmeg.

3   Coat same skillet with cooking spray and heat on medium-high. Once skillet is hot, pour egg mixture into skillet. Let egg mixture set slightly. Tilt pan, carefully lift edges of omelet with spatula, and allow uncooked portion to flow underneath cooked portion. Cook about 2 to 3 minutes or until eggs are set.

4   Spoon spinach-shrimp mixture onto half of the omelet. Sprinkle with grated cheese. Carefully loosen omelet with spatula, then fold in half. Cook for 1 minute or until cheese is melted. Slide omelet onto a plate, cut in half.

MAKES 2 SERVINGS

NUTRITIONAL ANALYSIS PER SERVING **243 calories** ▪ 39 percent fat (total fat 10 g, saturated fat 3.8 g) ▪ 6 percent carbohydrate (1.6 g fiber) ▪ 55 percent protein.

A

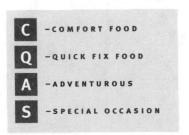

C —COMFORT FOOD

Q —QUICK FIX FOOD

A —ADVENTUROUS

S —SPECIAL OCCASION

Appetizers, Snacks, and Quick Fixes

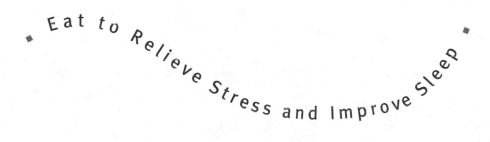

Eat to Relieve Stress and Improve Sleep

EACH OF US experiences tension in different ways and for different reasons, but we all know exactly what a friend means when she says, "I'm stressed out!" Besides tight shoulders, irritability, or a clenched jaw, day-in and day-out stress undermines our ability to sleep, wreaks havoc on our eating habits, wears down our immune systems, leading colds and disease, and even turns hormones and nerve chemicals topsy-turvy, causing weight gain, memory loss, and depression.

Stress, sleep, and diet are intertwined. For example:

- Well-nourished people handle stress and sleep better than people who neglect their diets.

- Stress upsets both nutritional status and sleep habits, while lack of sleep and/or nutrients is a stress in itself, aggravating the stress response, raising the levels of stress hormones, interfering with blood sugar regulation, and increasing the chances of illness down the road.

- People often forgo adequate sleep when they are stressed because they can't sleep. Or they cut back on zzzz's to extend their working hours.

- During maxed-out times, it's common to fall into eating habits that interfere with a good night's sleep. Add daily hassles to a body already marginally nourished, and it's likely you won't have the reserves to handle stress. Disease, premature aging, and infection can result.

- Finally, many sleep disturbances, such as sleep apnea and snoring, are caused by excess body weight brought on by stress, and are resolved when people adopt healthy eating habits that help them lose the extra pounds.

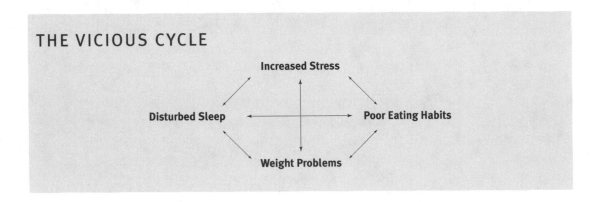

THE VICIOUS CYCLE

Increased Stress

Disturbed Sleep ← → Poor Eating Habits

Weight Problems

In short, what you eat (or don't eat) affects how well you sleep and handle stress, and whether or not stress makes you sick. It's a good idea to go into the stress war nutritionally well armed, rather than assuming you can make up for lost time once the battle begins.

Stress, Hormones, and Weight Gain

While their nutritional needs are at an all-time high, stressed-out people make the worst food choices. They chow down hamburgers, sausage pizza, French fries, and other foods high in fat, sugar, and calories. Women, in particular, turn to the sweet-and-creamy foods, such as chocolate, ice cream, and cookies. It's no surprise that these stress-triggered diets lack the nutrients the body needs to handle stress, but oversupply calories, which pack on the pounds.

Stress leads to weight gain for reasons other than food choices. The stress hormone—cortisol—encourages the body to accumulate fat, especially around the middle where it does the most harm, increasing the risk for heart disease, diabetes, high blood pressure, and other ills.

The issue here is chronic, not temporary, stress. A single bout of stress—say, you swerve to avoid a collision on the highway—causes cortisol levels to rise instantly and then return to normal. Cortisol is meant for these occasional short-lived stresses, and it was designed specifically as an "in case of emergency" hormone. In contrast, chronic stress is an unnatural state for the body that jams cortisol levels into high gear. That's where problems start.

One function of cortisol is to help the body replenish calories after a stressful experience, such as running away from an attacker, and to store those calories in the abdomen for future use. Cortisol triggers both a hike in insulin levels (insulin is a hormone that further increases appetite and fat storage) and a drop in serotonin levels (low levels of this nerve chemical increase depression, irritability, and cravings for sweets). Cortisol is useful for the occasional worry, but chronic stress bathes the body in a flood of cortisol that leads to an around-the-clock, insatiable appetite, typically for sweets and fatty foods. It also unleashes an army of free radicals that damages cells in the body and brain. You literally stew in your own juices.

Weight gain, even obesity, is strongly linked to chronic stress. In fact, nibbling, gnawing, and eating are common in all animals under stress and may be ways to release pent-up tension. Researchers at Louisiana State University found that stressed animals chew and gnaw more than calm animals, while studies on uptight people show they are more likely to chew their nails, smoke cigarettes, dive into the cookie jar, and drink more alcohol than are carefree people. The need to nosh is a strong predictor of substantial weight gain in people, according to a study from the University of Helsinki in Finland. The trick is to nibble on healthful, low-fat snacks, like the ones you'll find in this section. The right foods will protect you from stress, not add insult to injury.

Stress = Nutrition Meltdown

Stress increases requirements for several nutrients, including the B vitamins, the antioxidants such as vitamins C and E, calcium, iron, magnesium, selenium, and zinc. A diet low in any or all of these nutrients only escalates stress-caused damage to the body. For example, low vitamin C further raises cortisol levels, aggravating the stress response. In contrast, diets loaded with vitamin C–rich foods lower cortisol levels and help people cope. The same chicken-and-egg scenario plays out with magnesium, a mineral flushed out of the body during stress and which aggravates the stress response when low. Magnesium also is important for normal sleep patterns. In short, if you want to cope and sleep better, stay healthy, and keep lean, then eat well prior to and during stress.

Eat to Cope and Sleep

Eating right when you're stressed out is simple if you plan ahead and make health a priority. To break the stress cycle:

- *Cut out caffeine.* A cup of coffee or tea is tempting when you're stressed or sleep deprived. But the caffeine in these drinks, or even a glass of cola or a chocolate doughnut, can linger in the system for up to 12 hours, amping up the stress response and keeping some people awake at night. If you are troubled by sleep problems, try eliminating caffeine. If you feel and sleep better after two weeks of being caffeine-free, avoid caffeine permanently. You can add a cup or two after the two-week trial, but cut back if insomnia returns.

- *Limit or avoid alcohol.* An occasional glass of wine is relaxing, but if you drink too much, you'll sleep less soundly and awake more tired. Alcohol suppresses a phase of sleeping called REM (Rapid Eye Movement), during which most dreaming occurs. Less REM is associated with more night awakenings and restless sleep. Avoid drinking alcohol within two hours of bedtime, and *never* mix alcohol with sleeping pills!

- *Keep supper light.* Big dinners make you drowsy, but they also interfere with a good night's sleep. Instead, eat your biggest meal by midafternoon and plan a light evening meal of about 500 calories. Include some chicken, extra-lean meat, or fish at dinner to help curb middle-of-the-night snack attacks.

- *Mild foods are best.* Spicy foods, as well as dishes seasoned with garlic, chilies, cayenne, or other hot spices, can cause nagging heartburn or indigestion, while the flavor-enhancer MSG (monosodium glutamate) causes vivid dreaming and restless sleep in some people. Ingesting gas-producing foods or eating too fast causes abdominal discomfort, which interferes with sound sleep. Avoid spicy foods at dinnertime, limit intake of gas-producing foods to the morning hours, and thoroughly chew food so you don't gulp air.

- *Drink water.* When tense, many people experience dry mouth, heart palpitations, and sweating, all caused by imbalances in the nervous system that are aggravated by dehydration. Aim for at least eight glasses a day.

- *Just say "no" to sugar.* Sweets send your blood sugar on a roller-coaster ride. You might enjoy the initial high, but not the deeper tiredness and anxiety that follow. Soothe a sweet tooth with fruit, yogurt, or a bowl of whole grain cereal, and skip the processed sugary items.

- *Focus on fiber.* Fiber-rich beans, fruits, vegetables, and whole grains keep you regular at a time when you otherwise might suffer from digestive upsets and constipation.

- *Eat regularly.* When you skip meals, you only accentuate the depression, anxiety, and fatigue brought on by daily hassles or lack of sleep. Stay focused, calm, and able to cope by eating small, frequent meals and snacks, starting with breakfast.

- *Mind your vegetables.* Fruits and vegetables are loaded with antioxidants to offset cortisol's harmful effects on the body and brain. Include at least two servings at every meal and one serving at every snack. For example, snack on Mango-Pineapple Salsa (page 35) with pita bread or dip baby carrots into Creamy Hummus Dip with Fresh Tomatoes and Basil (page 39).

Snack When Stressed

Forget the three-meals-a-day rule and go for small, frequent meals and snacks when stressed. Skip meals, and you are likely to binge later. Eat small, frequent snacks, and you provide your body with a regular supply of high-quality fuel, while sidestepping the urge to overeat later in the day. Include daily one or two of the snack ideas in this section, such as a salsa or dip along with raw vegetables, as your midmorning and midafternoon snacks.

Before bedtime, choose a light evening snack as a natural alternative to sleeping pills. A high-carbohydrate snack, such as toast and jam, triggers the release of serotonin, the brain chemical that aids sleep. According to preliminary studies, a light carbohydrate-rich snack before bedtime helps some people sleep longer and more soundly. A glass of warm milk contains the building block for serotonin (i.e., the amino acid tryptophan) but is too high in protein for that building block to enter the brain. The warm liquid does soothe, relax, and provide a feeling of satiety, which might help facilitate sleep.

Need something to bite into or a way to release that tension in your jaw? Try chomping on baby carrots, apple slices, jicama sticks, raw green beans, or other crunchy vegetables dunked in any of the dips in this section, and skip the urge to snack on chips and fatty snack items.

Finally, medicate with movement. Exercise every day to "burn" up the stress hormones and relax the body for a good night's sleep. Numerous studies have found that people who exercise daily have lower stress levels than sedentary people. Exercise raises levels of natural morphinelike compounds called endorphins, chemicals in the brain that keep you calm.

All of the appetizers and snacks in this section are designed with flavor and stress-busting nutrition in mind, allowing you to get the biggest nutritional bang for your bite and to protect your body from the ravages of stress.

12 QUICK-FIX SNACKS

1. **THE EUROPEAN SNACK:** Top a slice of toasted nut bread with 1 ounce low-fat cheese and slices of a Granny Smith apple. Serve with ice water or orange juice.

2. **SWEET 'N' CREAMY:** Spread fat-free whole wheat crackers with fat-free cream cheese and top with mango chutney. Serve with calcium-fortified soymilk.

3. **VEGGIE DIP:** Munch on raw vegetables (bell peppers, broccoli, baby carrots, zucchini) dipped in fat-free ranch dressing. Serve with sparkling apple juice.

4. **HEALTHY DIPPERS:** (1) Cut whole wheat bagels into thin strips and bake at 350° for 5 minutes or until crisp; (2) split whole wheat pitas and cut each half into 8 wedges, place on a baking sheet, and bake at 400° for 8 minutes or until crisp; or (3) cut corn tortillas into 8 wedges, place on baking sheet, and bake at 350° for 9 minutes or until crisp.

5. **APPLE SNACKS:** Drizzle apple wedges with nonfat caramel sauce.

6. **CRUNCHY, CHEWY, SWEET:** Almonds stuffed into dates or pitted dried plums are a mood pleaser and alternative to candy bars.

7. **MINI-TOMATO BOWLS:** Fill hollowed-out cherry tomatoes with tuna salad, hummus, or leftover couscous.

8. **CELERY LOGS:** Stuff fresh crisp celery stalks with light Boursin cheese spread.

9. **1-MINUTE SNACK:** Top half of a toasted whole wheat bagel with 1 tablespoon fat-free strawberry cream cheese.

10. **SHRIMP ON CUCUMBER ROUNDS:** Dollop each slice of cucumber with fat-free cream cheese, add a cooked shrimp, and top with purchased cocktail sauce.

11. **FRUIT TORTILLA:** Spread fat-free cream cheese and a little all-fruit jam on a heated tortilla, fill with fresh fruit such as peach slices and strawberries, and roll into a burrito.

12. **SALT 'N' CRUNCH:** Top a whole wheat cracker with fat-free cream cheese, a slice of a Granny Smith apple, and a bread-and-butter pickle slice.

Mango-Pineapple Salsa

This sweet and spicy salsa goes well on firm fish, such as halibut or sea bass, as well as grilled shrimp. As an appetizer, serve with baked tortilla chips or thin slices of apple.

1 whole mango, peeled, pitted, and chopped into cubes

½ cup fresh pineapple, chopped into small cubes

¼ cup fresh cilantro, chopped

⅓ cup red onion, diced

⅓ cup red bell pepper, diced

1 clove garlic, minced

2 tablespoons canned diced chilies, drained

2 tablespoons fresh lime juice

salt (optional)

1   Combine all ingredients in medium bowl.

2   Cover and refrigerate for 1 hour before serving.

MAKES 2 CUPS OR 4 SERVINGS

NUTRITIONAL ANALYSIS PER SERVING 54 calories ▪ 4 percent fat (total fat ‹ 0.5 g, saturated fat 0 g) ▪ 91 percent carbohydrate (2 g fiber) ▪ 5 percent protein.

Avocado-Lime Salsa

This refreshing salsa goes well as a topping on tacos, burritos, wraps, scrambled eggs, or as a dip for baked tortilla chips.

MOOD TIP

Avocados are high in fat, but the fat is heart- and body-friendly monounsaturated fat. Research shows that including some of these fats in the diet (from nuts, seeds, olives, or avocados) helps with weight loss, possibly because they are so satisfying that we eat less later in the day.

1 large avocado, peeled, pitted, and chopped

½ cup tomato, diced

¼ cup red onion, diced

¼ cup corn (best if pan-seared until toasted)

2 tablespoons fresh cilantro, chopped

1 tablespoon fresh lime juice

1 tablespoon canned chilies, drained and diced

salt, to taste

1   Combine all ingredients in medium bowl.

2   Cover and refrigerate for 1 hour before serving.

MAKES 2 CUPS OR 4 SERVINGS

NUTRITIONAL ANALYSIS PER SERVING **102 calories** ▪ **64 percent fat (total fat 7.2 g, saturated fat 1 g)** ▪ **30 percent carbohydrate (2.5 g fiber)** ▪ **6 percent protein.**

Artichoke Dip

The buffet isn't complete without a few good dips. This one is fat-free yet tastes just like full-fat.

Serve with raw vegetables, whole grain crackers, or whole wheat pita triangles.

1 (14-ounce) can water-packed artichoke hearts, drained, finely chopped, and squeezed through strainer to remove excess fluid

¾ cup fat-free cream cheese

1 clove garlic, minced

¼ cup fat-free mayonnaise

¼ teaspoon freshly ground white pepper

salt substitute, to taste

1   In a medium bowl, blend all ingredients.

2   Combine a third of the mixture in a blender. Return to bowl and combine with mixed ingredients. Serve immediately or refrigerate before serving.

MAKES 9 SERVINGS OF 3 OUNCES EACH

NUTRITIONAL ANALYSIS PER SERVING 58 calories ▪ 3 percent fat (total fat ‹ 0.5 g, saturated fat 0 g) ▪ 48 percent carbohydrate (2.3 g fiber) ▪ 49 percent protein.

S

Black Bean Dip with Pita Wedges

A spicy, low-fat snack packed with complex carbohydrates, this dip is great for a party or an early afternoon snack.

3 cups from recipe for Black Beans with Cumin and Chipotle Peppers (page 154)

1 teaspoon lemon juice

¼ cup fat-free sour cream (optional)

1 tablespoon fresh cilantro, chopped

¼ cup salsa (optional)

1 package of whole wheat pita bread, sliced into 6 wedges per pita

1   In a food processor, puree black bean recipe and lemon juice.

2   Add some sour cream if mixture is too thick.

3   Spoon into a festive bowl, sprinkle with chopped cilantro or dollop with sour cream and salsa!

4   Serve with the pita wedges warm or at room temperature.

MAKES 6 SERVINGS

NUTRITIONAL ANALYSIS PER SERVING **242 calories** ▪ **14 percent fat (total fat 3.8 g, saturated fat ‹ 1 g)** ▪ **69 percent carbohydrate (9 g fiber)** ▪ **17 percent protein.**

C

Creamy Hummus Dip
with Fresh Tomatoes and Basil

Homemade hummus is easy to make and takes only seconds in a food processor. The result is a fresh, tasty hummus with much better flavor than store-bought versions. Try it for lunch with pita wedges and red bell pepper slices. It is especially good in the summer with fresh garden tomatoes. One serving supplies almost 3 milligrams of iron and lots of magnesium, folic acid, and B vitamins.

---

1 (15-ounce) can garbanzo beans (chick peas), rinsed and drained

1 tablespoon fresh lemon juice

2 tablespoons olive oil

2 cloves garlic, minced

pinch of cayenne pepper

¼ cup green onions, sliced thinly (green part only)

salt and pepper, to taste

1 large vine-ripe tomato, diced

2 tablespoons fresh basil, chopped

1   In a food processor, blend garbanzo beans, lemon juice, and enough water to make smooth. Add olive oil, garlic, cayenne, green onions, blend quickly to mix.

2   Spoon into a festive bowl. Season with salt and pepper.

3   Arrange diced tomatoes on top of mixture, sprinkle with fresh basil.

4   Serve with crusty bread, crackers, or toasted pita wedges.

MAKES 8 SERVINGS OF ½ CUP EACH

NUTRITIONAL ANALYSIS PER SERVING **182 calories** ▪ **28 percent fat (total fat 5.7 g, saturated fat ‹ 1 g)** ▪ **55 percent carbohydrate (6 g fiber)** ▪ **17 percent protein.**

C

Low-Fat Chunky Guacamole

Do you love guacamole but don't like the fat and calories? Try this chunky version that substitutes green peas for most of the avocado yet retains the taste and texture of the original. It has half the calories of traditional guacamole and almost 85 percent less fat (and almost no saturated fat!). Use it as a dip for baked tortilla chips, or heat up a whole wheat tortilla and fill with low-fat cheddar cheese, fresh cilantro, and a serving of this yummy guacamole for a quick-fix snack.

1½ cups frozen green peas, thawed

1 small, ripe avocado, peeled, pitted, and cut into chunks

2 tablespoons fat-free mayonnaise

1 tablespoon fresh lemon juice

¼ teaspoon cumin

¼ teaspoon chili powder

2 cloves garlic, minced

salt, to taste

1 tablespoon diced green chilies

½ cup mild or medium commercial salsa

2 tablespoons onion, diced

1 medium tomato, diced (approximately ⅔ cup)

1   In a food processor or blender, combine peas, avocado, mayonnaise, lemon juice, cumin, chili powder, garlic, and salt. Process until thoroughly blended but not completely smooth. Stop and scrape sides if needed.

2   Transfer pea mixture to medium bowl, stir in green chilies, salsa, onion, and tomato.

3   Cover and refrigerate for 1 to 2 hours to allow flavors to blend. Will keep refrigerated for up to 2 days.

MAKES APPROXIMATELY 2½ CUPS

NUTRITIONAL ANALYSIS PER ¼ CUP **49 calories** ▪ **42 percent fat (total fat 2.3 g, saturated fat < 0.5 g)** ▪ **45 percent carbohydrate (2 g fiber)** ▪ **13 percent protein.**

Grilled Polenta Rounds with Tomato Caponata

Precooked, ready-to-eat rolled polenta makes this appetizer easy to prepare. Serve as an hors d'oeuvre or as a light lunch along with a tossed salad. The caponata can be made two days in advance and stored in the refrigerator.

1½ tablespoons olive oil

1 medium eggplant, unpeeled and diced

1 small onion, chopped

½ green bell pepper, chopped

2 cloves garlic, minced

1 (14.5-ounce) can Italian tomatoes, chopped

1 teaspoon honey

1 teaspoon dried oregano

½ teaspoon dried rosemary, crushed

½ teaspoon red pepper flakes

⅛ teaspoon ground nutmeg

2 tablespoons balsamic vinegar

2 tablespoons capers, drained

1 package (18-ounce) precooked, ready-to-eat rolled polenta (basil-garlic flavored preferred)

cooking spray

Heat grill to medium-high or use a stovetop skillet to grill.

1   Warm oil in a large saucepan over medium heat. Add eggplant, onion, bell pepper, and garlic. Sauté until tender, about 5 minutes.

2   Add remaining ingredients, except for polenta. Bring to a boil, reduce heat, and simmer for 15 minutes. Remove from heat, cover, and cool. Set aside.

3   Slice precooked polenta into 12 slices. Spray both sides of polenta with a small amount of cooking spray.

4   Place polenta rounds on grill or stovetop skillet. Cook until brown on each side, about 1 to 2 minutes per side.

5   Place warm polenta rounds on a serving tray, spoon caponata on each slice, and serve. Save any leftover caponata for another use.

MAKES 12 APPETIZERS

NUTRITIONAL ANALYSIS PER APPETIZER **123 calories** ▪ **30 percent fat (total fat 4.1 g, saturated fat 1.7 g)** ▪ **58 percent carbohydrate (2.8 g fiber)** ▪ **12 percent protein.**

Roasted Corn Salsa

This colorful, refreshing side dish complements any meal or snack and is especially good with salmon, halibut, or grilled chicken. It can also can be served as an appetizer or snack with warm whole wheat tortillas.

3 cups corn, fresh or frozen

2 teaspoons olive oil

½ red bell pepper, finely diced

1 jalapeño pepper, seeded and minced

1 small tomato, chopped

juice and grated rind of 1 lime

juice and grated rind of 1 small orange

½ teaspoon cumin

¼ teaspoon salt

¼ cup fresh cilantro, chopped

Preheat oven to 350°.

1   In a medium bowl, toss corn and olive oil.

2   Spread corn on a large baking sheet. Roast for 10 minutes. Let cool.

3   Meanwhile, mix the remaining ingredients in a medium bowl. Add roasted corn. Toss well. Serve immediately or refrigerate for up to 2 days.

MAKES 3 CUPS

NUTRITIONAL ANALYSIS PER ¼ CUP **45 calories** ▪ **22 percent fat (total fat 1 g, saturated fat 0 g)** ▪ **67 percent carbohydrate (1.5 g fiber)** ▪ **11 percent protein.**

Q

Toasted Crostini with Brie, Spicy Shrimp, and Peach Chutney

Spicy, but with a hint of sweetness, the brie in this appetizer adds a creamy mellow finish. The peach chutney gives it a final kick.

---

1 (8-ounce) loaf of baguette-style French bread

¾ pound (at least 20) medium-sized shrimp, peeled and deveined

1 (4.5-ounce) round of brie cheese, cut into 20 small squares

⅓ cup peach chutney

MARINADE

1 tablespoon canned chipotle pepper in adobo sauce, finely minced

1 tablespoon adobo sauce (from same can of chipotle peppers)

2 tablespoons honey

1½ teaspoons brown sugar

Heat oven to 425°. Soak skewers in cold water for 30 minutes prior to grilling.

1   Cut French bread into 20 (½-inch-thick) slices. Place on ungreased baking sheet. Bake for about 4 minutes per side or until crisp and light brown on both sides. Remove from oven. Set aside on a plate.

2   In a medium bowl, whisk together all ingredients for the marinade.

3   Add clean, dry shrimp to marinade and toss to coat. (You can cover and refrigerate for up to 2 hours at this stage.)

4   Remove shrimp from marinade. Arrange in a single layer on a flat baking sheet. Bake for 3 to 4 minutes or until shrimp is just opaque. (Don't overcook.) Keep warm.

5   Top each slice of crostini with a piece of brie cheese and spread with a knife. Top with 1 to 2 cooked shrimp. Place on a large baking sheet. Bake until brie has melted, about 1 to 2 minutes.

6   Remove from oven, dollop each crostini with peach chutney. Arrange on a platter and serve hot.

MAKES ABOUT 20 APPETIZERS

NUTRITIONAL ANALYSIS PER APPETIZER **87 calories** ▪ **25 percent fat** (total fat 2.4 g, saturated fat 1.2 g) ▪ **48 percent carbohydrate** (0.5 g fiber) ▪ **27 percent protein.**

Thai-Grilled Prawns with Coconut Dipping Sauce

Sweet, hot, and creamy is the flavor adventure this appetizer adds to any buffet or snack. For a main course, serve over rice along with Green Beans and Toasted Slivered Almonds (page 216).

MOOD TIP

Coconut contains saturated fat, but it's a different type than is found in artery-clogging meat or fatty dairy products. The saturated fats in coconut are primarily short (artery-clogging fats are long) and are more likely to be used for energy than stored as body fat or packed into arteries.

FOOD TIP

Fresh lemongrass should be firm and pale to light green. Avoid stalks that are dry or yellow. Cut off the spiky green top and eliminate any woody core. Then use the tender heart of the stalk for cooking.

MARINADE

½ cup light coconut milk

1 teaspoon curry powder

1 teaspoon fish sauce or soy sauce

1 stalk lemongrass, trimmed and sliced into 2-inch pieces

1 teaspoon sugar

¼ cup fresh cilantro, minced

1 pound medium-sized prawns, cleaned and deveined (tiger prawns work well)

12 bamboo skewers (presoaked in cold water for 30 minutes)

SAUCE

3 tablespoons peach chutney

3 tablespoons light coconut milk

½ teaspoon curry powder

1 teaspoon fresh ginger, peeled and minced

pinch of cayenne (more for spicier flavor)

1   To prepare marinade: In a small saucepan, place coconut milk, curry, fish sauce, and lemongrass. Simmer over medium heat for 5 minutes, stirring frequently. Remove from heat, stir in sugar and cilantro. Pour into a bowl. Set aside to cool.

2   In a large plastic Ziploc bag, pour in cool marinade and prawns, and seal. Distribute marinade well, covering prawns. Place on a plate. Chill for 30 minutes or up to 1 hour.

3   Preheat grill. Remove prawns from marinade. Weave prawns onto skewers. (Several will fit on 1 skewer.)

4   Grill the prawns over a hot grill for about 2 minutes on each side. Try to keep skewers flat to grill more evenly.

5   Dipping sauce: In a small bowl, add all dipping sauce ingredients, mix well to combine. Cover and refrigerate until ready to use. Take out 15 minutes before use or store, covered, in refrigerator for 3 days.

6   To serve, place on a platter with dipping sauce in the center.

MAKES 8 APPETIZER SERVINGS

NUTRITIONAL ANALYSIS PER SERVING **80 calories** ▪ 19 percent fat (total fat 1.7 g, saturated fat 1 g) ▪ **20 percent carbohydrate (0 g fiber)** ▪ **61 percent protein.**

Tomato Chutney with Ginger

Serve this chutney with an entrée, cold as a party dip, as a spread for sandwiches, or on crostini.

1 tablespoon olive oil

2 shallots, minced

2 tablespoons fresh ginger, peeled and minced

1 clove garlic, minced

⅓ cup cider vinegar

1 (14-ounce) can stewed tomatoes, chopped

2 tablespoons brown sugar

2 tablespoons honey

1 teaspoon ground cumin

½ teaspoon ground cinnamon

¼ to ½ teaspoon cayenne

pinch of cardamom

1   Add oil to a medium saucepan and sauté shallots, ginger, and garlic for 2 minutes over medium heat.

2   Add vinegar, continue to cook for an additional minute.

3   Stir in all remaining ingredients. Reduce heat and simmer for approximately 20 minutes or until mixture is thick. Stir frequently.

4   Cool. Serve at room temperature. Chutney will keep in an airtight container in the refrigerator for up to 4 days.

MAKES 1¼ CUPS, OR 5 SERVINGS OF ¼ CUP EACH

NUTRITIONAL ANALYSIS PER SERVING **97 calories** ▪ **25 percent fat** (total fat 2.7 g, saturated fat 0 g) ▪ **71 percent carbohydrate** (1.7 g fiber) ▪ **4 percent protein**.

A S

Bruschetta with Baked Mediterranean Marinara and Goat Cheese

This delectable, attractive appetizer has an authentic rich tomato-olive flavor. Creamy goat cheese adds depth and balance to the spicy-sweet base. If you can't find this slightly upscale tomato sauce (in a jar) with other commercially prepared tomato sauces, use any thick tomato sauce that has olives, onions, peppers, and basil. The sauce and bread can be prepared the day before and stored in a Ziploc plastic bag.

---

2 cups commercial tomato sauce (Mediterranean olive with sun-dried tomatoes)

1 tablespoon balsamic vinegar

1 tablespoon honey

½ teaspoon crushed red pepper flakes

1 baguette, cut diagonally into 1-inch slices (20 slices total)

cooking spray

1 (4-ounce) log of goat cheese with fine herbs, sliced into 1-inch rounds

garnish with dried thyme or rosemary

Preheat oven to 425°.

1   In a medium saucepan, place the first 4 ingredients. Mix well. Simmer, uncovered, over medium heat for 5 minutes.

2   Place baguette slices on a baking sheet. Spray both sides of bread with cooking spray. Bake until light brown, about 8 minutes, turning once during cooking time. Remove from oven, let cool.

3   Pour sauce into a small, round baking dish, a 3-cup au gratin ramekin, or a pair of 1½ cup custard-style ramekins. Place sliced goat cheese on top of sauce. Sprinkle with dried thyme or rosemary.

4   Bake for 10 minutes or until cheese is golden brown.

5   Remove from oven. Spoon about 1 tablespoon sauce and cheese on each toasted baguette slice. Serve hot.

MAKES 20 APPETIZERS

NUTRITIONAL ANALYSIS PER APPETIZER 47 calories ▪ 39 percent fat (total fat 2 g, saturated fat 1 g) ▪ 41 percent carbohydrate (0 g fiber) ▪ 20 percent protein.

Q

Caramelized Leek Tart with Apples and Blue Cheese

As an appetizer or light lunch, this tart goes well with a tossed salad and a glass of Chardonnay.

cooking spray

1 preprepared Pillsbury pie crust (unfold, fill, and bake)

2 teaspoons olive oil

1 medium sweet onion, thinly sliced, then cut in half

2 leeks (white part only), halved lengthwise, thinly sliced

½ teaspoon salt

¼ teaspoon cracked pepper

2 teaspoons balsamic vinegar

1 teaspoon brown sugar

½ cup crumbled blue cheese

1 cup liquid egg substitute (equivalent to 4 whole eggs)

1 cup fat-free half-and-half

1½ teaspoons dried thyme

2 medium apples, peeled, seeded, and thinly sliced (use any combination of apples)

nutmeg

Preheat oven to 425°. Coat a 10-inch tart pan with cooking spray.

1   Unfold pie crust into tart pan. Gently press dough to cover bottom and sides of pan. Bake for 10 minutes or until crust is light brown. Remove from oven. Set aside. Reduce oven temperature to 350°.

2   In a large, nonstick skillet, warm olive oil over medium heat. Add onions, leeks, salt, and pepper. Sauté for about 10 minutes, stirring occasionally until golden brown. Add balsamic vinegar and brown sugar. Stir well, then spoon caramelized onion mixture evenly on the bottom of tart crust. Add crumbled blue cheese to cover onion mixture. Set aside.

3   In a medium bowl, whisk together egg substitute, half-and-half, and thyme. Pour into tart pan. Place sliced apples on top of tart mixture, starting along outer edge and working toward center of tart in a circular pattern. Overlap apples where necessary. Continue layering apples until tart surface is covered with apples. Sprinkle with nutmeg.

4   Bake for 25 minutes or until center of tart is firm.

5   Cool for 5 minutes. Serve warm or at room temperature.

MAKES 8 SERVINGS

NUTRITIONAL ANALYSIS PER SERVING **251 calories** ▪ **43 percent fat (total fat 12 g, saturated fat 5 g)** ▪ **44 percent carbohydrate (1.7 g fiber)** ▪ **13 percent protein.**

Rice Cakes Layered with Low-Fat Peanut Butter, Toasted Wheat Germ, Bananas, and Honey

This snack is great for hungry kids after school. Other nut butters, such as cashew, almond, and hazelnut, are alternatives to peanut butter.

---

4 salt-free rice cakes (Quaker brand is tasty)

8 teaspoons low-fat peanut butter

4 teaspoons toasted wheat germ

1 banana, peeled and thinly sliced

4 teaspoons honey

raisins (optional)

1   Layer each rice cake with 2 teaspoons peanut butter, 1 teaspoon wheat germ, and several slices of banana.

2   Drizzle with honey.

3   Sprinkle with raisins, if desired.

MAKES 4 SERVINGS

NUTRITIONAL ANALYSIS PER SERVING **154 calories** ▪ **26 percent fat (total fat 4.4 g, saturated fat 1 g)** ▪ **64 percent carbohydrate (1.7 g fiber)** ▪ **10 percent protein.**

Mexican Five-Layered Spread

This version of a popular spread contains less than half the calories and 10 percent of the fat found in the original, yet the pleasure, taste, and texture remain the same. A great appetizer, snack for the kids, or accompaniment to a buffet. The Low-Fat Chunky Guacamole (page 40) goes well with this snack.

⅔ cup commercial salsa

⅓ cup tomatoes, diced

4 tablespoons fresh cilantro, diced

1 (8-ounce) can fat-free
refried beans

½ cup fat-free sour cream

½ cup reduced-fat cheddar cheese, grated

¼ cup green onions (tops only),
thinly sliced

baked tortilla chips

1   In a medium bowl, mix salsa, tomatoes, and cilantro. Set aside.

2   Spread beans evenly over the bottom of a 9-inch pie pan. Spread sour cream evenly over beans. Spread salsa mixture over sour cream. Sprinkle cheese evenly over salsa. Top with green onions.

3   Serve immediately with chips or cover and refrigerate for up to 24 hours.

MAKES 4 SERVINGS

NUTRITIONAL ANALYSIS PER SERVING **116 calories** ▪ **13 percent fat (total fat 1.7 g, saturated fat ‹ 1 g)** ▪ **55 percent carbohydrate (4.8 g fiber)** ▪ **32 percent protein.**

C Q

Slow-Roasted Tomatoes and Pesto on Polenta Pizzas

Use leftover Slow-Roasted Tomatoes with Garlic and Herbs (see page 221), and this appetizer or snack takes only minutes to make. It keeps well and can be reheated, too.

cooking spray

1 tube precooked polenta (sun-dried tomato garlic is especially good), cut into 12 rounds

12 slices of leftover Slow-Roasted Tomatoes with Garlic and Herbs

6 teaspoons commerical pesto

¼ cup low-fat mozzarella cheese, grated

Preheat oven to 425°. Coat a cookie sheet with cooking spray.

1   Place polenta rounds on cookie sheet. Top each round with 1 slice of tomato, ½ teaspoon pesto sauce, and 1 teaspoon cheese.

2   Bake until cheese melts and begins to brown, approximately 10 minutes.

3   Cool for 2 to 3 minutes, then transfer with a spatula to serving platter.

MAKES 12 APPETIZERS

NUTRITIONAL ANALYSIS PER APPERTIZER **60 calories** ▪ **25 percent fat (total fat 1.7 g, saturated fat 0.6 g)** ▪ **59 percent carbohydrate (1.2 g fiber)** ▪ **16 percent protein.**

Q

Chili-Spiced Shrimp Spring Rolls

Assembling these rolls is a snap, once you get the hang of rolling the delicate rice paper around the yummy insides. They are also delicious dipped in Thai peanut sauce. Make the rolls ahead of time to save last-minute rushing.

FISH SAUCE

1 small jalapeño pepper, minced

2 teaspoons sugar

1 clove garlic, minced

juice from ½ lime

2 tablespoons fish sauce (*nam pla*)

⅛ teaspoon fresh mint leaves, minced

4 tablespoons water

SPRING ROLLS

cooking spray

2 tablespoons chili sauce

1 teaspoon chili powder

1 pound medium shrimp, shelled and deveined

12 (9-inch) round rice papers

3 cups romaine lettuce leaves, spines removed and cut into ½-by-3-inch strips

1 cucumber, peeled, seeded, and cut into toothpick strips

¼ cup green onions, diced

12 large fresh mint leaves, sliced into thin strips

⅔ cup fresh cilantro, chopped

2 tablespoons jalapeño pepper, seeded and minced

1½ cups mung bean sprouts

Preheat oven to 425°. Line a cookie sheet with tinfoil and coat with cooking spray.

1   To prepare sauce: Mash jalapeño pepper with sugar into a paste with a mortar and pestle. Add garlic and mash into paste. Add lime juice, fish sauce, mint leaves, and water. Stir well. Set aside. (Sauce will keep for 24 hours.)

2   Mix chili sauce and powder in a small bowl. Add shrimp and stir to coat thoroughly. Place on cookie sheet and bake for 5 minutes or until shrimp are pink and cooked through. Remove from oven and place shrimp on plate lined with a paper towel.

3   Fill a 9-inch pie pan with warm water. Dunk 1 sheet of rice paper into warm water. Leave in the water only long enough for paper to begin to soften but still retain some firmness. (If paper softens too much, it is too fragile to roll.) Shake off excess water and lay paper flat on a clean work surface. Place a few strips of lettuce on the end of the paper closest to you, leaving about 1 inch on either side. Add 4 strips of cucumber, some green onions, mint leaves, cilantro, a pinch of jalapeño pepper, a few mung sprouts, and 2 shrimp. Fold sides of paper over vegetables, then gently and tightly roll paper into a cylinder. Place on serving platter. Repeat process 11 times.

4   Serve immediately with fish sauce or cover and refrigerate for up to 5 hours.

MAKES 12 SPRING ROLLS

NUTRITIONAL ANALYSIS PER ROLL AND SAUCE **79 calories** ▪ **9 percent fat (total fat 0.8 g, saturated fat 0 g)** ▪ **50 percent carbohydrate (1.2 g fiber)** ▪ **41 percent protein.**

S A

Cranberry Chutney

This spread can be used on turkey sandwiches or chicken quesadillas, as a topping for fat-free cream cheese with whole grain crackers, or as an accompaniment to roast pork, turkey, or chicken.

½ cup tart apple (Granny Smith), peeled and chopped

½ cup yellow raisins

½ cup onion, diced

¼ cup sugar

¼ cup Splenda

½ cup white vinegar

½ cup celery, diced

½ cup apple juice

1 teaspoon ground cinnamon

1 teaspoon ground ginger

dash of ground cloves

1 (12-ounce) bag fresh or frozen cranberries

1 Combine all ingredients in a medium saucepan over medium-high heat.

2 Bring to a boil, reduce heat, and simmer, uncovered, for 30 minutes or until sauce thickens. Stir occasionally.

MAKES 8 SERVINGS OF APPROXIMATELY ⅓ CUP EACH

NUTRITIONAL ANALYSIS PER SERVING **96 calories** ▪ **2 percent fat (total fat ‹ 0.5 g, saturated fat 0 g)** ▪ **95 percent carbohydrate (3 g fiber)** ▪ **3 percent protein.**

Q

Bite-Size Lettuce Wraps

This appetizer makes a lovely display and can be assembled ahead of time or served in individual bowls so that guests prepare their own portions. (Prepare a few wraps beforehand so guests have a sample to copy.) Each wrap has its own unique taste and provides a small mouthful of flavor blast. You can make this appetizer a day or two in advance, since even the sauce will keep for several days as long as it is refrigerated.

½ cup flaked coconut

SAUCE
1 jar hoisin sauce

½ teaspoon toasted coconut

1 rounded teaspoon fresh ginger, peeled and minced

a few drops of hot sauce

WRAPS
½ cup fresh ginger, peeled and minced

4 limes, cut into 8 pieces each

⅔ cup green onions, diced (white and light green parts only)

½ cup dry-roasted peanuts, chopped

½ cup salted sunflower seeds

50 palm-sized, cup-shaped lettuce leaves (Boston, butter, or fresh baby spinach)

Preheat oven to 350°.

1   Spread coconut on a cookie sheet and bake until golden brown. Remove from oven and set aside to cool.

2   To prepare sauce: Place in a blender hoisin sauce, ½ teaspoon toasted coconut, minced ginger, and hot sauce to taste. Blend until smooth. Transfer sauce to a nonstick saucepan and heat over medium heat until just about to simmer, stirring frequently. Remove from heat and refrigerate until ready to use.

3   Arrange in individual bowls or separate heaps on a serving platter: the coconut, ginger, limes, onions, peanuts, and sunflower seeds. Arrange the lettuce leaves on a separate deep serving bowl and provide a brush.

4   To assemble wraps: Brush a small dab of sauce onto a leaf and sprinkle coconut, ginger, onions, peanuts, and sunflower seeds into the center of leaf. Squeeze a few drops of lime juice on top and fold lettuce to form a bite-size wrap that can be popped into the mouth in one bite.

MAKES APPROXIMATELY 50 WRAPS

NUTRITIONAL ANALYSIS PER WRAP **36 calories** ▪ **50 percent fat (total fat 2 g, saturated fat < 0.5 g)** ▪ **40 percent carbohydrate (0.5 g fiber)** ▪ **10 percent protein.**

Shrimp and Roasted Green Pepper Seviche

Vary this recipe by using diced roasted asparagus instead of green pepper and add more or less serrano chilies, depending on your preference for spiciness. Save yourself time by using pre-cooked and shelled medium shrimp and roasting the green peppers the day before.

cooking spray

2 green peppers, stemmed, seeded, and quartered

$\frac{1}{2}$ pound, medium-size shrimp, unpeeled (approximately 20 shrimp)

$\frac{1}{2}$ cup red onion, finely diced

$\frac{1}{3}$ cup fresh lime juice

2 tablespoons champagne vinegar

$\frac{1}{2}$ teaspoon fresh thyme leaves

$\frac{1}{4}$ teaspoon dried oregano

1 tablespoon serrano chilies, finely diced

3 plum tomatoes, diced and drained

2 tablespoons fresh cilantro, diced

1 avocado, peeled, seeded, and diced

salt, to taste

Preheat oven to 400°. Coat a cookie sheet with cooking spray.

1   Place green peppers on cookie sheet, spray them with cooking spray and roast until peel begins to separate from flesh and peppers are soft, turning once during roasting. Remove from oven. When cool, peel as much of the skin away as possible and dice. (Will make approximately 1 cup total.) Set aside.

2   In a medium saucepan, bring 1 quart water to a boil. Add shrimp, remove from heat, drain off liquid, cover, set aside to allow shrimp to finish cooking (approximately 15 minutes). Transfer to cookie sheet to cool. Peel and devein shrimp and cut into $\frac{1}{2}$-inch pieces.

3   In a large bowl, place shrimp, red onion, lime juice, vinegar, thyme, oregano, and chilies. Cover and set aside at room temperature for 1 hour to allow flavors to blend.

4   Add roasted green peppers, tomatoes, cilantro, and avocado to shrimp and toss gently. Season with salt.

5   Transfer to a serving bowl and serve with baked tortilla chips.

MAKES APPROXIMATELY 10 SERVINGS OF $\frac{1}{2}$ CUP EACH

NUTRITIONAL ANALYSIS PER SERVING 72 calories ▪ 42 percent fat (total fat 3.3 g, saturated fat 0.5 g) ▪ 29 percent carbohydrate (1.4 g fiber) ▪ 29 percent protein.

C —COMFORT FOOD

Q —QUICK FIX FOOD

A —ADVENTUROUS

S —SPECIAL OCCASION

Lunchables
and Sandwiches

Midday Energy Boosters

EVEN IF YOU eat a great breakfast and pack your briefcase, purse, or glove compartment with healthful snacks, you still need to refuel midday for both your mood and your energy level. What you eat is as important as when. Make the right choices, and you're likely to glide through the afternoon in a good mood with lots of energy and ability to concentrate. A few wrong choices could set you up for a siesta rather than an action-packed afternoon, as well as an after-dinner binge.

The Power Lunch

You need to eat and you need to eat well at the midday meal, but that doesn't mean lunch must take hours of preparation. Basically, you want lunch to be light in both calories and fat. A low-fat meal that supplies about 500 calories helps you stay alert through the afternoon hours, boosts energy, and fills you up without filling you out. Heavy or calorie-packed meals at this time of day will leave you feeling sluggish, both mentally and physically.

Lunch should also supply a balance of quality carbohydrates (whole grains, starchy vegetables, or legumes) and protein-rich foods (lean meat, chicken breast, fish, legumes, or nonfat milk products). The carbs fuel your brain and body throughout the afternoon hours, while protein helps you feel full longer, so you are less likely to reach for a candy bar or bag of chips. Don't make the mistake of focusing solely on carbs. A high-carbohydrate lunch, such as a plate of pasta with marinara sauce and a tossed salad, raises serotonin levels in the brain, which leaves you relaxed and perhaps a bit sleepy. Combine carbohydrates and protein—with a Black Bean Burrito, Grilled Turkey Reuben on Dark Rye, or a Grilled Cheese, Tomato, and Roasted Yellow Pepper Sandwich—and you curb the serotonin effect and raise levels of energizing chemicals such as dopamine and norepinephrine. This leaves you feeling alert and ready to concentrate.

Midday Fat: Don't Overdo It

Carb-loving brain chemicals in the morning entice us to want waffles, toast, and pancakes for breakfast, but by afternoon, another brain chemical is at the helm of our appetite center and encourages us to eat fatty foods. Like neuropeptide Y (NPY), discussed in the "Breakfast and Breads" section, galanin is a chemical produced in the hypothalamus, the appetite center of the brain. Galanin ensures that we get ample long-term fuel—that means fat. Unlike NPY levels, which drop after we eat a bowl of cereal or any carb-rich food, the more fat we eat, the more galanin we produce. Have a light lunch—such as Prawn and Asparagus Lettuce Wraps with Hoisin Sauce or Chicken Salad Pitas with Red Pepper and Dill served with a fruit salad—and galanin levels are satisfied, but sustained at low levels. Go for the drive-through special of a cheeseburger and French fries or have a tossed salad smothered in high-fat dressing, and galanin levels remain high, possibly leading to cravings for more fatty foods later in the day. It's a vicious cycle: Galanin encourages us to eat fatty foods, and the more fatty foods we eat, the greater the rise in galanin. The only way to break the cycle is to eat fat in moderation, not in excess, especially from midday through bedtime.

The Importance of Regular Meals

You've already heard the rationale behind eating frequent mini-meals and snacks throughout the day. This eating style not only helps sidestep a host of mood problems, from fatigue to irritability, but also aids in weight loss and the prevention of medical conditions such as heart disease, diabetes, and hypertension. For example, a study from the Faculty of Medicine in Toulouse, France, found that body weight decreased the most in men who divided their food intake into several small meals and snacks throughout the day compared with men who ate the same calories but in fewer meals. Researchers at the University of Michigan School of Public Health report that women who divide their food intake into several little meals and snacks throughout the day are leaner with less body fat than are women who eat the same calories but pack them into two or three big meals. In fact, the more little meals and snacks the women ate (up to six a day), the lower their body fat.

"It makes sense that the body is better adapted to small doses of fuel and nutrients all day long than trying to handle a glut of food every so often," says Sharon Edelstein, Sc.M., research scientist at George Washington University in Washington, D.C., and the lead researcher on a study that linked snacking with a lower risk for disease. Our ancestors evolved by grazing—not gorging—on nuts, berries, roots, and very lean wild game. Feasts were rare and probably occurred only when someone in the tribe slew a large animal. In short, our bodies were designed for nibbling on high-fiber, low-fat foods, not the "gorge 'n' fast" eating style of modern society.

Common sense is also backed by scientific know-how. "Nibbling, compared to gorging on big meals, helps improve cholesterol metabolism and keep insulin levels low," says David Jenkins, M.D., a professor of medicine and nutritional science and the director of the Risk Factor Modification Center at St. Michael's Hospital in Toronto.

Why nibbling aids fat metabolism is poorly understood. One theory proposes that large, infrequent meals set up a feast-or-fast scenario where the body stores more incoming calories as fat as a safeguard against what it perceives as a famine. As a result, fat-building enzymes in fat tissue might be activated after a big meal, thus potentially placing a person at greater risk of weight gain. In contrast, dividing the same calories into five or more little meals and snacks encourages the body to "burn" the food for immediate energy rather than store it in the hips and thighs.

In addition, body heat production after a meal, called diet-induced thermogenesis, might be higher following multiple little meals than it is with a few big meals, so more calories are wasted as heat rather than are stored as body fat. "The secret to triggering the thermogenic effect," says C. Wayne Callaway, M.D., an associate clinical professor of medicine at George Washington University in Washington, D.C., "is to consume enough calories at each meal to get the burn off of calories." Dr. Callaway suggests that consuming approximately 25 percent of the day's total calories at each meal could increase thermogenesis by up to 25 percent.

The benefits of little meals extend beyond your waistline. Dr. Jenkins reports that nibbling lowers blood cholesterol, LDL-cholesterol, and insulin levels, and improves insulin sensitivity: "We've noted beneficial changes in blood lipids and insulin levels within weeks of initiating a nibbling style of eating." Dr. Jenkins notes that the trickle-down effect on health is a lowered risk of diabetes, heart disease, and possibly even cancers of the colon and breast.

Finally, eating at consistent times each day curbs hunger and prevents overeating later in the day. People who spread their food intake into little meals are more satisfied, consume up to 27 percent fewer calories, and have an easier time managing their hunger compared with people who skip meals or eat a few big meals.

But wait. Before you race to the vending machine with a license to binge, keep in mind that unplanned nibbling can make or break your weight-management efforts, mood, and health. The secret is not to add more meals to your usual diet, but to divide your current food intake into five or six little meals, including a healthful lunch, while emphasizing fiber and nutrients and deemphasizing fat, sugar, and calories.

12 QUICK-FIX LUNCHES

No time to think about recipes or food prep? Here are a dozen five-minute lunch ideas, most of which travel well in a brown bag.

1. **PEANUT BUTTER CANDY SANDWICH:** Mix equal parts peanut butter, toasted wheat germ, and honey. Spread on 2 slices of whole wheat bread. Serve with soymilk and a fruit salad.

2. **QUESADILLAS:** Place tortillas on a heated skillet or griddle and top with grated, low-fat cheese, chopped green onions, grated carrots, salsa, and another tortilla. Cook until lightly brown on both sides. Cut into wedges and serve with additional salsa, Low-Fat Chunky Guacamole (page 40), or fat-free sour cream.

3. **BEAN 'N' VEGETABLE BURRITO:** Fill a flour tortilla with black beans, low-fat cheese, and any favorite vegetables (chopped red or green onion, chopped red bell pepper, tomato slices, grated carrots, corn, etc.). Roll up tortilla and top with salsa, Low-Fat Chunky Guacamole (page 40), and/or fat-free sour cream.

4. **VEGGIE PIZZA:** Top commercial pizza crust (Boboli) with: (a) commercial pizza sauce, grated low-fat mozzarella cheese, packaged sliced mushrooms, and leftover vegetables or (b) sliced tomatoes, sliced red onion, Gorgonzola cheese, and fresh basil. Bake at 425° for 10 minutes or until cheese melts and bubbles.

5. **CHICKEN MANGO SANDWICH:** Spread hoisin sauce on a slice of sourdough bread and layer roasted chicken, mango slices, a thin slice of red onion, and cilantro. Top with sourdough bread, press down, and slice diagonally in half. Serve with a spinach salad.

6. **FRUIT SANDWICH:** Spread 2 tablespoons fat-free ricotta cheese on a slice of whole wheat bread, top with fresh peaches, pineapple, or sliced mango and a dash of nutmeg or cinnamon. Broil until cheese bubbles. Serve with a tossed salad or nonfat milk.

7. **VEGGIE SANDWICH:** Spread 2 tablespoons fat-free cream cheese on a slice of whole wheat bread, layer with cucumber and tomato slices and sprouts, and top with a second slice of bread. Serve with nonfat milk, soymilk, or fruit juice.

8. **HOT DOG:** Cook a fat-free hot dog and wrap in a whole wheat bun. Serve with baby carrots and fruit.

9. **CURRIED CHICKEN SANDWICH:** Mix half of a 5-ounce can of white chunk chicken with curry powder, dry mustard, diced celery, lemon juice, and fat-free mayonnaise. Spread on 2 slices of whole wheat bread. Serve with apricot nectar or other fruit juice.

10. **BLT:** Layer 2 slices of turkey bacon, lettuce, tomato slices, and fat-free mayonnaise on whole wheat toast.

11. **NUT BREAD SPREAD:** Mix fat-free cream cheese, chutney, and grated orange peel. Spread on nut bread. Serve with orange slices and nonfat milk.

12. **SPICED-UP TUNA:** Mix tuna with nonfat mayonnaise, curry powder, dried cranberries, and chopped green onions. Spread between 2 slices of your favorite bread and serve with a tossed salad and soymilk.

Ironing Out Fatigue

If you're a woman battling fatigue midafternoon, look to your iron intake, not a cup of coffee, for the solution. As many as 80 percent of exercising women and 20 percent of women in general are iron deficient.

Iron is critical to fighting fatigue. As a component of hemoglobin in the blood and myoglobin within the cells, iron is the key oxygen carrier in the body. When iron levels decrease, the tissues become oxygen starved, resulting in fatigue, poor concentration, and reduced work performance.

Compared with men, women have almost twice the daily iron requirement but consume half as much food. Fergus Clydesdale, Ph.D., a professor who heads the Department of Food Science at the University of Massachusetts in Amherst, says a well-balanced diet supplies approximately 6 milligrams of iron for every 1,000 calories. Based on this ratio, women must increase their average intake from 2,000 calories to at least 3,000 calories daily to meet their daily requirement of 15 to 18 milligrams. (Iron requirements are as high as 25 milligrams a day for women with heavy menstrual losses or who use intrauterine devices for birth control.)

Limiting meat in an effort to cut back on saturated fat adds to the iron shortage. There are basically two types of dietary iron:

1. The iron in meat, called "heme" iron.

2. The "nonheme" iron in plants, such as dried beans, whole grains, and dark green vegetables.

As much as 30 percent of dietary heme iron is absorbed, compared with only 2 to 7 percent of nonheme iron. That means you must eat 4 to 15 times as many servings of kidney beans (at two-thirds of a cup per serving) to match the iron absorbed from 3 ounces of red meat. Jan Johnson-Shane, Ph.D., R.D., an associate professor of nutrition at Illinois State University who has studied the beneficial effect of red meat on iron status, says, "If the serving is small, say three ounces, then extra-lean red meat is an excellent source of iron while still falling within the guidelines of a low-fat diet."

With high requirements for and low intakes of iron, most women during the childbearing years should consume several servings daily of iron-rich foods and maximize iron absorption by including vitamin C–rich foods, such as a tossed salad, steamed vegetables, or a glass of orange juice, at every meal. Women who eat fewer than 2,500 calories a day (or who have a blood test called the serum ferritin that shows their iron levels have fallen below 20 micrograms/liter) might consider taking a daily multiple vitamin that contains 18 milligrams of iron. Severe iron deficiency will require a higher-dose prescription supplement. Lunches in this section that are especially high in iron include: Chicken Salad Pitas with Red Pepper and Dill (2.1 milligrams/serving), Grilled Cheese, Tomato, and Roasted Yellow Pepper Sandwich (3.2 milligrams/serving), and Sesame Salmon Sandwich (4 milligrams/sandwich). Also check out the "Entrée" section for the following iron-rich meat dishes (all supply approximately 3.0 milligrams/serving): Grilled Asian Flank Steak with Wasabi Cream Sauce, Individual Meat Loaves with Fresh Thyme, and Classic Chicken Pot Pie.

Watch Out for the Midday Quick Fix

A candy bar or a cup of coffee is a quick pick-me-up, but you're probably undermining your energy level if you are fueling your day with sugar and caffeine. Granted, a cup of coffee revs the nervous system, focusing your concentration, improving your reaction times, and energizing your mood. However, overdo it by drinking more than two or three cups a day, and the first symptom of caffeine withdrawal is fatigue. If you are riding the caffeine roller coaster of highs and lows by drinking coffee, tea, or colas throughout the day, you will experience an improvement in sustained energy when you cut back on or cut out these caffeine-rich beverages.

Another word of warning when it comes to coffee and tea: These beverages, both caffeinated and decaffeinated, contain compounds called tannins that reduce iron absorption by up to 90 percent. Drink a cup of coffee or glass of iced tea with lunch, and you miss out on most of the iron in the meal. Sip these drinks between, not with, meals.

Sugary foods also provide a quick energy jolt, followed by a more serious energy drop, which forces you to return for another sugar fix, setting up another vicious cycle. Larry Christensen, Ph.D., who conducted research at the University of South Alabama on the effects of sugar and caffeine on depression, found that many people unresponsive to other therapies showed marked improvement in both fatigue and depression when they cut out sugar and/or caffeine.

All of the recipes in this section are based on the guidelines for a healthy lunch; they are light and low-fat. Most are extra-rich in iron, and all should be served with other energy-boosting foods, such as a salad or bowl of soup, not with coffee, tea, or soft drinks.

Black Bean Burritos

These burritos are great for lunch and snacks, or freeze for later use.

1 recipe for Black Beans with Cumin and Chipotle Peppers (page 154)

10 (8-inch) whole wheat tortillas, warmed

2 cups reduced-fat Monterey or cheddar cheese, grated

4 cups lettuce (any leaf lettuce or baby spinach), shredded

2 cups tomato, chopped

½ cup fat-free sour cream

½ cup commercial salsa

¼ cup fresh cilantro, chopped

1   Spread ⅓ to ½ cup prepared and heated black bean mixture on edge of each warm tortilla.

2   Sprinkle with cheese, lettuce, tomato, a dollop of sour cream, and salsa. Then sprinkle with cilantro.

3   Roll up, gently, folding edges in. Serve immediately or wrap up and refrigerate for a lunch.

MAKES 10 BURRITOS

NUTRITIONAL ANALYSIS PER BURRITO **326 calories** ▪ **28 percent fat** (total fat 10 g, saturated fat 5 g) ▪ **53 percent carbohydrate** (9 g fiber) ▪ **19 percent protein**.

C

Chicken Salad Pitas with Red Pepper and Dill

Use leftover roast chicken to make these simple and tasty pita sandwiches.

1 cup leftover roasted chicken breast, skinned and diced

⅓ cup red bell pepper, diced

3 tablespoons green onion, diced

2 tablespoons mayonnaise

2 tablespoons fat-free mayonnaise

¼ teaspoon dill

salt and pepper, to taste

2 whole wheat pita breads

leaf lettuce

1   In a medium bowl, mix ingredients through salt and pepper.

2   Cut pita breads in half. Stuff a quarter of the chicken salad into each pita half. Stuff pitas with lettuce and serve.

MAKES 4 SERVINGS

NUTRITIONAL ANALYSIS PER SERVING 295 calories ▪ 30 percent fat (total fat 9.8 g, saturated fat 2 g) ▪ 21 percent carbohydrate (2.1 g fiber) ▪ 49 percent protein.

Q

Minted Lamb Pockets with Honey Yogurt Dressing

A light and healthy lunch option using low-fat yogurt and fresh mint.

MINTED LAMB

½ pound ground lamb

½ cup onion, finely chopped

1 apple, peeled, seeded, and diced

3 tablespoons fresh mint, minced

½ teaspoon ground cinnamon

⅛ teaspoon ground nutmeg

½ teaspoon salt

2 tablespoons balsamic vinegar

3 whole wheat pita breads, sliced in half

DRESSING

¼ cup plain, nonfat yogurt

2 teaspoons honey

1   In a nonstick skillet, over medium-high heat, cook lamb for 5 minutes or until no longer pink, stirring frequently to break into small pieces. Drain lamb and place in a large bowl. Set aside.

2   In same skillet, add onion and sauté until translucent, about 3 to 4 minutes. Add apple and sauté for 2 minutes. Remove from heat. Place in bowl with lamb.

3   Add remaining ingredients, except pita bread, to lamb mixture. Mix well.

4   To make dressing, mix yogurt and honey in a small bowl. Set aside.

5   Spoon lamb mixture into pita pockets. Dollop with dressing.

MAKES 6 POCKET SANDWICHES

NUTRITIONAL ANALYSIS PER POCKET SANDWICH **196 calories** ▪ **37 percent fat (total fat 8 g, saturated fat 3 g)** ▪ **40 percent carbohydrate (2.4 g fiber)** ▪ **23 percent protein.**

A

Grilled Cheese, Tomato, and Roasted Yellow Pepper Sandwich

A wonderful twist on the classic grilled cheese and a great way to sneak extra vegetables into your day (one sandwich supplies two servings of vegetables). Roast the peppers ahead of time, and this sandwich takes only 12 minutes from start to finish. You can also freeze these sandwiches once cooked, then microwave to reheat. If you can't find sun-dried tomato paste at your grocery store, increase the tomato paste to 3 tablespoons. You can substitute tart apple slices for the tomato for a crunchy, sweet flavor.

FOOD TIP

You probably never will use an entire can of chipotle peppers at one meal. After opening a can, freeze the remaining peppers in individual freezer bags for later use.

1 tablespoon sun-dried tomato paste

2 tablespoons tomato paste

1 teaspoon canned chipotle pepper, diced

2 teaspoons honey

6 slices French or sourdough bread

6 ounces low-fat cheddar cheese, grated

3 firm medium tomatoes, sliced thin

3 thin slices red onion

1 yellow pepper, seeded, sliced into 6 slices, and roasted*

½ cup cilantro, chopped

cooking spray

Heat nonstick skillet or griddle.

1   Blend pastes, chipotle pepper, and honey. Spread 1 tablespoon mixture on one side of all 6 slices of bread.

2   Divide half of cheese equally and place on 3 slices of bread, paste side up. Top with tomatoes, red onion, roasted yellow pepper, cilantro, and second half of cheese. Top with remaining 3 slices of bread, paste side inward.

3   Coat skillet or griddle with cooking spray and arrange 3 sandwiches. Cook until each side of bread is golden brown, approximately 5 minutes per side. Serve warm.

MAKES 3 SANDWICHES

NUTRITIONAL ANALYSIS PER SANDWICH **312 calories** ▪ **18 percent fat (total fat 6 g, saturated fat 3 g)** ▪ **56 percent carbohydrate (4 g fiber)** ▪ **26 percent protein.**

*To roast yellow pepper, place on cookie sheet sprayed with cooking spray. Bake at 425° turning occasionally, approximately 15 minutes, until skin begins to bubble and turn brown in places. Pepper should be tender, but still firm.

Veggie Bagel Bites

Make this bagel sandwich for lunch, a light dinner, or an afternoon snack for the kids. It also makes a great appetizer. Slice into quarters, pierce with a toothpick to pile high on a plate for individual nibbles.

---

4 tablespoons fat-free cream cheese

4 whole wheat bagels, halved

4 thick slices of tomato

½ cucumber, thinly sliced

4 thin slices red onion

1 cup alfalfa sprouts

1   Spread cream cheese on 4 bagel halves (1 tablespoon per half). Top cream cheese with the remaining vegetables. Cover with the remaining bagel halves.

2   Slice each bagel into quarters. (If necessary, use a toothpick to hold sandwiches in place.)

MAKES 4 SERVINGS OR 8 HALF SERVINGS

NUTRITIONAL ANALYSIS PER FULL SANDWICH **186 calories** ▪ **5 percent fat (total fat 1 g, saturated fat 0 g)** ▪ **73 percent carbohydrate (6.6 g fiber)** ▪ **22 percent protein.**

Q

Prawn and Asparagus Lettuce Wraps with Hoisin Sauce

Flavor for few calories, these wraps are good alone or served with steamed rice. Skip the lettuce and wrap the prawn mixture into rice sheets for a quick spring roll.

FOOD TIP
Hoisin sauce, a sweet-and-spicy Asian condiment made with soybeans, spices, and garlic, can be found in the Asian section of your grocery store.

½ pound medium-size prawns, peeled and deveined

2 teaspoons sesame oil

3 cloves garlic, chopped

2 tablespoons fresh ginger, peeled and diced

¼ cup green onions, chopped

1 large red bell pepper, stemmed, seeded, and diced

¼ pound asparagus, trimmed and diced

2 teaspoons soy sauce

¼ cup hoisin sauce

1 head butter lettuce, washed and dried

1   Chop prawns into small pieces. Set aside.

2   Warm oil in a large nonstick skillet over medium-high heat. Add garlic, ginger, and green onions and toss in oil. Add red pepper and asparagus and continue to stir-fry for 3 minutes. Add prawns and soy sauce and stir for 2 minutes or until prawns turn pink. Remove from heat.

3   Transfer prawn mixture to medium serving bowl. Place bowl in the middle of a large platter and arrange lettuce leaves around the bowl. Serve with hoisin sauce. To eat, spread a little hoisin sauce on lettuce leaf, place a spoonful of prawn mixture on top, wrap lettuce leaf around, and eat with fingers.

MAKES 4 SERVINGS

NUTRITIONAL ANALYSIS PER SERVING **117 calories** ▪ **29 percent fat (total fat 3.7 g, saturated fat ‹ 1 g)** ▪ **26 percent carbohydrate (1.6 g fiber)** ▪ **45 percent protein.**

Sesame Salmon Sandwich

This tasty sandwich is quick to make and loaded with omega-3 fats; B vitamins; vitamins A, E, and C; and most minerals. By using leftover salmon from last night's dinner, you save even more time. Serve with a Mango-Lemon Daiquiri (page 269), and you've met just about all your vitamin and mineral needs (except calcium and iron) for the entire day!

MOOD TIP

People who regularly eat fish show less loss of mental function as they age compared with people who eat more vegetable oils and fried foods during their lives, according to a study from the National Institute of Public Health in the Netherlands.

2 teaspoons hoisin sauce

1 teaspoon soy sauce

¼ teaspoon toasted sesame oil

1 teaspoon fresh ginger, peeled and grated

pinch of red pepper flakes

4 ounces salmon fillet, skin removed

1 teaspoon sesame seeds

salt and pepper, to taste

cooking spray

2 slices sourdough bread

1 tablespoon red onion, thinly sliced

1 plum tomato, sliced

½ cup spinach leaves, washed, stemmed, and patted dry

1 Mix hoisin sauce, soy sauce, sesame oil, ginger, and red pepper flakes in a small bowl. Set aside.

2 Sprinkle salmon fillet with sesame seeds, salt, and pepper. Place in sprayed skillet, cover, and sauté over medium heat until fish is cooked through, approximately 3 to 4 minutes per side, depending on thickness of fish.

3 Spread hoisin mixture evenly on one side of both slices of bread. Top with salmon, onion, tomato, and spinach. Top with other slice of bread, press down gently, and slice diagonally in half.

MAKES 1 SANDWICH

NUTRITIONAL ANALYSIS 417 calories ▪ 36 percent fat (total fat 16.8 g, saturated fat 3.7 g) ▪ 35 percent carbohydrate (4.2 g fiber) ▪ 29 percent protein.

Toasted Whole Wheat Bagels with Brie and Strawberries

For a change of pace, try this quick and yummy lunch. For a special occasion, serve with Pecan, Tart Apple, and Dried Cherry Salad (page 123).

---

2 ounces brie cheese, thinly sliced

2 whole wheat bagels, sliced in half and lightly toasted

4 strawberries, chopped

4 teaspoons honey

2 teaspoons slivered almonds

Preheat oven to broil.

1   Arrange slices of brie evenly on toasted bagel halves. Top with strawberries, drizzle with honey, and sprinkle with almonds.

2   Place on a baking sheet. Broil until brie starts to melt; watch closely. Serve hot.

MAKES 4 SERVINGS OF ½ BAGEL EACH

NUTRITIONAL ANALYSIS PER SERVING **158 calories** ▪ **28 percent fat (total fat 5 g, saturated fat 2.6 g)** ▪ 57 percent carbohydrate (3.7 g fiber) ▪ 15 percent protein.

Q

Gourmet Pizza with White Clam Sauce, Spinach, Garlic, and Fresh Tomatoes

This pizza goes especially well with Baby Greens and Orange Salad with Pecans and Celery Seed Dressing (page 133).

---

1 (10-ounce) container light Alfredo sauce

1 (6.5-ounce) can chopped clams, drained

2 cloves garlic, minced

1 cup fresh spinach, finely chopped

2 tablespoons low-fat Parmesan cheese, grated

1 tablespoon cooking sherry

1 (14-ounce) premade pizza crust (such as Boboli)

½ cup low-fat mozzarella cheese, shredded

1 cup tomatoes, diced

Preheat oven to 425°.

1   In a medium bowl, combine ⅔ cup light Alfredo sauce (save the rest for another pizza or other use), clams, garlic, spinach, Parmesan cheese, and cooking sherry. Stir to mix.

2   Pour sauce on pizza crust, spreading evenly and leaving a 1½-inch border around crust. Sprinkle with mozzarella cheese, then tomatoes.

3   Place pizza on a flat baking sheet and bake for 20 minutes or until center is bubbly hot and crust edges are golden brown. Remove from oven. Let rest several minutes. Slice into 8 wedges and serve.

MAKES 8 SERVINGS

NUTRITIONAL ANALYSIS PER BURRITO **264 calories** ▪ **30** percent fat (total fat **8.8 g,** saturated fat **3.6 g**) ▪ **46** percent carbohydrate (**1.4 g** fiber) ▪ **24** percent protein.

A

Quinoa Tabbouleh with Fresh Mint

Quinoa replaces the more traditional bulgur wheat in this tabbouleh.

FOOD TIP

Quinoa (pronounced KEEN-wa) is a birdseed-shaped, mild-flavored grain that was called "the mother grain" by the Incas. Quinoa is one of the only grains rich in protein and is also a good source of magnesium, copper, and potassium. Quinoa supplies about 5 milligrams of iron for every cup. It usually is well tolerated by people who are allergic or intolerant to wheat.

1 cup quinoa, cooked according to package directions and chilled

1 tomato, diced

1 cup fresh parsley, minced

½ cucumber, peeled and diced

¼ cup green onions, thinly sliced

1 tablespoon olive oil

3 tablespoons fresh lemon juice

2 cloves garlic, minced

¼ teaspoon salt

¼ cup mint leaves, minced

lettuce leaves

1 whole wheat pita, sliced into 4 wedges

1 lemon, sliced into 4 wedges

1   In a medium salad bowl, combine chilled quinoa, tomato, parsley, cucumber, and green onions. Mix well and set aside.

2   In a small bowl, whisk together oil, lemon juice, garlic, and salt. Pour into quinoa mixture and mix well. Stir in mint leaves. Cover and refrigerate for at least ½ hour (or up to 24 hours) to develop flavors.

3   To serve: Cover 4 salad plates with fresh salad greens of choice. Spoon tabbouleh salad evenly on plates. Place pita and lemon wedge on the side of each plate and serve.

MAKES 4 SERVINGS

NUTRITIONAL ANALYSIS PER SERVING **248 calories** ▪ **22 percent fat (total fat 6.1 g,** saturated fat 0.8 g) ▪ **65 percent carbohydrate (3 g fiber)** ▪ **13 percent protein.**

Turkey Burgers with Caramelized Onions

A great summer lunch on the barbecue served with Sesame-Ginger Coleslaw (page 121) or Sweet Potato Chutney Salad (page 122). In the winter, broil these burgers and serve with Roasted Beet Salad with Orange Vinaigrette (page 131) and Baked Lima and Butter Beans in a Thick BBQ Sauce (page 223). Add a teaspoon of Dijon mustard to the ground turkey for more flavor and moisture.

---

cooking spray

1 pound ground turkey breast

⅓ cup sun-dried tomatoes, drained and diced

⅓ cup roasted red bell pepper, drained and diced

¼ cup onion, diced fine

1 tablespoon dried basil

½ teaspoon cumin

salt and pepper, to taste

3 tablespoons Dijon mustard

3 tablespoons fat-free mayonnaise

½ onion, thinly sliced

2 teaspoons sugar

2 tablespoons red wine vinegar

salt and pepper, to taste

⅓ cup fat-free chicken broth

4 whole wheat hamburger buns

lettuce leaves (optional)

Spray a cookie sheet with cooking spray.

1   In a large bowl, mix turkey, tomatoes, red pepper, onion, basil, cumin, salt, and pepper. Form into 4 patties, pat to ¾-inch thickness, and place on cookie sheet. Cover with plastic wrap and refrigerate for 1 hour (or up to 5 hours).

2   Place mustard and mayonnaise in a small mixing bowl, blend well, and set aside.

3   Heat broiler or barbecue grill to medium-high.

4   Spray large nonstick skillet with cooking spray and place over medium-high heat. Add sliced onion and sauté until soft and beginning to brown, about 8 minutes. Add sugar, vinegar, and salt and pepper, to taste. Reduce heat to low and simmer for 10 minutes or until onions are golden brown. Add chicken broth, a tablespoon at a time as needed to keep onions from sticking (you might not need the entire ⅓ cup). Remove from heat and set aside.

5   Broil or grill turkey burgers until cooked through, approximately 6 minutes per side. Set buns facing down on grill or facing up under broiler for 1 minute or until lightly toasted.

6   Spread mustard-mayonnaise mixture on bottom of 4 bun halves (1½ tablespoons per half). Lay burgers over mixture. Top with onions, lettuce (if desired), and the other bun halves. Serve warm.

MAKES 4 BURGERS

NUTRITIONAL ANALYSIS PER BURGER **303 calories** ▪ **14 percent fat (total fat 4.7 g,** **saturated fat < 1 g)** ▪ **43 percent carbohydrate (3 g fiber)** ▪ **43 percent protein.**

S

Tofu Cakes in Sweet Ginger Sauce

This spicy vegetarian lunch goes well with Coconut Rice with Ginger and Cardamom (page 194) or Asian Cucumber Salad (page 140).

MOOD TIP

Soy foods, such as tofu, contain estrogen-like compounds, called phytoestrogens, that help offset fluctuations in women's natural estrogen, possibly helping to curb the symptoms of PMS and menopause.

1 (14-ounce) package of firm tofu, rinsed and patted, dry

5 teaspoons brown sugar

½ cup fat-free chicken broth

3 tablespoons light soy sauce

4 tablespoons onion, minced

2 cloves garlic, minced

1 rounded tablespoon fresh ginger, peeled and minced

pinch of red pepper flakes

3 tablespoons green onions, diagonal-sliced thin

1   Slice block of tofu into ½-inch-thick slices (each slice will be approximately 3 inches by 2 inches by ½ inch). Set on a plate lined with paper towels to soak up extra moisture.

2   Place sugar in a medium nonstick skillet over medium heat. Let sugar melt and turn slightly brown, stirring frequently. Add chicken broth, reduce heat to low, and mix until sugar is completely dissolved. Add soy sauce, onion, garlic, ginger, and pepper flakes, increase heat to medium-high and stir until mixture comes to a gentle boil.

3   Lay tofu slices on top of soy mixture, reduce heat, and simmer uncovered for 7 minutes. Flip tofu slices, cover with some of the sauce, and continue to simmer for an additional 5 minutes. When tofu is heated through and sauce has thickened slightly, remove from heat.

4   Transfer tofu and sauce to a small platter, sprinkle with green onions, and serve immediately.

MAKES 4 SERVINGS

NUTRITIONAL ANALYSIS PER SERVING **181 calories** ▪ **41** percent fat (total fat 8 g, saturated fat 1 g) ▪ **24** percent carbohydrate (0.7 g fiber) ▪ **35** percent protein.

California-Style Roasted Veggie Burrito

Make these burritos ahead of time, wrap tightly in plastic wrap, and store in the refrigerator for a quick-fix lunch at home or on the go. Try experimenting with different roasted vegetables, including parsnips, carrots, eggplant, and mushrooms. In the summertime, you can grill the vegetables on the barbecue, instead of roasting, to add an even richer flavor.

---

cooking spray

¾ cup commercial salsa

¼ cup tomato, chopped

2 tablespoons fresh cilantro, chopped

2 zucchinis, washed, dried, and cut into 8 long, thin strips

2 red bell peppers, stemmed, seeded, and cut into large sections

1 small sweet potato, peeled and cut into 4 strips

4 10-inch tortilla wraps (garlic and herb, spinach, or tomato all work well)

1 cup canned black beans, rinsed and drained

1 cup cooked instant brown rice

Preheat oven to 400°. Spray a cookie sheet with cooking spray.

1   Blend salsa, tomato, and cilantro in a small bowl. Cover and refrigerate.

2   Place zucchini, peppers, and sweet potato strips on cookie sheet and roast for 20 minutes or until zucchini is tender, peppers are beginning to brown, and potato is tender but firm. Turn twice during roasting to prevent burning. Remove from oven and take off skins from peppers.

3   Lay a tortilla on a flat surface. Spread ¼ cup black beans, ¼ cup brown rice, 2 zucchini strips, a quarter of the red peppers, 1 strip of sweet potato, and ¼ cup salsa along middle of tortilla. Tightly roll tortilla into a burrito and wrap in plastic wrap to compact burrito and allow it to form a roll. Repeat this step for remaining burritos. Refrigerate until ready to serve (up to 24 hours). Can be served cold or warmed in the microwave.

MAKES 4 SERVINGS

NUTRITIONAL ANALYSIS PER SERVING **305 calories** ▪ **15** percent fat (total fat 5 g, saturated fat 1 g) ▪ **44** percent carbohydrate (2.5 g fiber) ▪ **41** percent protein.

Q

Grilled Turkey Reuben on Dark Rye

One bite and you become a reformed corned beef Reuben fan. Not only is this turkey Reuben lower in fat and salt, it is moist. Be sure to ask for "oven-baked" turkey breast, sliced very thin at your local deli. Also, request that your cheese be sliced very thin. You will be surprised how high a pile of turkey sliced "very thin" can be, compared with thick-sliced turkey.

4 tablespoons reduced-fat Thousand Island dressing

8 slices dark rye bread

½ pound oven-baked turkey breast, sliced very thin

¼ pound low-fat Swiss cheese, sliced very thin (Alpine Lace cheese is especially good)

1 cup sauerkraut, drained

1 medium tomato, sliced thin

cooking spray

1   Spread 1 tablespoon of Thousand Island dressing on each of 4 slices of bread. Set aside.

2   Arrange turkey, cheese, sauerkraut, and tomato evenly on the remaining 4 slices of bread. Top with the Thousand Island slices of bread. Press firmly together.

3   Spray a large nonstick skillet or griddle with cooking spray. Heat to medium-high. Spray sandwiches with cooking spray when ready to place in skillet. Grill until brown and crisp; turn once. May need to press down each side with a spatula, to heat through. If sandwiches are not hot in middle, microwave on high for 1 minute each. Serve immediately.

MAKES 4 SANDWICHES

NUTRITIONAL ANALYSIS PER SANDWICH **288 calories** ▪ **29 percent fat (total fat 9.3 g, saturated fat 2.4 g)** ▪ **44 percent carbohydrate (5 g fiber)** ▪ **27 percent protein.**

C

Build-Your-Own Fish Tacos

Build-your-own tacos are a great lunch for a crowd. Serve with Avocado-Lime Salsa (page 36), Low-Fat Chunky Guacamole (page 40), and Classic Lemonade (page 278).

cooking spray

juice of 1 large lemon

1 teaspoon chili powder

1 teaspoon paprika

½ teaspoon dried oregano

1 pound fillet of sole

salt

1 tablespoon canned jalapeño pepper, diced

1 tablespoon fresh lemon juice

⅔ cup commercial salsa

2 tablespoons onion, minced

3 tablespoons fresh cilantro, chopped

1 cup tomato, diced and drained

3 cups cabbage, shredded

⅔ cup fat-free sour cream

1 large avocado, peeled, pitted, and sliced into 12 thin slices

12 corn tortillas

Heat broiler. Line a cookie sheet with tinfoil and coat with cooking spray.

1   In a pie pan, mix lemon juice, chili powder, paprika, and oregano. Dip sole briefly into lemon mixture, covering both sides, and place on cookie sheet. Salt lightly. Broil until cooked through, approximately 3 minutes. Remove from oven. When cool, break into large chunks and place in medium bowl. Gently stir in jalapeño pepper and lemon juice. (If you like a spicier taste, add an extra tablespoon of jalapeño pepper.) Set aside.

2   In a medium bowl, mix salsa, onion, and cilantro. Set aside.

3   Place tomatoes, cabbage, sour cream, and avocado in separate serving bowls. Set aside.

4   Heat a nonstick griddle to medium-high. Place tortillas on griddle and warm, turning once.

5   Fill each tortilla with 1 ounce of the fish mixture, ¼ cup cabbage, 1 tablespoon of tomatoes, 1 tablespoon of salsa, 1 slice of avocado, and 1 tablespoon of sour cream.

MAKES 12 TACOS

NUTRITIONAL ANALYSIS PER TACO **149 calories** ▪ **23 percent fat (total fat 3.8 g, saturated fat ‹ 1 g)** ▪ **50 percent carbohydrate (3 g fiber)** ▪ **27 percent protein.**

S

Roasted Veggie Focaccia Layered with Eggplant, Roasted Peppers, Portabello Mushrooms, Feta Cheese, Arugula, and Garlic Balsamic Vinaigrette

VINAIGRETTE

1 tablespoon olive oil

2 tablespoons balsamic vinegar

2 large cloves garlic, minced or pressed

1 teaspoon sugar

1 teaspoon Italian seasoning or basil

FOCACCIA

cooking spray

1 medium eggplant, sliced into ½-inch-thick slices

2 medium portabello mushrooms, cleaned, with stems removed

¼ teaspoon salt

¼ teaspoon pepper

1 cup roasted peppers (from commercial jar of roasted peppers), rinsed, patted dry, and sliced into thick strips

½ cup arugula salad greens

¼ cup feta cheese, crumbled

1 (9-inch) purchased focaccia bread round (rosemary-onion works well)

Preheat oven to 425°. Cover a large, flat baking sheet with foil and spray with cooking spray.

1 In a small bowl, whisk together all vinaigrette ingredients. Set aside.

2 Arrange eggplant slices and whole mushrooms in a single layer on baking sheet. Sprinkle with salt and pepper. Drizzle about 1 tablespoon vinaigrette over eggplant and mushrooms. (Save the remaining vinaigrette for later.) Place vegetables in oven. Roast for 15 minutes or until golden brown and tender. Remove from oven. Set aside.

3 Meanwhile, place roasted peppers, arugula, and feta cheese in separate bowls.

4 Remove portabello mushrooms from baking sheet and slice into ½-inch strips. Set aside.

5 Slice focaccia in half horizontally. Place one layer of eggplant on bottom half. Add several sliced mushrooms, drizzle with about 1 teaspoon vinaigrette. Top with a sprinkle of feta cheese and arugula. Continue layering process until all ingredients are used. Cover with top half of focaccia. Press down firmly. Place back on foiled baking sheet. Bake for 10 minutes or until bread is golden brown and crispy.

6 Remove from oven. Slice into quarters and serve hot.

MAKES 4 SANDWICHES

NUTRITIONAL ANALYSIS PER SANDWICH **329 calories** ▪ **26 percent fat (total fat 9.5 g, saturated fat 3.5 g)** ▪ **60 percent carbohydrate (9 g fiber)** ▪ **14 percent protein.**

A

Northwest Sushi Roll-Ups with Smoked Salmon

The unique culinary cuisine in the Pacific Northwest is renowned for its salmon, wild mushrooms, and world-famous vineyards. Serve this lunch with a white wine from Oregon.

2 ounces light cream cheese

1 teaspoon cream-style horseradish

2 cups cooked rice (white or brown), warm or cold

1 cup carrots, peeled and grated

1 cup cucumber, diced very small (use a hothouse brand—seedless)

3 tablespoons seasoned rice vinegar

3 tablespoons water

2 teaspoons fresh ginger, peeled and minced

1 teaspoon Splenda

8 small whole wheat or white tortillas (7 inches by 7 inches)

4 ounces smoked salmon, broken into large pieces (or 4 ounces fresh grilled salmon)

1   In a small bowl, combine cream cheese and horseradish. Mix well. Set aside.

2   In a medium bowl, combine rice, carrots, and cucumber. Mix well. Set aside.

3   In a small bowl, whisk together rice vinegar, water, ginger, and Splenda. Pour into rice mixture. Stir well. (Can be prepared up to 24 hours in advance; cover and store in refrigerator.)

4   To prepare sushi roll-ups: Place 1 tortilla on a 10-inch square of plastic wrap. Spread 1 teaspoon of cream cheese mixture over tortilla. (Don't worry about getting mixture on edges, since you will cut them later.) Spread about ⅓ cup rice mixture evenly on inner third of tortilla. Place several pieces of smoked salmon down center of rice mixture. Beginning at closest edge to you, roll tortilla firmly and tightly over rice-salmon mixture. Continue to roll until completed. Use clean plastic wrap underneath to wrap the sushi roll-up tightly. Repeat process until all wraps have been completed. Refrigerate overnight or at least 4 hours.

5   To serve, trim off edges, cut rolls into 8 slices, and serve.

MAKES 8 SERVINGS

NUTRITIONAL ANALYSIS PER SERVING **173 calories** ▪ **14 percent fat (total fat 2.7 g, saturated fat 1 g)** ▪ **70 percent carbohydrate (3.5 g fiber)** ▪ **16 percent protein.**

Toasted Tomato and Fresh Basil on Sourdough

Jeanette's brother "the Chef" has declared this to be the ultimate use and taste for a fresh-picked vine-ripened tomato.

---

2 tablespoons fat-free or reduced-fat mayonnaise

4 thick slices sourdough bread, toasted

2 medium vine-ripened tomatoes, cored and cut into 4 slices each

½ cup fresh basil leaves, rinsed, dried, with stems removed

1 teaspoon olive oil mixed with 1 teaspoon balsamic vinegar

salt and pepper, to taste

1   Spread 1 tablespoon mayonnaise on 2 slices toasted bread. Place 4 slices tomatoes and ¼ cup fresh basil leaves on each slice of bread with mayonnaise. Drizzle with olive oil–balsamic mixture. Season with salt and pepper.

2   Top with remaining slices of toasted bread, cut in half, and serve.

MAKES 2 SANDWICHES

NUTRITIONAL ANALYSIS PER SANDWICH **199 calories** ▪ **19 percent fat** (total fat 4.2 g, saturated fat < 1 g) ▪ **69 percent carbohydrate** (3.7 g fiber) ▪ **12 percent protein**.

1-2-3 Sloppy Joes

This low-fat version of the traditional Sloppy Joe goes great with a tossed salad.

FOOD TIP

This comfort-food lunch for kids and adults has been prized in American culture for decades because it is both inexpensive and nourishing. The origin of the Sloppy Joe might be Sioux City, Iowa, where the "loose-meat sandwich" was first seen on the menu.

2 teaspoons canola oil

1 small onion, diced (approximately ⅔ cup)

2 cloves garlic, minced

1 pound ground turkey breast

1 (12-ounce) jar chili sauce

2 tablespoons brown sugar

6 whole wheat hamburger buns, lightly toasted

1   In a medium nonstick skillet, warm oil over medium heat. Add onion and garlic and sauté until translucent, approximately 5 minutes.

2   Add turkey to skillet and stir, breaking up clumps, until cooked through, approximately 7 minutes. Add chili sauce and sugar to skillet, stir, and cook until heated through, approximately 3 minutes.

3   Spoon turkey mixture over bottom halves of buns, top with remaining halves, and serve immediately.

MAKES 6 SLOPPY JOES

NUTRITIONAL ANALYSIS PER SLOPPY JOE **302 calories** ▪ **15 percent fat (total fat 5 g, saturated fat ‹ 1 g)** ▪ **55 percent carbohydrate (2 g fiber)** ▪ **30 percent protein.**

Chicken and Peanut Wraps

Make extra wraps for quick lunches later in the week. Cover them tightly with plastic wrap, and they will keep in the refrigerator for two days. Or prepare all the ingredients, refrigerate, and make a wrap as you go.

6 tablespoons reduced-fat peanut butter

4 teaspoons fresh ginger, peeled and minced

2 cloves garlic, minced

4 tablespoons fresh lime juice

8 teaspoons soy sauce

¼ teaspoon red pepper flakes

¼ cup green onion, chopped

8 ounces cooked chicken breast, shredded

½ cup fresh cilantro, chopped

1 cup red bell pepper, stemmed, seeded, and sliced into thin strips

1 apple, peeled, cored, and sliced into thin strips

1 cup lettuce, sliced into strips

4 (12-inch) tortilla wraps (garlic herb or spinach are both good)

1 In a medium bowl, blend peanut butter, ginger, garlic, lime juice, soy sauce, and pepper flakes.

2 Stir the green onion, chicken, and cilantro into peanut sauce. Blend well.

3 Spoon a quarter of the peanut-chicken mixture onto a tortilla. Top with a quarter of the red pepper, apple, and lettuce. Roll up and serve.

MAKES 4 WRAPS

NUTRITIONAL ANALYSIS PER WRAP **366 calories** ▪ **28 percent fat (total fat 11.4 g, saturated fat 2.7 g)** ▪ **42 percent carbohydrate (5 g fiber)** ▪ **30 percent protein.**

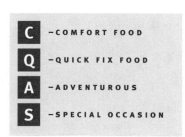

C –COMFORT FOOD
Q –QUICK FIX FOOD
A –ADVENTUROUS
S –SPECIAL OCCASION

Soups and Stews

Emotional Eating

- Does a bag of chips help calm you down?

- Do you graze from the refrigerator after putting the kids to bed?

- After an exhausting week, do you reward yourself with a half gallon of ice cream?

- Do cookies help ease your troubled mind when you're frustrated or angry?

- Do you head for the kitchen when you're bored or lonely?

If so, you're not alone. Most people have at one time or another eaten to soothe their moods. Some people feed their feelings once in a while, others every day. We eat to curb anger, frustration, or when unhappy. We eat for companionship when lonely or jealous. We eat to feel better about ourselves after being criticized or ignored, or when our feelings have been hurt. We use food as a tranquilizer when we're anxious or as a mood elevator when we're depressed. We eat for fun when happy, excited, nervous, or with friends. Some of us eat for frivolous reasons (e.g., to soothe daily hassles), and some of us eat to numb unresolved traumas, violence, or neglect in our past.

It's a Chemical Thing

There's nothing wrong with an occasional snack to soothe a mood. In fact, the marriage of emotions and food is as basic to our natures as breathing. Our first lesson in life is to associate food with love. As babies, the most powerful comforter when we were distressed was food, so it makes sense that as adults we continue to turn to that source of comfort. Grabbing a cookie is one way to reexperience a feeling of security, home, or a safe place.

A hormone called oxytocin hard-wires this connection into the brain. Oxytocin is released in the new mother right after her baby is born. It stimulates milk production and helps strengthen the mother-child bond. While this chemistry is useful in the early months of life, limited evidence suggests that elevated levels of oxytocin in adults might cloud the distinction between physical hunger and feeling lonely or in need of love, which then could lead to overeating and possibly weight gain.

Other chemicals in the body also nudge us to nosh. A chemical in the brain called serotonin regulates our moods and our appetites. When serotonin levels are high, we feel good, calm, and satisfied; when they are low, we feel irritable, moody, tense, anxious, even depressed, and we crave carbohydrate-rich foods—in particular, sweets. And rightfully so. These are the very foods that raise serotonin levels and help us feel better. It doesn't take too many trips to the cookie jar to unconsciously learn to self-medicate with sweets when we are down in the dumps.

The Diet Connection

Restrictive diets contribute to emotional eating. "People who diet or eat fewer calories than they need are semi-starving themselves, and this places them at particular risk for uncontrolled emotional eating," warns Bruce Arnow, Ph.D., a clinical psychologist and associate professor of psychiatry at Stanford University Medical Center.

Repeated dieting also teaches a person to replace internal cues of real physical hunger with external signals, such as eating at certain times or eating only certain foods. This numbs you to the hunger response. Once a person loses the ability to recognize physical hunger, it is easy to mistake emotional discomfort, such as feeling lonely or depressed, for hunger. Consequently, dieters often eat for reasons other than just needing fuel, which can lead to weight gain. "It's amazing how much food a person can consume when eating in response to feelings like depression or loneliness, rather than physical hunger," says Barbara Rolls, Ph.D., at Pennsylvania State University. "It's essential that we learn to listen to our bodies, eat only when physically hungry, stop when comfortably full, and find nonfood ways to sooth our emotions."

Stuff It

Turning to food for something other than physical nourishment only trades one problem for another. Curling up with a bag of cookies temporarily solves boredom, but at a cost. As long as you're eating, the cookies provide a sense of comfort and reassurance; they soothe the inner ache or divert your thoughts from uncomfortable issues. In the long run, you pack on the pounds, and you're left feeling ashamed, guilty, and mad at yourself. "A red flag that emotional eating has become a problem is when you notice it has become a pattern to turn to food when you are anxious, depressed, or frustrated. This is especially a problem when you start to gain weight," says Gayle Timmerman, Ph.D., R.N., an associate professor in the School of Nursing at the University of Texas and the lead researcher on a National Institutes of Health–funded study on bingeing, deprivation, and dieting.

Emotional eating seldom drives you to eat broccoli. "Emotional eaters choose fatty, sugary foods, such as ice cream, cookies, chips, or doughnuts," says Dr. Arnow. You're also more likely to mend a mood with hamburgers, pizza, or chocolate than with chard or tofu. Powering down these high-fat and sugar items means that people who eat to stuff emotions are likely to end up overweight, while people who learn to handle their emotional eating lose weight.

In short, the kitchen shouldn't be your psychiatrist's couch or emotional-management center. If eating to soothe emotions is getting in the way of enjoying life or maintaining your weight, you must find a way to comfort yourself with something other than food or at least choose foods that nurture your health and mood, rather than stuff them.

Check In

Emotional eaters need alternative coping skills. "People who develop habits of turning to food every time things go wrong, program themselves for emotional eating," says Dr. Arnow. "If they anticipate that they are likely to overeat later, they starve themselves early in the day, which of course can lead to a binge."

What can you do instead?

- Eat regular meals, rather than skipping meals and overeating later.

- Stop yourself before a snack and check in with your emotions. In fact, several times a day, ask yourself how you are feeling. Are you mad, happy, sad, calm, angry, frustrated, excited, hungry, or what? Ask yourself what you need. Do you need a hug, a breath of fresh air, a good talk with a friend, or a snack? Many times your cravings are for something other than food. In those cases, do something to feel better, rather than unconsciously grab a bag of chips. For example, a brisk walk or a bike ride will do much more for relieving frustration than eating a stale doughnut in the employees' lounge.

- Remind yourself that food won't make you feel better. Believe it or not, that simple strategy actually works. In one study, people who were feeling down in the dumps ate less when told that fatty snacks wouldn't improve their moods.

- Dr. Timmerman recommends you develop a list of five things you will do before you eat, such as call a friend or take a 20-minute walk. "This helps diffuse the urge to eat," she adds.

- Don't deprive yourself. If you are craving a piece of cake and that is exactly what you want and need, serve yourself a small piece and enjoy every bite. Just do it consciously, not emotionally.

- Minimize the damage of emotional eating by substituting nutritious, or at least low-calorie, foods that will still leave you feeling satisfied. "If you turn to sweet-and-creamy foods when you are down in the dumps, try sugar-free, fat-free pudding; if you go for the chips, keep baked chips on hand," recommends Dr. Timmerman. Stocking the kitchen with only healthy comfort foods is the first step in stopping the emotional eating cycle.

Comfort Foods

We often reach for favorite comfort foods when we need a little emotional pick-me-up. They taste best on dreary, damp days and are what we yearn for when lonely. Comfort foods make us feel better, safer, and loved. They warm our tummies and calm our hearts.

Each of us has our own personal stash of favorite comfort foods, often stemming from childhood memories. There usually is a little of "Mom's home cooking" in the equation. My mom often served hot tea sweetened with milk and sugar along with cinnamon toast when I was sick as a child. Today, the smell of cinnamon is comforting to me, and I enjoy nothing better than a cup of tea on a winter's day. For many Americans, comfort food is synonymous with meat loaf and mashed potatoes, peanut butter and jelly sandwiches, ice cream, a special cake or batch of cookies, beef stew, macaroni and cheese, apple pie, or chicken and noodles. Soup is almost always on people's list of comfort foods. A study from the University of Illinois found that 40 percent of comfort foods were old-time favorites, such as soup.

Caloric Density: The Case for Soups and Stews

If you are in need of a comfort fest, your best bet is a hot cup of soup or bowl of stew. These foods are most likely to satisfy your mood and your taste buds, while filling you up, not out. That's because they are "calorie-dilute."

Caloric density ranks foods by calories per gram. Calorie-dense foods, such as refined grains, processed snack foods, or greasy fast foods, supply a hefty dose of calories for every gram, while calorie-dilute foods, such as fruits, vegetables, whole grain pasta, and legumes, supply few calories for the same weight.

THE LOWDOWN ON CALORIC DENSITY

Caloric density is calculated by dividing the calories in a food by its weight in grams. A good-mood diet is based on foods with low-caloric density. The more calorie-dense foods in your diet, the more likely you will gain weight. Here are a few foods, ranked from high to low caloric density.

FOOD	CALORIES	CALORIES/GRAM
Oil (1 tablespoon)	120	8.8
Cheddar cheese (1 ounce)	110	4.0
Glazed doughnut (2 ounces)	180	3.5
French fries (5 ounces)	450	3.1
Cheese pizza (3½-ounce slice)	310	3.0
Ice cream (1 cup)	340	1.8
Broiled fish (6 ounces)	200	1.2
Yogurt, fruit, low-fat (8 ounces)	230	1.0
Oatmeal, cooked (1 cup)	150	0.6
Apple (1)	90	0.6
Carrot, raw (1)	30	0.4
Broccoli, cooked (½ cup)	21	0.3
Spinach, raw (1 cup)	10	0.2

So what does this have to do with feeling full? According to studies conducted by Dr. Rolls, people stop eating when they have consumed a given weight or volume of food, regardless of its calories. "When we gave people either 300, 450, or 600 ml drinks that contained the same calories, the people who drank the greatest volume ate less a half hour later," says Dr. Rolls. In short, you will fill up on a certain volume of food, but a pound of potato chips will add 2,427 calories to your diet, while a pound of blueberries supplies only 254 calories. Put another way, three bite-size chocolate chip cookies weigh only an ounce, contain 144 calories, and do little to fill you up. Or you can pig out on four cups (32 ounces) of Garden Tomato Soup with Fresh Basil for the same calories and feel full all afternoon.

Ounce for ounce, foods weigh the most when they're packed with water and fiber, which could be the reason why calorie-dilute, fiber-rich soups and stews fill us up on fewer calories, keep us feeling satisfied between meals, and help us lose weight, while calorie-dense foods high in fat and/or sugar spur us to eat more. Researchers at the University of Sydney created a "Satiety Index" by asking people to consume 38 common foods and then measure their hunger and food intake for the two hours following the meals. The researchers found that people consumed fewer calories, yet felt more satisfied, after eating fiber-rich, water-packed foods, such as cooked oatmeal or pasta, oranges, and beans, than when they ate high-fat, fiber-poor croissants, cake, doughnuts, or candy.

Soups and stews are satisfying because they are some of the best sources of water and fiber, and, therefore, weigh a lot. One study found that people who ate a bowl of soup at the beginning of a meal cut back on calories in the rest of the meal, whereas cheese and crackers did not rein in appetites. In another study from Pennsylvania, women were asked to eat a 270-calorie "first course" before lunch that consisted of either a chicken-rice casserole, the same casserole served with 10 ounces of water, or the casserole made into a soup by adding 10 ounces of water. Only the women who ate soup cut back on calories for the rest of the meal, and they stayed full longer throughout the day than the other women.

The trick is to make calorie-dilute foods, such as soups and stews, the basis of a meal plan, not the whole diet. (Hint: Soup-only diets don't work, but soup added to a healthful diet does.) You'll get larger portions for the same calories by switching from Swedish meatballs to broth-based or chunky vegetable soup as an appetizer. Cream-based soups fit the bill only if they are thickened with potatoes or fat-free half-and-half, not real cream.

The best thing about using caloric density in preparing meals is that cutting calories doesn't mean you are famished all day. Just the opposite. Have a hefty serving of one of the stews or soups in this section for lunch, and you'll feel warm and satisfied all afternoon. What a great way to comfort and nourish yourself at the same time! Every section in this cookbook provides other traditional comfort foods that have been given a low-calorie face-lift.

12 QUICK-FIX SOUPS

1. **PMS SOUP:** Calcium helps curb the symptoms of premenstrual syndrome (PMS). You can enrich most canned soups by using nonfat milk instead of water.

2. **VEGGIES À LA CAMPBELLS:** Add leftover vegetables to canned vegetable soup or a can of carrots or corn to beef barley soup.

3. **INSTANT CREAMED SOUPS:** Puree leftover vegetables and add to canned vegetable beef soup.

4. **CHUNKY TOMATO SOUP:** Heat canned tomato soup with nonfat milk, toss in dried Japanese wasabi peas or edename (green soybeans).

5. **BATCH IT:** Make a double batch on the weekend of any of the recipes in this section and use throughout the week for lunches and dinners.

6. **PUREE TO SOUP:** Add fat-free half-and-half or nonfat milk to leftover Creamy Cauliflower Puree (page 225) and reheat in microwave.

7. **SOUP TO STEW:** Add frozen potatoes O'Brien to a can of vegetable soup to turn a soup into a thick stew.

8. **QUICK CREAM OF MUSHROOM SOUP:** Dilute a can of low-fat cream of mushroom soup with fat-free half-and-half or nonfat evaporated milk and add fresh sliced mushrooms.

9. **CHILLED FRUIT SOUP:** Peel and seed a mango and puree in blender. Add a little orange juice, nonfat evaporated milk, and a dash of nutmeg or cinnamon. Chill and serve.

10. **CREAM OF ASPARAGUS SOUP:** Puree a can of asparagus, add nonfat milk or fat-free half-and-half, salt, pepper, and spices to taste. Heat in microwave and serve.

11. **INSTANT CLAM CHOWDER:** To a can of clam chowder, add fat-free half-and-half or nonfat evaporated milk and extra canned clams. Serve with a tossed salad and crusty bread.

12. **MORE SOUP TO STEW:** Add leftover chicken and frozen peas to commercial chicken noodle soup.

Smoky Sweet Potato 'n' Corn Chowder

If you like a spicy bite to your soup, add an extra chipotle pepper.

2 teaspoons olive oil

⅔ pound turkey ham, skinned and diced

⅔ cup red bell pepper, diced

½ green bell pepper, diced

2 cups yellow onions, diced

3 medium sweet potatoes, peeled and cut into ¾-inch cubes

1 (26-ounce) can fat-free chicken broth

2 teaspoons "Better Than Bouillon" Chicken Base (optional)

1 canned chipotle chili, diced

1 (16-ounce) bag of frozen corn

1 cup nonfat milk or ½ cup nonfat milk and ½ cup fat-free half-and-half

cilantro, chopped (optional)

1   Warm oil in a large saucepan over medium heat. Cook turkey ham until heated through. Add peppers and onion and continue cooking, stirring frequently, until onion is tender, approximately 10 minutes.

2   Add sweet potatoes, chicken broth, bouillon, and chipotle chili to pot, cover, and simmer for 15 minutes or until potato is cooked but still firm.

3   Add corn and heat through. Just before serving, add milk. Serve and garnish with cilantro if desired.

MAKES 6 SERVINGS OF 2 CUPS EACH

NUTRITIONAL ANALYSIS PER SERVING **259 calories** ▪ **17 percent fat (total fat 5 g, saturated fat 1 g)** ▪ **57 percent carbohydrate (5 g fiber)** ▪ **26 percent protein.**

A

Garden Tomato Soup with Fresh Basil

Every year I plant too many tomato plants. This soup is a great solution, since it uses 14 cups of fresh tomatoes! If you want a sweeter taste, add a teaspoon or two of sugar toward the end of the cooking period. Serve with quesadillas or Green and Red Chunky Salad with Oregano (page 125).

FOOD TIP

Looking for other ways to use up those garden tomatoes? Here are a few solutions: (1) slice tomatoes, drizzle with olive oil and sprinkle with salt; (2) make a sandwich with tomato slices, turkey bacon, arugula, and avocado; (3) serve slow-roasted beefsteak tomatoes drizzled with olive oil as a side dish; (4) garnish grilled fish with diced tomatoes; or (5) sauté diced tomatoes and serve with eggs, toast, and orange juice for breakfast.

MOOD TIP

Research from Pennsylvania State University found that tomato soup and chunky vegetable soups help curb appetite, so people eat less at the same or next meal.

1 teaspoon olive oil

2 cups yellow onion, chopped

7 cups tomatoes, chopped (about 2 pounds)

1 (49-ounce) can fat-free chicken broth

2 tablespoons "Better Than Bouillon" Chicken Base (optional)

3 cloves garlic, minced

7 cups tomatoes, diced

salt and pepper, to taste

⅓ cup fresh basil leaves, chopped

Parmesan cheese, grated (optional)

1   In a large saucepan, warm oil over medium heat. Add onions and sauté for 5 minutes or until tender, stirring frequently. Add 7 cups chopped tomatoes and stir until heated through. Add chicken broth and bouillon, bring to a gentle boil, reduce heat, and simmer for 45 minutes or until stock is reduced to about 8 cups.

2   In batches, blend stock in a blender until creamy. Return to saucepan and add garlic and 7 cups diced tomatoes, salt, and pepper. Bring to boil, reduce heat, and simmer for 15 minutes.

3   Remove soup from heat, stir in basil, and adjust seasonings. Sprinkle individual bowls with grated Parmesan if desired. If you don't plan to eat all the soup at one sitting, mix some of the basil only into the portion to be eaten immediately. Reheat leftovers and add the rest of the basil at a later time.

MAKES 8 SERVINGS OF APPROXIMATELY 1¾ CUPS EACH

NUTRITIONAL ANALYSIS PER SERVING **116 calories** ▪ **19 percent fat** (total fat 2.4 g, saturated fat ‹ 1 g) ▪ **60 percent carbohydrate** (5 g fiber) ▪ **21 percent protein.**

A

Pumpkin-Corn Soup with Creamy Lime-Ginger Sauce

This rich autumn soup takes only 30 minutes to make, yet it is filling and warm on a cool autumn evening. Tastes great with corn bread and a salad (Sesame-Ginger Coleslaw on page 121 would be a great accompaniment). This soup is especially high in beta-carotene and iron, and supplies hefty doses of B vitamins, calcium, magnesium, vitamin E, and selenium.

SOUP

1 (16-ounce) bag of frozen corn

3 cups fat-free chicken broth

3 cloves garlic, minced

1 tablespoon "Better Than Bouillon" Chicken Base (optional)

salt and pepper, to taste

1 (29-ounce) can pumpkin

2 tablespoons brown sugar

SAUCE

¼ cup fresh lime juice

1 tablespoon fresh ginger, peeled and grated

½ cup fat-free sour cream

lime peel, finely grated

1 Steam corn until hot. In batches, place corn in blender with enough chicken broth to puree until smooth. Run through sieve and discard skins.

2 In a large nonstick saucepan, place corn-and-stock juice, remaining chicken broth, garlic, chicken base, and salt and pepper. Cook over medium heat, stirring occasionally until mixture comes to a boil. Reduce heat and add pumpkin and sugar. Stir and heat through, about 15 minutes.

3 To prepare sauce: In a small saucepan, heat juice and ginger over medium heat to disperse ginger. In small bowl, pour juice through sieve to remove ginger. Add sour cream and blend thoroughly.

4 To serve, drizzle 1 tablespoon of sauce over each bowlful of soup, then run a fork sideways though cream. Sprinkle lightly with finely grated lime peel.

MAKES 4 SERVINGS OF 2 CUPS EACH

NUTRITIONAL ANALYSIS PER SERVING **248 calories** ▪ **8 percent fat (total fat 2.2 g,** saturated fat ‹ 1 g)** ▪ **75 percent carbohydrate (10 g fiber)** ▪ **17 percent protein.**

Black Bean Chili with Chicken

Move over traditional red bean chili, black beans are here to stay. This recipe will satisfy the chili connoisseur. Fresh hot corn bread with honey is the perfect complement to this meal.

FOOD TIP

A bonanza of soluble fiber, black beans help keep blood sugar levels on an even keel, staving off hunger and helping to maintain energy levels throughout the day.

1 recipe for Black Beans with Cumin and Chipotle Peppers (page 154)

4 (4-ounce) skinless, boneless chicken breasts, boiled and diced

2 (10-ounce) cans Mexican diced tomatoes and green chiles

½ teaspoon ground cinnamon

2 teaspoons canned chipotle peppers in adobo sauce, diced (or 1 teaspoon crushed dried chipotle peppers)

1 cup water

low-fat cheddar cheese, grated (optional)

baked tortilla chips, crushed (optional)

lime wedges (optional)

1   In a large soup pot, over medium-high heat, place all ingredients except for cheddar cheese, tortilla chips, and lime wedges. Bring to a boil, then reduce heat to medium low and simmer for 20 minutes.

2   Spoon chili into soup bowls.

3   Place low-fat cheddar cheese and crushed tortilla chips into separate bowls and use as chili's toppings. Use the lime wedges to squeeze juice into chili for added zest.

MAKES 10 SERVINGS OF APPROXIMATELY 1 CUP EACH

NUTRITIONAL ANALYSIS PER SERVING **207 calories** ▪ **16 percent fat (total fat 3.7 g, saturated fat < 1 g)** ▪ **51 percent carbohydrate (7 g fiber)** ▪ **33 percent protein.**

C

Posole Soup

Prepare yourself for a real treat if you haven't discovered this traditional Mexican soup. It screams with authentic flavor and the aroma is heavenly. Simple and quick to make. For a vegetarian meal, leave out the chicken.

---

2 (15.5-ounce) cans Great Northern beans, undrained

1 (15.5-ounce) can hominy, undrained

2 (14.5-ounce) cans Mexican stewed tomatoes, undrained

1 (28-ounce) can diced Italian plum tomatoes, undrained

1 (11-ounce) can whole kernel yellow corn, undrained

1 (7-ounce) can diced green chilies

2 teaspoons ground coriander

1 teaspoon fresh orange rind, grated

1 teaspoon hot chili powder

½ cup orange juice

2 bay leaves

2 cups of water

2 cups white chicken meat, diced or shredded

¼ cup fresh cilantro, chopped

1   Combine all ingredients except cilantro in a large soup pot or Dutch oven. Bring to a boil. Cover, reduce heat, and simmer for 20 to 30 minutes, stirring occasionally. Discard bay leaves.

2   Add cilantro, stir to mix. Add more water or tomatoes if soup is too thick.

3   Ladle into bowls.

MAKES 10 SERVINGS OF APPROXIMATELY 1½ CUPS EACH

NUTRITIONAL ANALYSIS PER SERVING **245 calories** ▪ **8 percent fat (total fat 2.2 g,** saturated fat ‹ 0.5 g) ▪ **67 percent carbohydrate (11 g fiber)** ▪ **25 percent protein.**

Old-Fashioned Country Vegetable-Beef Stew

I grew up on this hearty stew, packed with carrots and other vegetables. This recipe makes enough to last all week for dinners, lunches, or snacks. Serve with biscuits, and you have a meal-in-one. Or freeze in smaller portions for use at a later date.

MOOD TIP

When you cook stews in cast-iron pots, the iron leeches out of the pot and into the food, significantly increasing the iron content of the meal. This is especially true for foods with a tomato base, such as this beef stew.

2 pounds extra-lean stew meat, trimmed and cut into 1-inch cubes

½ cup all-purpose flour

½ teaspoon paprika

¼ teaspoon salt

1 tablespoon canola oil

32 ounces 99 percent fat-free beef broth

1 tablespoon "Better Than Bouillon" Beef Base (optional)

1 (15-ounce) can tomato sauce

3 large bay leaves

4 cups yellow onions, chopped

6 cloves garlic, minced

4 cups celery, chopped in 1-inch chunks

8 cups carrots, peeled and chopped into 1-inch chunks (about 14 carrots)

½ pound mushrooms, washed and sliced thick

½ pound white or red potatoes, cut into large chunks

salt and pepper, to taste

1   In a medium plastic bag, add meat, flour, paprika, and salt. Shake to coat meat thoroughly.

2   Heat oil in large Dutch oven (preferably cast iron). Place floured meat in pan and cook over medium heat to brown, turning frequently, about 10 minutes. Add broth, bouillon, tomato sauce, and bay leaves. Stir, cover, and simmer for 1 hour (or longer if time allows, up to 3 hours).

3   Add onion and garlic to meat and cook, covered, another 20 minutes.

4   Add celery, carrots, and mushrooms. Cook for 20 minutes.

5   Add potatoes and mix to cover with stew broth. Cover pan and continue to simmer until potatoes are tender, approximately 25 minutes. Season with salt and pepper.

MAKES 18 CUPS

NUTRITIONAL ANALYSIS PER CUP **177 calories** ▪ **17 percent fat** (total fat 3.3 g, saturated fat 1 g) ▪ **50 percent carbohydrate** (4.1 g fiber) ▪ **33 percent protein.**

Heartwarming Winter Vegetable Soup

This hearty soup is quick to make and chock-full of yummy vegetables. It's a meal in itself served with warmed bread.

FOOD TIP
Have you ever added a tablespoon, not the recommended teaspoon, of salt to a recipe? To rescue an oversalted soup or stew, add a quartered raw potato, a dash of sugar, or even a little tomato paste to temper the saltiness. Throw out the potato before serving.

1 teaspoon olive oil

1 cup turkey ham, cut into ½-inch cubes

1 medium onion, chopped (about 1½ cups total)

4 cloves garlic, minced

1 cup celery, diced

2 bay leaves

2 cups winter squash, peeled, seeded, and cubed (acorn, butternut, kabocha, or hubbard squash)

1 cup carrots, peeled and sliced in thin rounds

2 yellow potatoes, peeled and cubed (about 2 cups total)

1½ teaspoons dried basil

¼ teaspoon cinnamon

1 (28-ounce) can stewed tomatoes, chopped

6 cups fat-free chicken broth

1 (15.5-ounce) can kidney beans, rinsed and drained

3 teaspoons fresh thyme leaves

½ package frozen chopped spinach

salt and pepper, to taste

1   Heat oil in a Dutch oven (preferably cast iron) over medium-high heat. Add turkey ham, onion, garlic, and celery, and sauté for 7 minutes or until onion is transparent. Add bay leaves, squash, carrots, and potatoes. Stir and continue to sauté for another 7 minutes.

2   Add basil, cinnamon, tomatoes, and broth. Bring to a boil, reduce heat, and simmer for 20 minutes or until vegetables are cooked through but not mushy.

3   Add beans, thyme, and spinach. Simmer for 5 minutes or until spinach is heated through. Season with salt and pepper.

MAKES 12 SERVINGS

NUTRITIONAL ANALYSIS PER SERVING **163 calories** ▪ **9 percent fat (total fat 1.6 g, saturated fat < 0.5 g)** ▪ **64 percent carbohydrate (6.7 g fiber)** ▪ **27 percent protein.**

C

Cioppino in a Robust Tomato Base, Infused with Fresh Fennel and Orange

This fish soup is a classic that has been revamped with fresh fennel and orange. The flavors linger long after the last bite.

FOOD TIP

Fennel is an aromatic herb similar in looks to dill. Both the root and the leaves have a mild licorice flavor. Fennel dates back to the ancient Greeks and Romans; the latter thought it aided weight loss.

2 tablespoons olive oil

2 fennel bulbs, sliced paper thin

2 leeks (white part only), sliced paper thin

1 large sweet onion, chopped

3 teaspoons dried oregano

1 teaspoon dried thyme

1½ teaspoons fennel seeds

½ teaspoon crushed red pepper flakes

1 (28-ounce) can crushed tomatoes with added puree

2 (8-ounce) bottles of clam juice

1 large orange, juice and rind

½ cup white wine or substitute with ½ cup orange juice

2 (6.5-ounce) cans chopped clams, plus liquid from 1 can only

1 pound uncooked medium-large shrimp, peeled and deveined

1 pound sea scallops, rinsed and patted dry

1 pound littleneck clams, cleaned

¼ cup fresh basil, chopped

1 Warm oil over medium heat in a heavy, large pot or Dutch oven.

2 Add next 7 ingredients (through red pepper flakes), sauté until tender, about 5 to 7 minutes.

3 Add tomatoes, clam juice, juice from orange and rind, and white wine. Increase heat and boil gently for 15 minutes. (This tomato base can be made the day before and stored in the refrigerator. When ready to use, heat to a gentle boil.)

4 Add clams and liquid from 1 can, shrimp, scallops, and littleneck clams. Cover pan, reduce heat, and simmer for 2 minutes or until shrimp is opaque. (Be careful not to overcook.)

5 Pour into soup bowls, sprinkle with fresh basil, and serve.

MAKES 8 SERVINGS

NUTRITIONAL ANALYSIS PER SERVING **331 calories** ▪ **17 percent fat (total fat 6.3 g, saturated fat ‹ 1 g)** ▪ **37 percent carbohydrate (5.4 g fiber)** ▪ **46 percent protein.**

Butternut Squash Soup with Cranberry Chutney and Roasted Pecans

It's time to get out those favorite soup bowls, light the candles, and prepare a simple mixed green salad to accompany this meal.

---

cooking spray

¼ cup pecans, chopped

1 teaspoon margarine or butter

1 medium sweet onion, diced

2 apples, peeled, seeded, and chopped

½ teaspoon ground nutmeg

3 cups fat-free chicken broth

1 medium butternut squash (about 1½ pounds), peeled, seeded, and cut into 1-inch cubes

½ cup light coconut milk

½ cup fat-free half-and-half

6 tablespoons commercial cranberry chutney, finely chopped

Preheat oven to 350°. Spray a cookie sheet with cooking spray.

1 Sprinkle pecans evenly over surface of cookie sheet. Bake for 3 to 5 minutes or until pecans are toasted. Remove and set aside.

2 In a large soup pot or Dutch oven, melt margarine or butter over medium heat, add onions, apples, and nutmeg. Cook and stir 3 minutes.

3 Add chicken broth and squash. Bring to a boil over high heat. Reduce heat to low. Cover and simmer 20 minutes, until squash is very tender.

4 Process squash mixture (in 2 batches) in a food processor until smooth.

5 Return squash mixture to pot. Add coconut milk, fat-free half-and-half. Stir well. (Add more chicken broth if the soup is too thick.) Heat until hot.

6 Ladle into soup bowls and dollop with 1 tablespoon cranberry chutney, sprinkle with toasted pecans, and serve hot.

MAKES 6 SERVINGS

NUTRITIONAL ANALYSIS PER SERVING **190 calories** ▪ **39 percent fat** (total fat 8.2 g, saturated fat 4.5 g) ▪ **51 percent carbohydrate** (4.3 g fiber) ▪ **10 percent protein**.

Creamy Artichoke Soup
with Roasted Hazelnuts

A great pot of soup will summon friends and family from miles away. This is the soup to do just that! Thick, velvety, yet delicately flavored. The roasted hazelnuts linger with unexpected savor.

cooking spray

4 tablespoons hazelnuts

4 large fresh artichokes, cleaned, stems cut even with bottom of artichoke. Slice ¼-inch off top of artichoke

3 cups water

4 cups fat-free chicken broth

4 tablespoons Wondra flour mixed with ⅓ cup water

1 cup fat-free half-and-half

1 tablespoon cooking sherry

salt and pepper, to taste

2 tablespoons fresh parsley, minced

Preheat oven to 350°. Coat a cookie sheet with cooking spray.

1   Place hazelnuts on cookie sheet. Toast for 5 minutes or until golden. Crush hazelnuts in food processor until very fine. Set aside.

2   Place artichokes snugly, upright, side by side in a large soup pot or Dutch oven. Add water, bring to a quick boil. Cover, reduce heat, and simmer about 30 to 45 minutes or until leaves easily pull apart from artichoke. Using tongs, remove artichokes from pot and cool. Do not discard artichoke water.

3   Add chicken broth and toasted hazelnuts to artichoke water and simmer over low-medium heat until you've completed steps 4 and 5.

4   While broth is simmering, remove leaves from each artichoke down to the choke and set aside. Using a knife or sharp-edged spoon, remove and discard the prickly, feathery choke to expose the artichoke heart. Place clean hearts in a bowl and set aside.

5   Gather artichoke leaves. Hold each leaf by its sharp tip, fresh side up. Scrape out the inner soft pulp, place in the bowl with the artichoke hearts. Repeat process with remaining leaves. Puree the leaf pulp and bottoms in a blender or food processor. (You may need to add ½ to 1 cup of reserved liquid from step 3 to help process.)

6   Add artichoke puree mixture to reserved liquid from step 3 and stir well. Bring soup to a gentle boil, add flour-water mixture. Stir until thickened. Reduce heat.

7   Stir in half-and-half, sherry, salt, and pepper. Garnish with parsley, and serve.

MAKES 6 SERVINGS

NUTRITIONAL ANALYSIS PER SERVING **149 calories** ▪ **27 percent fat** (total fat 4.5 g, saturated fat ‹ 1 g) ▪ **49 percent carbohydrate** (4.7 g fiber) ▪ **24 percent protein.**

C A

Hearty Lamb and Barley Stew

Scotch broth is the technical name for this delicious stew, but broth it is not! This stew is thick and creamy, with just a hint of cinnamon to complement the tender flavor of lamb. A great dish to serve on St. Patrick's Day. To round out the dish, serve with a tossed salad and whole grain bread.

1 tablespoon olive oil

2 small lamb loin chops (approximately 1 pound), trimmed of all fat

salt and pepper, to taste

1 onion, chopped

2 celery stalks, chopped

3 carrots, peeled and chopped

1 leek (white part only), sliced thinly

2 cloves garlic, minced

6 cups water

1 tablespoon "Better Than Bouillon" Beef Base

2 bay leaves

1 cinnamon stick

⅔ cup pearl barley

1 teaspoon fresh thyme leaves, chopped

1 teaspoon fresh rosemary, chopped

salt and pepper, to taste

1   Heat oil in a large soup pot or Dutch oven. Salt and pepper chops, add to pot, and cook over medium heat until brown on both sides, approximately 3 minutes per side. Remove from pot.

2   Add onions, celery, carrots, leek, and garlic to the pot. Sauté until tender for 5 to 7 minutes or until onions are translucent.

3   Add water, beef base, bay leaves, cinnamon, barley, thyme, rosemary, and lamb chops to pot. Bring to a boil, reduce heat to low, and simmer uncovered for 45 minutes or until broth thickens. (If stew becomes too thick, add more water.)

4   Remove lamb chops, cinnamon, and bay leaves. Let chops cool, then remove meat from bone and cut into small pieces. Return lamb to pot. Season with salt and pepper. Heat through, ladle into bowls, and serve. This soup tastes especially good the next day.

MAKES 6 SERVINGS

NUTRITIONAL ANALYSIS PER SERVING **173 calories** ▪ **22 percent fat (total fat 4 g, saturated fat < 1 g)** ▪ **60 percent carbohydrate (5.6 g fiber)** ▪ **18 percent protein.**

Lentil Soup with Hot Italian Sausage

Hot Italian sausage and fresh spinach give this soup its distinctive flavor and appeal. Add a tossed salad and Crusty French Bread (page 18) to complete this hearty meal!

2 tablespoons olive oil

1 cup sweet onion, diced

½ cup carrots, peeled and diced

½ cup celery, diced

1½ cups lentils, rinsed

5 cups fat-free chicken broth

2 cups stewed tomatoes, chopped with juices

⅓ pound hot Italian sausage, browned and well drained

1 bay leaf

1 teaspoon each: dried thyme, basil, fennel seeds (crushed)

½ teaspoon salt

2 cups fresh spinach, chopped

1 cup fat-free half-and-half

1   In a large soup pot or Dutch oven, warm oil over medium heat. Add onion, carrots, and celery. Sauté until soft, about 5 minutes.

2   Add lentils, chicken broth, tomatoes, sausage, and all seasonings including salt. Bring to a boil, reduce heat to medium-low, and simmer for 40 minutes or until lentils are soft.

3   During last 5 minutes of cooking, add spinach and half-and-half, stir well, and continue to cook until spinach is wilted, about 3 minutes. (If soup is too thick, add more chicken broth or half-and-half.) Serve immediately.

MAKES 8 SERVINGS

NUTRITIONAL ANALYSIS PER SERVING **283 calories** ▪ **29 percent fat (total fat 9 g, saturated fat 2.3 g)** ▪ **44 percent carbohydrate (6.4 g fiber)** ▪ **27 percent protein.**

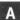

Wild Rice and Mushroom Soup with Fresh Herbs

For variety, use a combination of exotic mushrooms that are available at many supermarkets, such as shiitake, portabello, or crimini. Using fresh herbs instead of dried herbs enhances this soup's earthy flavor.

2 tablespoons olive oil

1 large yellow onion, chopped

2 stalks celery, chopped

½ cup carrots, peeled and chopped

5 cups fresh mushrooms, cleaned, stemmed, and sliced

3 tablespoons all-purpose flour

5 cups fat-free chicken broth

2 cups cooked wild rice

1 cup fat-free half-and-half

1 tablespoon marsala cooking wine

1 tablespoon fresh marjoram leaves

1 tablespoon fresh sage, finely chopped

1 tablespoon fresh thyme leaves

salt and pepper, to taste

1   In a large saucepan or Dutch oven, warm oil over medium-high heat. Add onion, celery, and carrots and cook for 5 minutes. Add mushrooms, cook 2 more minutes. (Add a little chicken broth if vegetables stick to pan.)

2   Sprinkle flour over vegetables, stir well to combine. Add chicken broth, cook and stir until mixture thickens, about 1 to 2 minutes.

3   Add wild rice, half-and-half, marsala, and herbs. Reduce heat to low, continue to cook for 5 minutes. Season with salt and pepper. Garnish with a sprinkle of fresh herbs and serve hot. (If soup is too thick, add more chicken broth or half-and-half.)

MAKES 8 SERVINGS

NUTRITIONAL ANALYSIS PER SERVING **153 calories** ▪ **26 percent fat** (total fat 4.4 g, saturated fat ‹ 1 g) ▪ **57 percent carbohydrate** (4.6 g fiber) ▪ **17 percent protein.**

C

Old-Fashioned New England Seafood Chowder

Traditionally made with cream and butter, this chowder savors the flavor but cuts the fat and calories to a fraction of the original. Serve with Crusty French Bread (page 18) and a tossed salad.

2 tablespoons butter

¼ cup carrots, peeled and grated

¼ cup celery, diced

¼ cup onion, diced

¼ cup red bell pepper, diced (optional)

3 tablespoons all-purpose flour

3½ cups low-fat (1 percent) milk

2 medium baker potatoes, peeled and diced (approximately 2½ cups)

salt and freshly ground pepper, to taste

1 cup fat-free half-and-half

1 pound cod fillet (or any white fish), cut into 1-inch chunks

½ pound shrimp meats, cooked

1   Melt butter in a medium saucepan over medium heat. Add carrots, celery, onion, and red pepper and sauté for 4 minutes or until onions are transparent.

2   Stir in flour. Gradually add milk, whisking continually to avoid clumping. Add potatoes, salt, and pepper. Bring to boil, reduce heat, and simmer, covered, for 20 minutes or until potato is cooked through but firm. Stir regularly to avoid burning on bottom.

3   Add half-and-half and cod, return to gentle boil, reduce heat, and simmer for 7 minutes or until cod is cooked through. Add shrimp and heat through, approximately 3 minutes. Adjust seasoning and serve.

MAKES 6 SERVINGS OF APPROXIMATELY 1½ CUPS EACH

NUTRITIONAL ANALYSIS PER SERVING **290 calories** ▪ **20 percent fat (total fat 6.4 g, saturated fat 3.6 g)** ▪ **38 percent carbohydrate (1 g fiber)** ▪ **42 percent protein.**

Minestrone with Spinach and Orzo Pasta

Spinach adds to the freshness of this hearty main-course Italian soup. For a twist, chop all ingredients small to complement the rice-shaped pasta. Feel free to experiment with different ingredients or with the amounts of ingredients to suit your taste.

---

1 tablespoon olive oil

1 cup yellow onion, diced

1 cup carrots, peeled and diced

2 celery stalks, diced

3 cloves garlic, minced

1 (28-ounce) can stewed tomatoes, diced

2 tablespoons tomato paste

8 cups fat-free chicken broth

1 teaspoon dried basil

1 teaspoon dried oregano

½ teaspoon freshly ground black pepper

4 cups fresh spinach, chopped

¼ cup fresh parsley, minced

½ cup orzo pasta

3 tablespoons fresh basil, minced

6 tablespoons freshly grated Parmesan cheese

1   In a large soup pot or Dutch oven, warm oil over medium-high heat. Add onion, carrots, celery, and garlic. Cover pot. Cook for about 6 minutes or until onion is translucent. Stir frequently. Add a little water or chicken broth if vegetables stick.

2   Add tomatoes, tomato paste, chicken broth, and seasonings. Cover and bring to a boil. Reduce heat to low and simmer for 20 minutes. Stir occasionally.

3   Uncover and increase heat to medium-high. Add spinach, parsley, and pasta. Cook until pasta is done, about 10 minutes. Add additional chicken broth if too thick.

4   Ladle into soup bowls and sprinkle with fresh basil and Parmesan cheese.

MAKES 8 SERVINGS OF APPROXIMATELY 1½ CUPS EACH

NUTRITIONAL ANALYSIS PER SERVING **171 calories** ▪ **26 percent fat (total fat 5 g, saturated fat 1.6 g)** ▪ **51 percent carbohydrate (4 g fiber)** ▪ **23 percent protein.**

C

Spicy Shrimp Gumbo over Couscous

This gumbo is thick enough to serve over hot, fluffy couscous. Serve with steamed broccoli or Petite Peas with Shiitake Mushrooms (page 226).

FOOD TIP

Gumbo, a southern regional dish, is a thick stew with a spicy Creole tomato base that typically includes fish, fowl, sausage, or a combination of the three. Okra, a vegetable often used in gumbos due to its delicate flavor and natural thickening ability, gives this stew its distinctive thick base.

2 tablespoons olive oil

1 medium onion, diced

¼ cup celery, diced

½ cup green bell pepper, diced

2 tablespoons all-purpose flour

3 (14-ounce) cans stewed tomatoes, chopped

1 (8-ounce) bottle clam juice

2 cups frozen okra, sliced

2 bay leaves

1½ teaspoons dried thyme

1½ teaspoons Cajun's Choice Creole seasoning

1 teaspoon paprika (regular or smoked)

¾ pound uncooked medium-size shrimp, peeled and deveined

salt and pepper, to taste

4 cups cooked couscous (prepared according to directions on package)

¼ cup fresh parsley, minced

1   In a large soup pot or Dutch oven, warm oil over medium heat. Add onion, celery, and bell pepper. Cook until tender, about 5 to 7 minutes. Cover pot to help sweat the vegetables.

2   Blend in flour and stir to thoroughly coat vegetables. Cook, stirring frequently, for 1 to 2 minutes until flour is golden brown.

3   Add remaining ingredients, except shrimp, parsley, and couscous. Bring ingredients to a boil, cover, and reduce heat to low. Simmer for 15 minutes, stirring frequently. Uncover pot and cook until base thickens, about 2 to 5 minutes.

4   Add shrimp and simmer until cooked through, approximately 3 minutes. If base is too thick, add any of the following: water, tomato juice, or clam juice. Season with salt and pepper.

5   Serve gumbo in soup bowls over small mound of couscous. Sprinkle with parsley.

MAKES 6 SERVINGS

NUTRITIONAL ANALYSIS PER SERVING **346 calories** ▪ **16 percent fat (total fat 6.1 g, saturated fat 1 g)** ▪ **61 percent carbohydrate (9 g fiber)** ▪ **23 percent protein.**

Chunky Chicken Noodle Soup

This soup is so creamy and full of vegetables that it's almost a stew, yet it has the rich flavor of the classic comfort-food soup.

---

1 (49.5-ounce) can fat-free chicken broth

1 pound skinless, boneless chicken breast

2 teaspoons olive oil

1¼ cups onion, diced

1½ cups carrots, peeled and diced

1 cup celery, diced

2 cloves garlic, minced

3 tablespoons all-purpose flour

½ teaspoon dried oregano

¼ teaspoon poultry seasoning

salt, to taste

1 tablespoon fresh thyme leaves

1 cup frozen green peas

2 cups cooked egg noodles

½ cup low-fat (1 percent) milk

½ cup fat-free half-and-half

1   Place 2 cups broth and chicken breast in a skillet, cover, and simmer over medium heat until chicken is just cooked through, turning once, for approximately 15 minutes. Set chicken aside to cool, then dice. Save broth.

2   In a large nonstick saucepan, warm oil over medium-high heat. Add onion, carrots, celery, and garlic and cook until onion is transparent, approximately 5 minutes. Sprinkle vegetables with flour, oregano, poultry seasoning, and salt. Toss to coat. Continue to stir gently for 1 minute.

3   Add broth from cooked chicken and remaining broth to vegetable mixture, cover, and reduce heat to medium. Gently simmer for 15 minutes or until carrots are tender. Add diced chicken, thyme, and peas and simmer for 2 minutes or until peas are heated through. Add noodles, milk, and half-and-half. Stir and heat until steaming but not boiling. Remove from heat and serve.

MAKES 8 SERVINGS

NUTRITIONAL ANALYSIS PER SERVING **215 calories** ▪ **17 percent fat (total fat 4 g, saturated fat 1 g)** ▪ **42 percent carbohydrate (3.2 g fiber)** ▪ **41 percent protein.**

C

Pasta Fagioli

Serve with a crisp green salad.

1 tablespoon olive oil

½ cup sweet yellow onion, chopped

½ cup carrot, finely chopped

½ cup celery, finely chopped

2 cloves garlic, minced

6 cups fat-free chicken broth

1 cup Ditali pasta (small tube-shaped pasta)

1 (9-ounce) can of red kidney beans, drained

1 (9-ounce) can of cannellini beans, drained

2 tablespoons basil, chopped

1 cup fresh spinach, chopped

salt and pepper, to taste

¼ cup low-fat Parmesan cheese, grated

1   In a heavy Dutch oven or saucepan, warm oil over medium heat. Add onion, carrot, celery, and garlic and sauté for 3 minutes.

2   Add chicken broth, bring to a boil, and add pasta. Cook for about 8 minutes or until pasta is done.

3   Add beans, basil, and spinach, reduce heat, and simmer until spinach is wilted. Season with salt and pepper. Add more chicken broth to increase volume of soup.

4   Ladle into soup bowls, sprinkle with Parmesan cheese.

MAKES 6 SERVINGS

NUTRITIONAL ANALYSIS PER SERVING **444 calories** ▪ **12 percent fat (total fat 5.9 g, saturated fat 1 g)** ▪ **64 percent carbohydrate (19 g fiber)** ▪ **24 percent protein.**

Beans, Greens, and Roasted Garlic Soup

Roast the garlic ahead of time, and this soup takes only about half an hour to prepare.

MOOD TIP

Kale is packed with more nutrients than any other vegetable. A half-cup serving supplies your entire daily requirement for beta-carotene and ample amounts of other mood-boosting nutrients, such as vitamin C, potassium, calcium, and iron.

1 head garlic

1 cup macaroni pasta or any small, tube-shaped pasta

1 tablespoon olive oil

2 large leeks

1 tablespoon fresh rosemary, diced

8 cups kale, washed and chopped

4 cups sweet potato, peeled and chopped into ½-inch pieces

7 cups fat-free chicken broth

1 tablespoon "Better Than Bouillon" Chicken Base (optional)

1 teaspoon dried basil

2 cans cannellini beans, rinsed and drained

salt and pepper, to taste

Heat oven to 425°.

1   Wrap garlic head in tinfoil and bake for 40 minutes or until soft. Remove from oven and cool. Remove cloves from papery shell and set aside.

2   Cook pasta in salted water according to directions on package and cook al dente. Drain and set aside.

3   In a large nonstick soup pan, warm oil over medium-high heat. Add leeks, rosemary, and roasted garlic cloves and sauté, stirring constantly, until leeks are transparent, approximately 5 minutes. Add kale and sweet potato, continue to stir for 5 minutes. Add chicken broth, chicken base, and basil. Return to a gentle boil, reduce heat, and simmer until potato is soft but firm, approximately 15 minutes.

4   Add beans and pasta to soup, season with salt and pepper, and heat through for 5 minutes. Serve hot.

MAKES 10 SERVINGS

NUTRITIONAL ANALYSIS PER SERVING **217 calories** ▪ **13 percent fat (total fat 3.2 g, saturated fat ‹ 1 g)** ▪ **64 percent carbohydrate (9.4 g fiber)** ▪ **23 percent protein.**

CaribBean One-Pot Stew

This one-dish stew is adapted from a recipe graciously provided by Bush's Best Beans. It is best garnished with chopped pineapple, sliced green onions, and chopped fresh cilantro. Serve with hot sauce if desired.

---

1 tablespoon olive oil

2 tablespoons fresh ginger, peeled and minced

4 cloves garlic, minced

¼ teaspoon jalapeño pepper, minced

1 cup celery, chopped fine

1 cup green bell pepper, stemmed, seeded, and chopped fine

2 cups onion, chopped fine

½ pound pork loin, trimmed and cut into ½-inch pieces

½ teaspoon cumin

½ teaspoon salt

¼ teaspoon freshly ground black pepper

3 cans (16-ounce) Bush's Best Dark Red Kidney Beans, rinsed and drained

1 (14.5-ounce) can diced tomatoes

1 (14-ounce) can fat-free chicken broth

1 cup frozen corn

1 pound sweet potato, peeled and cut into ½-inch cubes

salt and pepper, to taste

1   In a large nonstick stockpot, warm oil over medium heat. Add ginger, garlic, and jalapeño, and sauté until soft, approximately 3 minutes. Add celery, green pepper, and onion, and cook until translucent, approximately 5 minutes. Remove from pot and set aside.

2   Season pork with cumin, salt, and pepper. Add to stockpot and brown on all sides, approximately 5 minutes.

3   Return cooked vegetables to pot and add kidney beans, tomatoes, broth, corn, and sweet potatoes. Bring to a boil, reduce heat, cover, and simmer for 20 minutes or until pork is tender and sweet potatoes are tender but still firm. Season with salt and pepper.

MAKES 8 SERVINGS

NUTRITIONAL ANALYSIS PER SERVING **322 calories** ▪ 16 percent fat (total fat 5.7 g, saturated fat 1.5 g) ▪ 58 percent carbohydrate (15 g fiber) ▪ 26 percent protein.

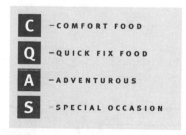

C –COMFORT FOOD

Q –QUICK FIX FOOD

A –ADVENTUROUS

S –SPECIAL OCCASION

Salads

Overcoming Overeating with Truly Tasty Foods

WHAT ARE YOUR favorite foods? Do you love steak sizzling on the grill or a chocolate chip cookie straight from the oven? Are your favorite foods the ones from childhood, like macaroni and cheese, creamed tuna, or homemade spaghetti? Whatever comes to mind, it's probably the taste above all else that ranks that food at the top of your list.

Taste is the number one reason why we choose the foods we do. No matter how good something is for you, how cheap it is, or how easy it is to get, if it doesn't taste good you're not going to eat it. If you like it, you'll eat it; if you don't, you won't.

Sounds simple. Yet under the surface, the process of taste is quite complex. What we choose to eat is rooted in the very essence of our being: chemicals in the nervous system relay messages back and forth between our brains and our mouths, and control appetite, memory, and mood.

Flavor: A Matter of Taste and Aroma

We eat because we are hungry, but it is the taste and aroma of food that make eating fun and enjoyable. Taste can be typecast into five basic qualities: salty, bitter, sweet, and sour are the original four. Umami is a recently identified taste that relates to the savoriness of food tied to an amino acid in meat and also found in the flavor-enhancer monosodium glutamate (MSG).

Taste receptors in your taste buds attach to nerves that send messages to your brain about the texture, temperature, and taste of the meal. One in every four of us is a "supertaster" and can pick up subtle off or bitter flavors that the rest of us don't taste. These supertasters have up to 60 times more taste receptors and are often turned off by common foods like broccoli or even desserts, saying they taste too bitter or too sweet.

Flavor is more than just taste or a few thousand nerves on your tongue firing at once. In fact, flavor is more about the nose than it is about the mouth. (Hint: Remember eating when you have a cold, when everything, from curried dishes to oatmeal cookies, tastes like cardboard?) Eighty percent of what we call flavor is really aroma. Those subtle smells from the complex mix of foods waft up the back of our mouths and trigger sensations, flavors, and even memories. The average person can detect 10 intensities each of 20,000 different odors.

Taste, Memories, and Emotions

Smells do more than just tickle our appetites and enhance the experience of eating. They are also one of the strongest links to emotions. Research from the Monell Chemical Senses Center in Philadelphia found that memories triggered by the aroma of food are more emotionally charged than memories triggered by any other cue, such as music or a picture.

This amazing ability to tie memories and emotions to aromas enhances the enjoyment of food and improves the taste of a glass of wine, a crisp salad, or a bowl of soup. It is also the basis of why each of us has a personalized list of comfort foods. If you ask yourself where you were or what you were doing last Tuesday, you might recall the day, but the details would be dry and unemotional. However, if you tie that memory to a candlelight dinner or the aroma of coffee while gossiping with your best friend, the memory will affect you deeply in an intimate and sometimes surprising way. Those memories stay in the brain your entire life. The smell of your mom's spaghetti can make you feel 10 years old again. The aroma of turkey roasting brings back images of Thanksgiving. Hot dogs smell like baseball games. No wonder taste is so important when it comes to the foods we choose!

12 QUICK-FIX SALADS

1. **APPLE 'N' NUT TOSSED SALAD:** Toss leaf lettuce with diced apples, chopped nuts, and fat-free vinaigrette dressing.

2. **MOCK WALDORF SALAD:** Combine chopped apples, chopped celery, chopped walnuts, dried cranberries, and cranberry-orange relish.

3. **PINEAPPLE COLESLAW:** Mix packaged coleslaw with drained pineapple chunks and low-fat commercial coleslaw dressing.

4. **SPINACH ORANGE SALAD:** Mix packaged baby spinach leaves with chopped red onion, drained mandarin oranges, chopped walnuts, and fat-free red wine vinaigrette dressing.

5. **MOCK TACO SALAD:** Mix packaged greens with drained black beans, corn kernels, chopped green onions, and chopped tomatoes. Top with a sprinkling of grated low-fat cheese and salsa.

6. **FALL FRUIT SALAD:** Drizzle peeled and sliced oranges, sliced red apples, and quartered figs with a mixture of apple juice concentrate, lime juice, cumin, and toasted pumpkin seeds.

7. **PEAR AND POMEGRANATE TOSS:** Seed and cube fresh pears, sprinkle with pomegranate seeds, and drizzle with lemon juice and fresh tarragon leaves.

8. **CRUNCHY CUCUMBERS:** Mix 1 thinly sliced cucumber, $1/2$ cup sliced mild onion, $1/3$ cup gourmet rice vinegar, and salt and pepper, to taste. Refrigerate for 2 hours.

9. **MARINATED VEGGIES:** Mix lightly steamed vegetables (broccoli, carrots, mushrooms, cauliflower, green beans, red pepper, etc.) with $1/4$ cup low-calorie Italian dressing. Marinate in the refrigerator for 1 hour or more.

10. **SHRIMP LOUIS:** Pour bagged lettuce into a bowl, top with slices of red onion, halved cherry tomatoes, a sliced hard-boiled egg, cooked shrimp meat, and low-fat Thousand Island dressing.

11. **BEET SALAD:** Sprinkle deli beets with feta cheese.

12. **FRESH SLICED TOMATOES WITH BASIL:** Slice 1 large tomato into 6 slices, drizzle with 1 teaspoon each of olive oil and balsamic vinegar. Sprinkle with $1/2$ teaspoon dried basil or 1 tablespoon fresh minced basil.

Sifting Fat from Flavor

We often equate flavor with foods that are high in fat, sugar, or salt. People are more likely to list hamburgers, chocolate, and chips than chard, oatmeal, and lentils on their favorite-foods lists. "We humans have a love affair with fat and sugar that dates back to our most ancient roots when these calorie-dense nutrients were in short supply. It is fat, beyond any other nutrient, that gives food the textures, aromas, and tastes that we desire most. Sugar, on the other hand, makes fat taste good," says Adam Drewnowski, Ph.D., a professor in the Departments of Epidemiology and Medicine at the University of Washington in Seattle.

Fat, sugar, and salt were scarce in our evolutionary past, so our ancient ancestors evolved complex appetite systems that drove them to eat foods rich in these nutrients when they were available. Fast-forward to the present, when greasy, sweet, and salty fast foods are everywhere. The battle of the bulge is a natural response to living in what Kelly Brownell, Ph.D., a professor of psychology at Yale University, calls a *toxic environment*. "We are exposed to an unprecedented supply of poor-quality food that is widely available, low cost, heavily promoted, and great tasting," says Dr. Brownell. The trick is to find ways to satisfy our ancient palates without packing on the pounds. That's where flavor can work in our favor.

The Yum Factor

Foods that are flavorful and that smell yummy are also the most satisfying. People report that they feel more full and satisfied on less food when they eat flavorful meals rather than bland diets. The more flavorful a meal, the more satisfying it is. "A wide variety of flavors are important to satisfy sensory needs," says Zoe Warwick, Ph.D., an associate professor of psychology at the University of Maryland. In her studies, people were more satisfied and less hungry when they ate savory meals, and at Duke University, people were most successful at dieting and weight loss when they ate flavor-packed foods.

It could be that we overeat salty chips and fries because our taste buds are craving flavor. "Many people need to experience taste and can't stop eating until that craving for flavor is satisfied," says Rosanne Gold, an award-winning chef and the author of *Little Meals*. Living on a sensory-monotonous diet where the only taste is sweet, salty, or greasy leaves our taste buds deprived of the thousands of other flavors and aromas on which our senses thrive. The trick here is to combine taste with health. "In the long run, satiety is enhanced and you're more likely to see weight loss when flavor, texture, and aroma are combined with a low-fat diet," says Dr. Warwick.

FLAVOR BOOSTERS, FAT BUSTERS

Bring out the flavors in your meals without using too much fat by following one or more of the following suggestions.

1. Use fresh herbs instead of dried herbs.

2. Select the most flavorful oils in cooking, such as sesame oil, walnut oil, extra-virgin olive oil, or a little butter. You will use less.

3. Drizzle a little olive oil or melted butter over a finished entrée. It will be the first taste that hits your taste buds, giving flavor for very little fat.

4. Use small amounts of intensely flavored cheese, such as Parmesan, Romano, Gorgonzola, or sharp cheddar, or sprinkle nuts, such as peanuts, pecans, or slivered almonds.

5. For a smoky "umami" taste, substitute turkey ham for bacon in recipes.

6. Tempt the eyes as well as the palate by picking foods with contrasting colors, serving foods on oversized plates so the plate's rim frames the meal, and always decorate with a garnish.

7. Buy super-fresh produce. Strong-tasting vegetables, such as broccoli and Brussels sprouts, get more pungent with age.

8. If some greens taste bitter, toss them with dried, canned, or fresh fruit to cut the bitter taste. Sprinkle bitter vegetables with salt or a salty condiment such as anchovies or olives.

9. For vegetable avoiders, add a dash of sugar to the steaming pot. Studies at the State University of New York at Buffalo found that people who typically don't like vegetables reported liking them more when they were accented with a 5 percent sugar solution. A sweet glaze made from soy sauce, sugar, garlic, and ginger also might work. Or try sprinkling vegetables with a butter substitute.

10. To make the most of flavor, don't use tobacco (smoking damages taste buds and blunts the taste of food), ask your physician if any prescribed medication will affect taste or smell, eat slowly to appreciate flavors, and seek medical help if you have a sudden loss of taste or smell.

A basic premise of this cookbook is that if we stimulate all the senses and excite even a fraction of our taste possibilities by combining sweet with bitter or sour, complementing various intensities of flavors, and capitalizing on the aroma of food, we will feel more satisfied on fewer calories, while loading up on the types of foods that soothe both our moods and our minds. You'll find this in all the recipes, from Smoky Sweet Potato 'n' Corn Chowder and Pan-Seared Asparagus with Gingered Onions to Very Berry Lemon Pancakes with Blueberry Sauce, Citrus-Scented Caramel Flan, and Grilled Halibut with Ginger-Mango Chutney. Interesting tastes and fragrant aromas tickle our palates, so we enjoy more and eat less. Researchers in Sweden and Thailand report that mood-boosting nutrients, such as iron, are absorbed up to 70 percent better when we enjoy the meal. All the more reason to maximize the dining experience with yummy flavors and aromas!

SALT SUBSTITUTES

If you believe the current trend in fast-food dining, then salt must be the only flavoring agent. Wrong! Stock your kitchen with any and all of the following ingredients that amplify flavor in cooking. Experiment with each. For example, maple flavoring is a traditional addition to oatmeal but also goes well with sweet potatoes.

- **NUTS:** Toasting nuts brings out the rich flavors.

- **GARLIC:** Great in pasta dishes, salad dressings, meats and fish, sautéed vegetables, and potato dishes.

- **MARINADES AND SALAD DRESSINGS:** Choose tangy or spicy low-fat or fat-free versions for meats, fish, vegetables, and salads.

- **FLAVORED VINEGARS AND OILS:** Use small amounts in salads, vegetables, meats, and fish.

- **SUN-DRIED TOMATOES:** Add to salads, pasta, and sauces.

- **EXTRACTS:** Almond, maple, vanilla, rum, coconut, and others are all fat-free and add great flavor to beverages, fruits, and more.

- **ORANGE AND LEMON PEEL:** Also called "zest," these finely grated peels can be added to fruits, breads and muffins, sauces for chicken or fish, and salad dressings.

- **FLAVORINGS:** Butter, garlic, bacon, and cheese flavorings add taste, but little fat, to vegetables, potatoes, pasta, and main dishes.

- **CHIPOTLE PEPPERS:** If chipotle is too spicy, try washing the pepper to remove seeds, then add a little of the sauce along with the chopped pepper to recipes. Or try powdered chipotle peppers from the spice section of your grocery store.

The Golden Rules of Salads

Salads are one of the most satisfying foods, according to numerous studies. Consequently, they are often the answer to everything from waistlines to health. Salads are especially suited to satisfying taste buds when a variety of textures, colors, aromas, and flavors are combined. But are those big bowls of rabbit food really calorie-free answers to a ravenous appetite and a surefire way to boost your mood and your health?

Yes and no. Crispy greens are one of life's little fat-free pleasures. However, many fatty concoctions are guzzled under the guise of "salad fixings." The fact that salad dressing is the number one source of fat in women's diets attests to the confusion over what is really a healthful salad and what is a fat-laden disaster. Here are a few survival skills that can help cut the fat, sodium, and sugar yet keep the taste, nutrition, and pleasure of a salad.

- *Heap your plate with greens, the greener the better.* Spinach is better than leaf lettuce, which is better than iceberg. Other raw-and-crispy "freebies" include: grated carrots, mushrooms, raw broccoli flowerets, alfalfa sprouts, tomatoes, radicchio lettuce, purple cabbage, cucumber, and sweet red pepper. Use avocado slices, nuts, and olives sparingly.

- *Focus on low-fat, protein-rich items.* Add one-half to two-thirds of a cup of beans, such as kidney, garbanzo and black beans, or black-eyed peas, lentils, and split peas. Other low-fat protein sources include sliced plain chicken or turkey breast or cooked egg white (whole egg contains more than a teaspoon of fat, while the white is fat- and cholesterol-free). Avoid luncheon meats, such as salami, ham, and pepperoni, which contain up to 60 percent fat calories and too much salt. Low-fat or fat-free cottage cheese is another healthy option and can be mixed with a low-calorie dressing to make less dressing go farther. Avoid the creamy cottage cheese that contains more than a teaspoon of fat for every half cup.

- *Skip the oil.* Just say no to anything mixed with oil, mayonnaise, cheese, or whipped cream. This includes potato or pasta salads, Mexican meat or cheese sauces, tuna mixed with mayonnaise, egg salad, macaroni and cheese, tartar sauce, and traditional Waldorf salad. A one-ladle serving of these foods could contribute up to three tablespoons of fat to the meal. Grated Parmesan is a tasty alternative when used sparingly (each tablespoon contains about a half teaspoon of fat), or try the low-fat and fat-free versions of Parmesan.

- *Be creative at home:*

    - Mix fruits and vegetables, such as raspberries in a spinach salad or mandarin oranges with butter lettuce.

- Use a teaspoon of toasted sesame oil, instead of a quarter cup of canola oil, for the dressing.

- Add strong flavors to the dressing, such as grated fresh ginger, cilantro, mustard, red pepper flakes, lemon peel, or roasted red peppers.

- The more you combine flavors, the more interesting the salad. Experiment with sweet, sour, and spicy flavors in salads. Add fresh mint leaves or grated lemon peel to a dressing or marinade.

- Think color. Mix oranges, greens, whites, and reds.

- *Choose accompaniments carefully.* Complement your salad with soup and whole grain bread. Broth-based soups packed with vegetables are best. A slice of whole wheat bread or a plain whole wheat bagel can add flavor without fat to the meal, but limit your intake of muffins or any baked item that has a shiny appearance, which is a red flag for too much fat or sugar.

- *Use low-fat dressings.* Remember that one small ladle of regular dressing at a salad bar supplies four teaspoons of fat and 170 calories. In essence, too much of the wrong dressing can transform four cups of low-fat vegetables into a 70 percent fat-calorie disaster! Choose low-calorie dressings and use them sparingly. Select watery versions, such as Italian and French, rather than thicker blue cheese and Thousand Island dressings, since they spread more evenly over the salad. Better yet, portion out a one-half-scoop serving into a separate container and lightly dip your fork into the low-calorie dressing first and then into the salad.

All of the salads in this section are graced with flavor, color, and enticing aromas, which help maximize enjoyment and cut back on fat and calories.

Sesame-Ginger Coleslaw

Compared with regular coleslaw, this slaw has 50 percent less calories and fat (most of that fat is healthful monounsaturated fat), no cholesterol, and twice the fiber. More important, it has twice the flavor and is rich in iron and folic acid, the B vitamin that boosts memory and reduces heart-disease risk. It takes less than 10 minutes to prepare and goes great with sandwiches or as a side salad along with fish or chicken for dinner.

MOOD TIP

As you enjoy this salad, notice the bouquet. This part of flavor comes from your nose, not your taste buds. You swallow and chew, and the air, with all the odors in it (in this case the blend of sweet fresh ginger and tart rice vinegar), is pumped up into your nose. The brain uses smell and taste together to create flavor.

3 tablespoons sesame seeds

4 cups of preshredded coleslaw mix or about ⅔ of a 16-ounce bag

⅔ cup green onions, sliced

3 tablespoons rice vinegar

1 tablespoon fresh ginger, peeled and grated

1 tablespoon sesame oil

1½ teaspoons sugar

salt and pepper, to taste

1   Toast sesame seeds in a nonstick skillet over medium heat until browned, about 4 minutes. Set aside.

2   Combine coleslaw mix and onions in a medium bowl.

3   Blend vinegar, ginger, oil, and sugar in a small bowl, pour over coleslaw-onion mixture, and blend thoroughly. Season with salt and pepper.

4   Let stand at least 5 minutes before serving (can be refrigerated up to 2 hours). Top with toasted sesame seeds just before serving.

MAKES 4 SERVINGS

NUTRITIONAL ANALYSIS PER SERVING 103 calories ▪ 60 percent fat (total fat 7.5 g, saturated fat 1 g) ▪ 29 percent carbohydrate (2 g fiber) ▪ 11 percent protein.

Sweet Potato Chutney Salad

This salad also works as a side dish for chicken or fish. It's colorful and chock-full of nutrients, with a subtle zing of flavor.

½ cup green onions, chopped in thin slices

½ cup chutney (Major Grey is best)

2 teaspoons sesame oil

2 teaspoons canola oil

2 tablespoons rice wine vinegar

salt and pepper, to taste

4 cups sweet potatoes, peeled and cut into 1-inch cubes (about 2 large sweet potatoes)

¼ pound green beans and yellow beans, trimmed and cut into 1½-inch lengths (about 1 cup)

¼ cup fresh cilantro, chopped

1   Combine onions, chutney, sesame and canola oils, vinegar, salt, and pepper in medium bowl. Set aside.

2   Steam potatoes until tender but still firm (about 10 to 12 minutes).

3   Steam beans until tender but still firm and bright green. Remove and place in ice to cool immediately. Once cool, remove from ice and drain.

4   Toss potatoes, beans, and cilantro in large bowl. Pour chutney sauce over top and toss.

MAKES 6 SERVINGS

NUTRITIONAL ANALYSIS PER SERVING **187 calories** ▪ **15 percent fat (total fat 3.2 g, saturated fat < 0.5 g)** ▪ **79 percent carbohydrate (5 g fiber)** ▪ **6 percent protein.**

Pecan, Tart Apple, and Dried Cherry Salad

The contrast of tart and sweet is accented by the light maple hint of dressing in this simple tossed salad. Serve with any chicken dish or as a meal at lunch. Don't be concerned about the total fat percentage. Since lettuce has almost no calories, all the calories come from healthy monounsaturated fats in the nuts and canola oil.

MOOD TIP
When people add a few nuts to their diet, they tend to eat less and have an easier time managing their weight, maybe because they feel more satisfied than when they eat only low-fat foods.

DRESSING

¼ cup maple syrup

¼ cup fat-free mayonnaise

3 tablespoons champagne vinegar

2 teaspoons sugar or maple sugar

2 tablespoons canola oil

salt and pepper, to taste

SALAD

½ cup pecan bits

1 tablespoon maple syrup

2 (5-ounce) bags of baby greens (about 18 cups lightly packed)

2 tart apples (such as Granny Smith), peeled, cored, and chopped

¾ cup dried cherries

1   To prepare dressing: In a blender, mix syrup, mayonnaise, vinegar, sugar, oil, salt, and pepper until creamy. Set aside.

2   Place pecans in a small bowl and drizzle with maple syrup. Toss and let stand for 10 minutes. Place on tinfoil in oven preheated to 350° for 10 minutes or until toasted. Remove and let cool.

3   Place greens in large bowl. Top with apples, cherries, and pecans.

4   Toss with dressing just before serving on chilled plates.

MAKES 8 SERVINGS

NUTRITIONAL ANALYSIS PER SERVING **185 calories** ▪ **40 percent fat (total fat 8 g, saturated fat ‹ 1 g)** ▪ **54 percent carbohydrate (3.7 g fiber)** ▪ **6 percent protein.**

A **S**

Sesame Salmon and Spinach Salad with Asian Vinaigrette

This salad is a meal in itself. Serve with Crusty French Bread (page 18) for lunch or dinner. Go easy on the dressing; it may be almost fat-free, but it's packed with flavor!

DRESSING

4 tablespoons green onions, thinly sliced

3 tablespoons rice wine vinegar

2½ tablespoons soy sauce

2 teaspoons sesame seeds

3 cloves garlic, minced

1 teaspoon dark sesame oil

1 tablespoon fresh lime juice

pinch of red pepper flakes

SALAD

1 teaspoon dark sesame oil

1 cup red onion, thinly sliced

1½ cups corn kernels (fresh is best, but frozen will do)

1½ cups Chinese pea pods, deveined and rinsed

16 ounces salmon fillet

1 teaspoon dark sesame oil

1 teaspoon sesame seeds

10 cups baby spinach, washed, stemmed, and patted dry

1 cup jicama, peeled and sliced into matchsticks

24 cherry tomatoes, halved

Preheat broiler.

1   To prepare dressing: Combine all ingredients and set aside for flavors to blend.

2   Warm 1 teaspoon sesame oil in large skillet over medium heat. Add onion and sauté for 8 minutes, stirring frequently. Add corn and pea pods and continue to sauté over medium heat, stirring frequently, for an additional 8 minutes or until corn kernels are toasted and pea pods are cooked but crispy. Set aside. (If you prefer, you can prepare this mixture ahead of time and reheat it just before serving.)

3   Rub salmon with 1 teaspoon sesame oil and sprinkle with 1 teaspoon sesame seeds. Place on foil-lined cookie sheet and broil for 4 to 5 minutes or until meat flakes easily with a fork (middle may be just barely done).

4   Divide spinach among 4 plates. Top with equal amounts of onion–pea pod mixture and jicama. Place on each plate 12 cherry tomato halves around sides of spinach and top salad with a quarter of the salmon. Drizzle with dressing to taste, approximately 2 to 3 tablespoons.

MAKES 4 SERVINGS

NUTRITIONAL ANALYSIS PER SERVING **365 calories** ▪ **31 percent fat (total fat 12.5 g, saturated fat 2 g)** ▪ omega-3 fats 2 g ▪ **35 percent carbohydrate (9.5 g fiber)** ▪ **34 percent protein.**

Green and Red Chunky Salad with Oregano

This easy vegetable side-dish salad is a great accompaniment to sandwiches and packs well in brown-bag lunches. You even can eat it with your fingers!

1 pound fresh green beans, washed and trimmed

⅓ cup red onion, diced

1 clove garlic, minced

2½ tablespoons red wine vinegar

1 teaspoon extra-virgin olive oil

salt and pepper, to taste

1 pound cherry tomatoes, cut into quarters

1½ teaspoons fresh oregano leaves, chopped

1   Steam green beans until tender but still crisp, approximately 10 minutes.

2   While beans are steaming, mix ingredients for vinaigrette: onion, garlic, vinegar, olive oil, salt, and pepper. Let sit for 10 minutes to blend flavors.

3   Put hot green beans in a large bowl and toss with vinaigrette mixture. Add tomatoes and oregano and toss again.

MAKES 4 SERVINGS AT APPROXIMATELY 1 GENEROUS CUP EACH

NUTRITIONAL ANALYSIS PER SERVING **79 calories** ▪ **17 percent fat (total fat 1.5 g, saturated fat 0 g)** ▪ **68 percent carbohydrate (5.6 g fiber)** ▪ **15 percent protein.**

Wild Rice and Roasted Vegetables with Thyme Vinaigrette

This rich and filling salad goes well with roast chicken, turkey, or pork. It is a beautiful addition to a holiday menu, too. If you have leftovers, make a 1-serving frittata by placing 1 cup of this rice-vegetable dish in a small frying pan along with 2 whipped eggs. Cover and cook over medium-low heat until eggs are cooked through, about 15 minutes. Salt, to taste.

FOOD TIP

Wild rice is called a rice because it is the seed of a cereal grass, but technically it is an aquatic grain, since it is the seed of a marsh grass that grows in the northern Great Lakes area. It has a hazelnut flavor, is dark brown in color, and is chewy. American Indians called wild rice mahnomen, *which means "gift of the gods."*

3 cups fat-free chicken broth (amount will vary depending on rice)

1 cup wild rice, rinsed

2 tablespoons olive oil

1 tablespoon champagne vinegar

1 tablespoon fresh thyme, chopped

1 clove garlic, minced

cooking spray

3 carrots, peeled and sliced diagonally into ½-inch slices

½ pound shiitake, crimini, or portabello mushrooms, stems removed and sliced into ½-inch slices

salt

1½ red bell peppers, stemmed, seeded, and cut into quarters

⅔ of a large yellow onion, cut into 1-inch wedges

Preheat oven to 425°.

1   To cook rice: In a medium saucepan, bring chicken broth to boil. Add rice, cover, return to boil, reduce heat, and simmer until rice is done, approximately 50 minutes (kernels crack, revealing the fluffy white interior). Amount of fluid will vary depending on rice; you may need to add additional broth or drain rice when done. (Makes approximately 3 cups of cooked rice.)

2   To prepare vinaigrette: In a small bowl, blend olive oil, vinegar, thyme, and garlic. Set aside.

3   While rice is cooking, roast vegetables: Spray a cookie sheet with cooking spray. Arrange carrots on one side and mushrooms on the other side. Spray with cooking spray and sprinkle with salt. Spray a second cookie sheet and arrange red peppers and onions on opposing sides, spray with cooking spray, and sprinkle with salt. Place both cookie sheets in oven. Roast vegetables for approximately 30 minutes or until tender, turning twice.

4   Drain rice if necessary, transfer to a medium bowl, and blend in vinaigrette. Add

vegetables while rice is still warm. Thoroughly stir and cover. Let sit for 10 minutes to allow flavors to blend and mushrooms to absorb some of the liquid. Serve at room temperature.

MAKES 6 CUPS

NUTRITIONAL ANALYSIS PER CUP **195 calories** ▪ **25 percent fat (total fat 5.4 g, saturated < 1 g)** ▪ **61 percent carbohydrate (5.4 g fiber)** ▪ **14 percent protein.**

S

Garbanzo Toss with Sun-Dried Tomatoes, Red Pepper, and Fresh Parsley

This light and flavorful salad goes well with any sandwich and is easy to pack for on-the-go lunches and snacks. For a quick sandwich, stuff a whole wheat pita with this yummy salad along with red or yellow pepper slices.

MOOD TIP
Ounce for ounce, red peppers have four times the vitamin C of oranges, plus a hefty dose of beta-carotene to protect your brain against damage from free radicals.

2 (15.5-ounce) cans garbanzo beans, drained and rinsed

⅔ cup fresh parsley, chopped

½ cup water or oil-packed sun-dried tomatoes, drained and thinly sliced

⅓ cup red bell pepper, diced

2 tablespoons fresh lemon juice

pinch of red pepper flakes

3 tablespoons olive oil

¼ teaspoon ground cumin

salt, to taste

1   In a medium bowl, combine all ingredients. Toss to blend.

2   Serve at room temperature. (Can be made the day before serving.)

MAKES 8 SERVINGS OF ½ CUP EACH

NUTRITIONAL ANALYSIS PER SERVING **252 calories** ▪ **34 percent fat (total fat 9.5 g, saturated fat 1 g)** ▪ **50 percent carbohydrate (7.8 g fiber)** ▪ **16 percent protein.**

Chili-Spiced Shrimp Salad with Mango-Pineapple Salsa

This salad is a meal in itself, served with bread sticks or a slice of Crusty French Bread (page 18).

Or accompany it with a sandwich or bowl of Heartwarming Winter Vegetable Soup (page 98).

½ pound raw large shrimp (approximately 1 dozen), peeled and deveined

1 teaspoon hot chili-sesame oil or chili paste

8 cups mixed baby greens, washed and dried

⅓ cup fresh lemon juice

2 teaspoons sesame oil

salt

Mango-Pineapple Salsa (page 35)

Preheat broiler.

1   Place shrimp in medium bowl and rub with chili-sesame oil. Let sit while broiler heats.

2   Place shrimp on foil-lined cookie sheet and place on middle rack of oven. Broil for 1 minute on each side or until shrimp are pink and cooked through.

3   Toss greens with lemon juice, sesame oil, and salt. Divide among 4 plates. Top greens on each plate with a quarter of the Mango-Pineapple Salsa and arrange 3 shrimp on top of salsa.

MAKES 4 SERVINGS

NUTRITIONAL ANALYSIS PER SERVING 167 calories ▪ 25 percent fat (total fat 4.6 g, saturated fat ‹ 1 g) ▪ 43 percent carbohydrate (3.7 g fiber) ▪ 32 percent protein.

Chicken Salad with Chutney and Toasted Coconut

Jazzed with crunch, tropical coconut and chutney flavors, and a light, creamy base, this mood-satisfying salad not only tantalizes your taste buds but also energizes your body, since it supplies an entire day's worth of some B vitamins and whopping amounts of iron, potassium, selenium, and zinc.

MOOD TIP

According to researchers at the Health Research and Studies Center in Los Angeles, raisins help regulate blood sugar levels without the rise and fall seen with more sugary snacks.

2 tablespoons coconut, shredded, already sweetened

3 tablespoons of your favorite chutney (mango is good)

2 tablespoons fat-free mayonnaise

2 teaspoons curry powder

2 cups cooked chicken, diced or shredded

1 pear, peeled, seeded, and diced

¼ cup golden raisins

4 cups mixed greens

2 tablespoons slivered almonds

Preheat oven to 300°.

1   Spread coconut in a single layer on a cookie sheet. Bake for 2 to 3 minutes, until starting to brown. Remove from oven and let cool. Set aside.

2   In a large bowl, combine chutney, mayonnaise, and curry. Stir to mix.

3   Add chicken, diced pear, and raisins. Toss gently to coat mixture.

4   Divide salad greens among 4 salad plates. Top greens on each plate with ½ cup chicken salad, then sprinkle with toasted coconut and slivered almonds.

MAKES 4 SERVINGS OF APPROXIMATELY 1½ CUPS EACH

NUTRITIONAL ANALYSIS PER SERVING **280 calories** ▪ **20 percent fat (total fat 6 g, saturated fat 1.9 g)** ▪ **33 percent carbohydrate (3.4 g fiber)** ▪ **47 percent protein.**

Roasted Beet Salad
with Orange Vinaigrette

A perfect salad to complement any meal at any time of the year. Beets are rich in iron and when roasted turn into sweet earthy jewels. The orange vinaigrette keeps the salad light and flavorful, while the crumbled blue cheese adds a tangy smooth aftertaste. This salad will have everyone talking beets, even those who say they don't like them! It supplies 61 percent of your daily requirement for vitamin C and ample amounts of vitamin E, folic acid, potassium, and B vitamins — nutrients that boost mood and brain power.

VINAIGRETTE
1/2 cup fresh orange juice

1 tablespoon grated orange peel

1 tablespoon shallots, peeled, sliced thinly, and chopped

2 teaspoons champagne vinegar

1/2 teaspoon sugar

3 tablespoons olive oil

SALAD
4 medium fresh beets

1 tablespoon olive oil

2 cloves garlic, minced

salt and pepper, to taste

5 cups mixed salad greens or 5 cups freshly cleaned spinach

2 tablespoons crumbled blue cheese

Preheat oven to 425°.

1   In a small bowl, combine all vinaigrette ingredients, whisk well. Put aside.

2   Cut off beet greens and discard (or use for another dish). Wash beets and pat dry. Slice in half, then into quarters. Toss with olive oil, garlic, salt, and pepper. Place beets in double-wrap aluminum foil. Close tightly. Place foil on cooking sheet and roast for 30 to 40 minutes or until tender. Let cool, then cut into bite-size pieces.

3   In a large salad bowl, toss green salad, beets, and vinaigrette. Arrange on 4 chilled salad plates and sprinkle with crumbled blue cheese.

MAKES 4 SERVINGS OF APPROXIMATELY 1½ CUPS EACH

NUTRITIONAL ANALYSIS PER SERVING **189 calories** ▪ **69 percent fat (total fat 14 g, saturated fat 2.7 g)** ▪ **24 percent carbohydrate (2.2 g fiber)** ▪ **7 percent protein.**

A

Greek Pasta Salad
with Red Wine Vinaigrette

This salad is great with a loaf of Crusty French Bread (page 18) and is high in B vitamins, vitamin C, magnesium, and trace minerals like copper, iron, manganese, and zinc. Whew! You probably feel better just making this salad!

VINAIGRETTE

⅓ cup red wine vinegar

¼ cup olive oil

2 cloves garlic, minced

2 teaspoons dried basil

1 teaspoon sugar

SALAD

1 pound farfalle (bow-tie pasta)

1 (6-ounce) bag prewashed baby spinach, chopped

12 cherry tomatoes, cut into quarters

½ red onion, thinly sliced

1 small cucumber, peeled, sliced 1 inch thick, then diced

¼ cup fresh parsley, chopped

3 tablespoons chopped olives

2 tablespoons capers, rinsed

¼ cup feta cheese, crumbled

1   Combine all vinaigrette ingredients, mix well, and set aside.

2   Cook pasta in a large pot according to directions on package, drain, and return pasta to pot.

3   Add spinach, tomatoes, onion, cucumber, parsley, olives, and capers. Mix to blend.

4   Pour vinaigrette over pasta, stir gently.

5   Transfer pasta salad to a large pasta bowl. Sprinkle with feta cheese. Cover and chill at least 1 hour or overnight. (If the dish is chilled overnight, you might need to drizzle it with a little olive oil and red wine vinegar, since pasta will absorb vinaigrette.)

MAKES 8 SERVINGS OF APPROXIMATELY 1 CUP EACH

NUTRITIONAL ANALYSIS PER SERVING **326 calories** ▪ **28 percent fat (total fat 10 g, saturated fat 2 g)** ▪ **60 percent carbohydrate (6 g fiber)** ▪ **12 percent protein.**

C

Baby Greens and Orange Salad with Pecans and Celery Seed Dressing

Fresh oranges with the sweetened celery seed dressing make this salad a great accompaniment to any entrée. Or serve at lunch with sandwiches or soups. If you want to cut the fat, reduce the pecans by half; then each serving will have 233 calories and 15 grams of fat.

1 cup pecan halves

1 tablespoon maple syrup

cooking spray

DRESSING

2 tablespoons fresh lemon juice

2 tablespoons shallots, minced

1 teaspoon dry mustard

2 tablespoons extra-virgin olive oil

1 teaspoon celery seed

1 tablespoon sugar

1 tablespoon red wine vinegar

¼ teaspoon salt

SALAD

2 medium navel or blood oranges

6 cups baby greens, washed and drained

½ cup red bell pepper, sliced into thin 1-inch-long strips

Heat oven to 350°.

1   Place pecans on tinfoil-lined cookie sheet. Bake for 5 minutes. Remove and toss with maple syrup in a small bowl. Spray tinfoil and return pecans to cookie sheet. Bake for 4 minutes or until golden brown. Remove from oven and set aside.

2   To prepare dressing: In a small bowl, whisk all dressing ingredients. Set aside for flavors to blend.

3   With a sharp knife, peel oranges, removing all rind and white pith. Separate sections and remove membrane when possible. Halve each section lengthwise.

4   In a large bowl, place baby lettuce, pecans, oranges, and red pepper strips. Toss with dressing to coat. Serve immediately.

MAKES 4 SERVINGS

NUTRITIONAL ANALYSIS PER SERVING **323 calories** ▪ **66 percent fat (total fat 23.6 g, saturated fat 2 g)** ▪ **28 percent carbohydrate (6 g fiber)** ▪ **6 percent protein.**

Red Rice and Kidney Bean Salad

This salad is a meal in itself or can be served as an accompaniment to any chicken or fish dish.

FOOD TIP

Arborio rice is a medium-grain Italian rice that cooks firm to the bite, or al dente. It works well in risotto and other classic Italian dishes.

2 cups fat-free chicken broth

1 cup white rice or arborio

2 teaspoons olive oil

1 cup onion, chopped

2 cloves garlic, minced

¼ red bell pepper, chopped

2 teaspoons chili powder

1 teaspoon dried oregano

salt, to taste

½ cup frozen green peas, thawed

1 can kidney beans, rinsed and drained

1 tablespoon fresh lemon juice

2 tablespoons fresh parsley, chopped

1   In a medium saucepan, bring broth to a boil, add rice, reduce heat, cover, and simmer until all liquid is absorbed and rice is soft but firm, approximately 25 minutes. Set aside.

2   While rice is cooking, heat oil in a medium pan over medium heat. Add onion, garlic, and red bell pepper and sauté until tender, approximately 5 minutes. Add chili powder, oregano, and salt. Blend well and add to rice mixture in last 15 minutes of cooking.

3   In a medium bowl, blend peas, beans, and lemon juice.

4   On a plate, arrange the rice on one side and the bean mixture on the other. Sprinkle with parsley and serve.

MAKES 8 SERVINGS

NUTRITIONAL ANALYSIS PER SERVING **234 calories** ▪ **10 percent fat (total fat 2.6 g, saturated fat ‹ 0.5 g)** ▪ **73 percent carbohydrate (6.4 g fiber)** ▪ **17 percent protein.**

Mandarin Toss with Mint-Lemon Dressing

This salad goes well with any chicken or fish entrée during any season, from winter through summer. Or serve at lunch with Minted Lamb Pockets with Honey Yogurt Dressing (page 66).

DRESSING
⅓ cup fresh lemon juice

1 teaspoon sugar

1 tablespoon Dijon mustard

2 cloves garlic, minced

3 tablespoons olive oil

⅓ cup fresh mint, finely diced

salt and pepper, to taste

SALAD
8 cups butter lettuce, washed, drained, and torn into bite-size pieces (or 1 bag of European blend lettuce)

4 mandarin oranges, peeled and sectioned, or 2 (11-ounce) cans mandarin oranges, drained

½ red bell pepper, stemmed, seeded, and cut into thin 1-inch-long strips

1   Place all dressing ingredients in a medium bowl and blend well with a whisk. Set aside so flavors will blend. (Dressing keeps in refrigerator for up to 2 days.)

2   Place lettuce in a large bowl, top with oranges and red pepper.

3   When ready to serve, pour dressing onto salad and toss gently. Serve immediately.

MAKES 6 SERVINGS OF APPROXIMATELY 1¼ CUP EACH

NUTRITIONAL ANALYSIS PER CUP **110 calories** ▪ **53 percent fat (total fat 6.5 g, saturated fat < 1 g)** ▪ **41 percent carbohydrate (1.5 g fiber)** ▪ **6 percent protein.**

Curried Couscous with Garbanzo Beans and Mandarin Oranges

This great summertime vegetarian salad can be served alone, on a bed of assorted greens, or as a cold side dish.

1 cup fat-free chicken broth

¼ cup orange juice

¼ cup dried currants

1 teaspoon olive oil

1 (5.7-ounce) box Near East Couscous mix (Mediterranean curry flavored)

½ cup canned garbanzo beans, drained and rinsed

½ cup canned mandarin orange segments, drained and chopped

½ cup water chestnuts, finely chopped

2 tablespoons green onions, finely sliced

DRESSING

3 tablespoons nonfat mayonnaise or nonfat yogurt

3 tablespoons orange juice

2 tablespoons mandarin orange juice (from can of orange segments)

1 teaspoon curry powder

½ teaspoon ground cumin

1   In a medium saucepan, combine chicken broth, orange juice, currants, olive oil, and contents of Mediterranean curry spice sack. Bring to a boil, stir in couscous. Cover, remove from heat, and let stand for 5 minutes, then fluff with a fork.

2   Place couscous in a medium salad bowl. Add garbanzo beans, oranges, water chestnuts, and onions. Stir and set aside.

3   In a small bowl, whisk together all the dressing ingredients. Pour dressing into couscous and mix well. Cover and refrigerate, preferably overnight to allow flavors to infuse the couscous. Stir gently before serving chilled. (Add some orange juice to moisten if couscous absorbs extra liquid while chilling.)

MAKES 5 SERVINGS

NUTRITIONAL ANALYSIS PER SERVING **259 calories** ▪ **7 percent fat (total fat 2 g, saturated fat 0 g)** ▪ **80 percent carbohydrate (6 g fiber)** ▪ **13 percent protein.**

Fresh Fruit Salad with Yogurt Dressing

Perfect for a hot afternoon luncheon, this fruit salad goes well with grilled halibut on a bed of spinach.

---

6 cups fresh mixed fruits, chopped (apples, bananas, berries)

1 cup fat-free strawberry or vanilla yogurt

¼ teaspoon almond extract

¼ teaspoon ground cinnamon

1 tablespoon sweetened coconut

1   Place fruit in a large salad bowl.

2   In a small bowl, mix yogurt, almond flavoring, and cinnamon.

3   Pour yogurt mixture over fruit. Toss well to coat. Sprinkle with coconut and serve.

MAKES 6 SERVINGS OF APPROXIMATELY 1 CUP EACH

NUTRITIONAL ANALYSIS PER SERVING **125 calories** ▪ **6 percent fat (total fat ‹ 1 g, saturated fat 0 g)** ▪ **86 percent carbohydrate (3.3 g fiber)** ▪ **8 percent protein.**

Q

Indonesian Rice Salad Medley

Refreshing, crisp, and colorful, this rice salad is flavored with tropical fruit. The healthy dressing is delicious with almost any rice salad. Look for the prepackaged tropical dried fruit medley in the baking section of your local supermarket, next to other dried fruits. Serve with Tandoori Chicken Made Simple from the recipe on page 170.

---

4 cups cooked basmati or jasmine rice, well chilled

1 cup tropical dried fruit medley

1 apple, cored and chopped with skin

½ cup fresh cilantro, chopped

½ cup red seedless grapes, sliced in half

¼ cup green onion, thinly sliced

2 tablespoons fresh mint, chopped

½ teaspoon salt or to taste

large lettuce leaves, one per serving

DRESSING

½ cup orange juice

2 tablespoons honey

2 teaspoons olive oil

1 teaspoon lime juice

½ teaspoon coriander

2 teaspoons fresh ginger, peeled and minced

1   In a large salad bowl, add all the rice ingredients in order (except salt). Set aside.

2   To prepare dressing: In a small bowl, whisk together orange juice, honey, olive oil, lime juice, and coriander. Add ginger and mix to combine.

3   Pour dressing over rice mixture. Mix well to moisten and combine ingredients. Salt, to taste.

4   To serve, arrange salad greens on small plates, spoon rice salad mixture on top. Rice salad can be refrigerated for several hours or overnight.

MAKES 8 SERVINGS

NUTRITIONAL ANALYSIS PER SERVING **227 calories** ▪ **6 percent fat (total fat 1.5 g, saturated fat 0 g)** ▪ **87 percent carbohydrate (2 g fiber)** ▪ **7 percent protein.**

Chicken Satay Chop Salad in Lettuce Parcels with Peanut Sauce

A fun, casual lunch salad, made of several small dishes to accompany the chicken and lettuce leaves.

SAUCE

½ cup light coconut milk

2 tablespoons reduced-fat peanut butter

¼ cup fresh cilantro, minced

1 tablespoon honey

2 teaspoons fresh ginger, peeled and minced

2 teaspoons shredded coconut

2 cloves garlic, minced

1 teaspoon each: cumin, corlander, lime juice, soy sauce, and sesame oil

½ teaspoon hot pepper flakes

SALAD

3 small skinless, boneless chicken breasts, cut into 1-inch strips

cooking spray

2 cups prepared coleslaw mix

1 head Boston lettuce leaves, washed, dried, separated

2 tablespoons roasted peanuts, chopped

2 tablespoons shredded coconut

¼ cup fresh cilantro, minced

1   In a small bowl, combine all sauce ingredients. Set aside.

2   In a large Ziploc plastic bag, add chicken strips and ¼ cup of sauce (set aside remaining sauce). Seal tightly. Turn to distribute evenly over chicken. Refrigerate for 20 minutes (up to 24 hours).

3   Coat grill with cooking spray. Heat grill to medium-high. Remove chicken from Ziploc bag. Place on grill, pour any remaining sauce from plastic bag over chicken. Close lid, cook chicken 2 to 3 minutes on each side or until no longer pink. Remove from grill. Chop chicken into 1-inch pieces, set aside. Keep warm.

4   In a medium bowl, add 2 cups coleslaw mix, chopped chicken, ⅓ cup reserved sauce (save the rest for dipping). Mix well. (Add a little more sauce if not moist enough.)

5   To serve, place a pile of lettuce leaves on a plate. Fill small bowls with leftover sauce, roasted peanuts, coconut, and cilantro. Put the bowl of chicken coleslaw next to small bowls of condiments.

6   To eat, place a small amount of chicken-coleslaw mix on a lettuce leaf. Sprinkle with roasted peanuts, coconut, cilantro, and wrap. Drizzle with sauce. Eat with fingers.

MAKES 4 SERVINGS

NUTRITIONAL ANALYSIS PER SERVING **225 calories** ▪ **43 percent fat (total fat 10.7 g, saturated fat 3.8 g)** ▪ **15 percent carbohydrate (2.4 g fiber)** ▪ **42 percent protein.**

A

Asian Cucumber Salad

Tangy, crispy, and easy to make, this Asian-inspired cucumber salad is a beautiful array of shredded colors that delicately float around thinly sliced cucumbers in a light rice vinegar dressing. Perfect for any meal.

2 large English cucumbers, peeled and thinly sliced

½ cup carrots, peeled and shredded

¼ cup red radish, shredded

¼ cup green onions (white and light green only), thinly sliced

½ cup rice wine vinegar

½ cup water

2 teaspoons fish sauce

3 teaspoons Splenda

1   In a medium salad bowl, mix cucumbers, carrots, radish, and green onions. Set aside.

2   In a small bowl, whisk together the remaining ingredients.

3   Pour vinegar dressing over cucumber mixture and toss to coat. Cover and refrigerate (up to 24 hours) until ready to eat.

MAKES 4 SERVINGS

NUTRITIONAL ANALYSIS PER SERVING **36 calories** ▪ **6 percent fat (total fat < 0.5 g, saturated fat 0 g)** ▪ **76 percent carbohydrate (2 g fiber)** ▪ **18 percent protein.**

Q

Wilted Spinach Salad with Warm Raspberry Vinaigrette and Toasted Hazelnuts

If you have a few calories to spare, sprinkle this salad with crumbled Gorgonzola cheese.

MOOD TIP

Spinach is rich in a phytochemical called lutein, which lowers the risk for age-related vision loss. Lutein levels in women fluctuate throughout the month, but it is unknown whether boosting levels will curb symptoms of PMS.

VINAIGRETTE

¼ cup raspberries (fresh or frozen)

¼ cup orange juice

1 tablespoon raspberry or red wine vinegar

1 tablespoon balsamic vinegar

1 tablespoon olive oil

2 tablespoons honey

SALAD

1 (10-ounce) bag baby spinach

¼ small red onion, thinly sliced

⅓ cup mushrooms, thinly sliced (any variety)

2 tablespoons hazelnuts, chopped and toasted*

4 tablespoons raspberries for garnish

1   Combine vinaigrette ingredients in a small food processor. Blend until smooth. Pour into a small saucepan. Heat over medium heat until vinaigrette mixture simmers. Remove from heat and keep hot.

2   In a large salad bowl, toss spinach, onion, and mushrooms.

3   Just before serving, drizzle hot vinaigrette over salad while tossing with a pair of tongs. (The vinaigrette needs to be hot enough to wilt the spinach and soften the leaves.) Divide salad evenly among 4 salad plates. Sprinkle with toasted hazelnuts and raspberries. Serve immediately.

MAKES 4 SERVINGS

NUTRITIONAL ANALYSIS PER SERVING **124 calories** ▪ **40 percent fat (total fat 5.5 g, saturated fat < 1 g)** ▪ **50 percent carbohydrate (3.2 g fiber)** ▪ **10 percent protein.**

*To toast hazelnuts, place them on tinfoil and bake at 350° until golden brown, approximately 10 minutes.

Low-Fat Caesar Salad

The blend of sour cream, Parmesan cheese, lemon, and garlic adds flavor without fat or calories to this quick-fix salad. Another fun way to serve this salad is to use whole Romaine lettuce leaves and dip them in a bowl of dressing. Or drizzle a small amount of dressing over whole lettuce leaves that are eaten with the fingers. The capers are optional, and for those not enamored with garlic, reduce to one minced clove.

DRESSING
½ cup fat-free sour cream

2 tablespoons low-fat mayonnaise

2 tablespoons Parmesan cheese, grated

2 tablespoons capers, rinsed and drained (optional)

1½ tablespoons lemon juice

2 cloves garlic, minced

¼ teaspoon coarsely ground pepper

SALAD
1 medium head Romaine lettuce, washed and chopped

several thin slices of red onion (optional)

1 cup fat-free seasoned croutons

1 teaspoon Parmesan cheese, grated (optional)

1   In a small bowl, combine all dressing ingredients. Stir well. Cover and refrigerate for 1 hour or overnight.

2   In a large salad bowl, combine lettuce and onions. Add dressing and toss to coat. Sprinkle with croutons and Parmesan cheese. Serve immediately.

MAKES 6 SERVINGS

NUTRITIONAL ANALYSIS PER SERVING **25 calories** ▪ **22 percent fat (total fat 0.5 g, saturated fat 0 g)** ▪ **43 percent carbohydrate (< 0.5 g fiber)** ▪ **35 percent protein.**

Q

 —COMFORT FOOD

 —QUICK FIX FOOD

 —ADVENTUROUS

—SPECIAL OCCASION

Entrées

Taming Out-of-Control Appetites

DO YOU HAVE a weakness for any one food? Do you pride yourself in eating moderately most of the time yet seem to have no limit when served pot roast, fried chicken, Mom's spaghetti, or some other favorite food? Do you eat just one potato chip, or do you eat the whole bag after the first taste? For me, it is pizza. I can't seem to find my limit and, if left unchecked, could probably eat an entire extra-large at one sitting.

Almost everyone faces an out-of-control appetite once in a while. (So my pizza problem isn't that far-fetched.) But why do our appetites run amok? Why can we eat an entire pan of brownies but balk at a small serving of chicken breast or spinach?

No one really knows exactly what triggers our appetites and causes some people to eat beyond basic hunger needs. A bunch of theories and a few facts have identified some of the puzzle pieces; yet the underlying reasons for overeating remain elusive and probably are a complex combination of factors. The good news? We do have some tried-and-true solutions to the problem. The entrées in this section, as well as the other recipes in this book, are based on those solutions.

Appetite versus Hunger

If the only reason we ate was because our stomachs were growling, meals would serve only to soothe physiological hunger and we would always refuse the second helping. Yet many of us often eat more than we need, whether we're hungry or not, and typically all the wrong stuff. In fact, overeating has become a national pastime. According to the U.S. Department of Agriculture's studies on Americans' eating habits, we now eat 300 calories more each day than we did a few decades ago. Combine gluttony with sloth, and—voilà—you have the current obesity epidemic.

Appetite is more than just hunger. Our appetite clocks are tickled by a wide array of chemicals in the brain, emotions, and social cues, as well as the sheer pleasure of eating and the culture in which we live. Confusion about what, when, and how much to eat is another contributor to out-of-control appetites. Our fondness for food is also a bit quirky: We favor foods our parents ate, and we eat less when watching ourselves eat, but more when we think a food is low in calories or fat, regardless of its actual content. The forces dictating our insatiable appetites seem endless.

Here's a quick course on how to tame the savage appetite beast.

Eat Less, Weigh More

Our nation's obsession with dieting aggravates out-of-control appetites. The more we jump on the fad-diet bandwagon, the more we eat and the fatter we get. Six out of every 10 people are now battling weight problems. The numbers rise every year.

Why? Besides the obvious effect fad diets have on your appetite-control chemistry (imagine what a low-carbohydrate diet must do to serotonin and NPY levels!), humans do not take well to deprivation. Tell yourself you will eat only three times a day, and you're hungry all day long. Make a vow to avoid chips, and it's the one food you want. Label grains as "bad," and you can't keep your hands off them.

Quick-weight-loss dieting also numbs the hunger response. People who have a long history of dieting lose the ability to recognize when they're hungry or full, so mistake any uncomfortable feeling, from boredom to anxiety, as a signal to eat.

Erratic eating habits also cripple our best efforts to choose nutritious foods. If you eat when you are comfortably hungry, you eat sensibly; if you wait until you are ravenous, you eat too much of the wrong stuff. "Many people skip meals thinking it's an easy way to cut calories," says C. Wayne Callaway, M.D., at George Washington University in Washington, D.C. "But the plan backfires and inevitably increases cravings for all the wrong foods, lowers resistance to snacking later in the day, and can increase the likelihood of overeating."

12 QUICK-FIX ENTRÉES

1. **GRILLED SALMON:** Mix honey, Dijon mustard, balsamic vinegar, and minced garlic in a small bowl. Rub on salmon steaks or fillets and grill for 3 minutes a side.

2. **HALIBUT VERA CRUZ:** Top grilled halibut (or any firm, white fish) with canned Mexican-style chopped tomatoes mixed with chopped fresh parsley and a dash of salsa.

3. **CARIBBEAN CHICKEN:** Flatten skinless, boneless chicken breasts. Rub with olive oil and jerk seasoning. Grill for 5 to 6 minutes per side or until done.

4. **QUICK PAELLA:** Prepare 1 box of yellow rice. Add 1 can Mexican stewed tomatoes, and ½ cup frozen green peas. Stir in up to 1 pound of any of the following or a combination: cooked shrimp, scallops, or turkey sausage cut into 1-inch slices.

5. **ONE-DISH TACOS:** Prepare 1 box of Mexican rice. Add 1 can of beans (kidney, black, or navy), 1 small can of diced green chilies, 1 cup shredded chicken, and 1 cup commercial salsa. Mix together until well combined. Spoon taco mixture in a large bowl, alongside a basket of warm tortillas. (Optional: small bowls of fat-free sour cream, lettuce, tomatoes, extra salsa.)

6. **PASTA PRONTO:** Cook fresh ravioli (found in the refrigerator section of the grocery store), top with bottled spaghetti sauce (such as Classico Tomato and Basil), and sprinkle with low-fat Parmesan cheese.

7. **CREAMED TUNA:** Make a white cream sauce with butter, flour, and nonfat milk. Flavor with a dash of Worcestershire sauce, paprika, salt, and pepper. Drain 1 large can of white albacore tuna and add to sauce. Serve over instant brown rice.

8. **INSTANT STIR FRY:** Slice chicken breast and sauté in canola oil. Add diced onion, minced garlic, and 1 package of frozen stir fry vegetables. Serve over instant brown rice.

9. **SHRIMP COCKTAIL:** Boil prawns in salted water with 2 bay leaves until pink, approximately 2 minutes. Serve with cocktail sauce, a tossed salad, and French bread.

10. **NACHOS:** Line a cookie sheet with foil. Spread baked tortilla chips evenly across cookie sheet, top with fat-free refried beans and grated low-fat cheese. Bake until cheese melts. Serve with fat-free sour cream, salsa, and chopped vegetables.

11. **LINGUINE WITH CLAMS:** Make a sauce combining minced garlic, clam juice, canned minced clams, chopped parsley, and a little white vermouth. Pour over cooked linguine and top with low-fat Parmesan cheese.

12. **BARBECUED CHICKEN:** Place chicken breasts or thighs in a heat-proof container. Pour commercial low-fat barbecue sauce over chicken and microwave for 10 minutes. Transfer to heated grill and complete cooking, until meat is cooked through. Serve with a tossed salad and microwaved baked potatoes.

Simple Steps

Weight gain did not become a widespread problem in the United States until the end of the 1970s. Prior to that time, people's weights had remained relatively stable. The steady increase in body fat results from small changes people make in their diets. For example, suppose you ate one extra corn chip every day at a cost of 14 calories. Over the course of 20 years (14 calories × 365 days × 20 years), you would consume an extra 102,200 calories, the equivalent of a 29-pound weight gain. Granted, most people haven't gained *that* much weight in the past three decades, but this does show how even small changes in what we eat can have profound effects on health.

The good news is that it takes only small changes in what we eat and how much we move to produce dramatic positive results in health and weight over time. For example, just giving up those chips (and not compensating by eating more of something else!) would produce a significant weight loss over the course of 30 years. Here are more easy answers to managing your weight and taming an out-of-control appetite.

- *Eat mindfully.* Pay attention to and enjoy every mouthful. Stop halfway through a meal, sit back, and listen to your body. If you still feel physically hungry, have a few more bites and listen again. Stop when you are comfortably full.

- *Watch portions.* We've become accustomed to gigantic servings. The recommended serving of grain is a 1-ounce bagel or half a cup of pasta, not the typical 5-ounce bagel served in most delis or the platter of pasta at restaurants. A serving of meat or fish is 3 ounces, not a 16-ounce steak that drapes over the plate. Pay attention to the recommended servings for each recipe in this book. If you stick with these serving sizes, you will feel satisfied, not stuffed.

- *Never socialize on an empty stomach.* We eat more when we dine with friends and family. So have a healthful snack before a party, serve reasonable portions, drink water to keep your hands busy at social gatherings, and split an entrée when dining out.

- *Don't mix alcohol with meals.* Even one drink opens the inhibition floodgates, leaving you more likely to overeat.

- *Give your favorite recipes a low-fat face-lift.* Make creamed sauces with cornstarch and low-fat milk instead of butter and whole milk. Use fat-free half-and-half instead of cream in recipes. Cut the fat by half or sauté in chicken broth. Double the amount of vegetables in a recipe to dilute the fat calories. The recipes in this book take advantage of every trick available to cut calories and maximize taste and nutrition.

WHAT'S A PORTION?

Here's a crash course on how to eyeball the accurate portions.

3 ounces of meat, chicken, fish	= palm of your hand
	= deck of cards
	= cassette tape
½ cup pasta, rice, oatmeal, potatoes, cooked vegetables, beans, canned fruit	= fist
	= tennis ball
	= tulip
1 cup cooked vegetables	= baseball
1-ounce bagel	= yo-yo
1 pancake	= compact disc
1 piece of fruit, medium-sized	= tight fist
1 ounce of low-fat cheese	= thumb
	= Ping-Pong ball
1 baked potato, medium-sized	= computer mouse
1 teaspoon of butter or oil	= postage stamp the thickness of finger
2 tablespoons salad dressing	= standard ice cube
1 cup low-fat milk or soymilk	= 2 wineglasses

- *Plan your entrées*. Since we center meals on an entrée, make sure the focus of your meals is nutritionally sound—low in fat and calories and rich in flavor, aroma, and texture. That's what you'll find in every entrée in this section.

- *Exercise*. "Daily physical activity shifts the body from energy excess to energy need, so what is considered overeating when you're sedentary is just fueling your body when you're fit," says Adam Drewnowski, Ph.D., at the University of Washington in Seattle. Exercise also balances our appetite-control chemicals, so it's no surprise that physically fit people are less prone to overeating than are couch potatoes.

Live to Eat or Eat to Live?

"Overeating would not be a problem if people ate platters of broccoli or zucchini," says Dr. Drewnowski. "The problem is we overeat foods high in calories from fat and sugar."

The whole issue of out-of-whack appetites comes down to focusing on real foods: fruits, vegetables, whole grains, legumes, extra-lean meats and fish, and calcium-rich foods. First fill your tummy with mangos, papayas, sweet potatoes, spinach, brown rice, black beans, seafood, nonfat yogurt, and other real foods found in the entrées in this section and the other recipes in this book. If there is room left over, turn to small portions of fattier fare, such as fried foods, cookies, snack foods, and full-fat recipes. You won't eat as much of these calorie-packed foods (in fact, you'll find with time that you prefer less-greasy foods). You will feel full longer, have more energy and a happier mood. You also will find that even when confronted with that plate of brownies, you'll be more likely to have just one, not the whole batch!

Grilled Halibut with Ginger-Mango Chutney

This chutney is so good you'll want to eat it plain! It also tastes great as a topping for grilled chicken breast or a firm, white fish, such as bass or shark. Make extra chutney and keep it in the refrigerator for up to one week to use as a topping on leftovers. It's also rich in vitamin C, vitamin A, folic acid, and iron!

CHUTNEY
cooking spray

2 cups red onion, finely chopped or minced

2 firm mangos, peeled, pitted, and cubed

1 cup tomato, chopped

3 tablespoons fresh ginger, minced

2 tablespoons garlic, minced

2 limes, juiced

3 tablespoons orange juice

¼ cup vermouth

3 tablespoons brown sugar

3 tablespoons rice wine vinegar

HALIBUT
4 (6-ounce) thick halibut fillets

olive oil cooking spray

coarse salt, to taste

freshly ground black pepper, to taste

1   To make chutney: Spray a large nonstick skillet with cooking spray, heat over medium heat. Add onion and sauté for 5 minutes, stirring occasionally. Add mango, tomato, ginger, and garlic and cook until heated through, about 7 minutes. Stir in lime juice, orange juice, vermouth, brown sugar, and vinegar. Bring to a gentle boil, reduce heat, and simmer for 15 minutes. Set aside.

2   Heat grill. Spray fish with olive oil spray and sprinkle with salt and pepper. Grill for 3 to 5 minutes on each side or until fish is flaky and no longer transparent throughout.

3   Top each serving of fish with ½ cup of chutney.

MAKES 4 SERVINGS

NUTRITIONAL ANALYSIS PER SERVING **364 calories** ▪ **11 percent fat (total fat 4.64 g, saturated fat < 1 g)** ▪ **46 percent carbohydrate (4.4 g fiber)** ▪ **43 percent protein.**

Crab and Veggie Cakes with Garlic-Chili Cream

Antioxidant-rich peppers and vegetables give this traditional dish an added boost. Make the sauce and cake batter ahead of time, then fry cakes for a quick 10-minute meal. Serve with a tossed salad and Crusty French Bread (page 18).

CREAM
½ cup fat-free mayonnaise
1 clove garlic, minced
3 teaspoons chili sauce
4 teaspoons fresh lemon juice

CAKES
cooking spray
⅓ cup red bell pepper, diced
¼ cup celery, diced
¼ cup red onion, diced
5 teaspoons canned chilies, diced
½ pound crabmeat, shredded

1 tablespoon fresh lemon juice
½ cup liquid egg substitute (equivalent to 2 whole eggs)
salt and pepper, to taste
1 cup bread crumbs
fresh parsley, chopped (optional)

1   Mix ingredients for garlic-chili cream, cover, and refrigerate for 1 hour to overnight.

2   Spray a nonstick medium skillet with cooking spray and place over medium heat. Add bell pepper, celery, onion, and chilies. Stir until onion is tender, about 5 minutes.

3   In a large bowl, mix pepper mixture, crabmeat, lemon juice, eggs, salt and pepper, and ¼ cup of garlic-chili cream. Add bread crumbs and toss until thoroughly mixed.

4   Form crab mixture into 4 (½-inch-thick) patties. (If you have the time, place patties on baking sheet, cover, and refrigerate for 1 hour or more.)

5   Spray a large, nonstick skillet and place over medium heat. Put cakes in skillet and cook until golden brown, about 8 minutes per side. Sprinkle with fresh parsley. Serve with remaining garlic-chili cream.

MAKES 4 SERVINGS

NUTRITIONAL ANALYSIS PER SERVING **220 calories** ▪ **14 percent fat (total fat 3.4 g, saturated fat ‹ 1 g)** ▪ **51 percent carbohydrate (1.7 g fiber)** ▪ **35 percent protein.**

C

Chicken with Mushrooms in Creamy Garlic-Pecan Sauce

Nut milk is a great alternative to heavy creams in recipes. Vary the thickness of the sauce by adjusting the amount of water you add to the ground nuts. You can replace some of the water with fat-free cream cheese or fat-free half-and-half for an even richer sauce. Try almonds or cashews instead of pecans for a change of flavor, too.

MOOD TIP

Adding nuts to the weekly diet could lower heart-disease risk by up to 50 percent, possibly because nuts contain health-giving compounds called polyphenolics. Nuts are also rich sources of vitamin E, fiber, magnesium, and potassium, as well as unsaturated fats and fiber, all of which help boost mood and lower heart-disease risk. For example, magnesium might help improve our ability to cope with stress.

¾ cup pecans

¾ cup water

1 teaspoon "Better Than Bouillon" Chicken Base (optional)

4 (4-ounce) skinless, boneless chicken breast halves

salt and pepper, to taste

cooking spray

⅓ cup green onions, chopped

3 cloves garlic, minced

6 cups mushrooms, sliced

fresh parsley, chopped

1   In a blender or food processor, finely grind pecans, scraping sides as needed. With blender running, add water and chicken base and continue to blend until mixture is smooth. Set aside.

2   Sprinkle chicken with salt and pepper and place in a large nonstick skillet coated with cooking spray. Cover and cook over medium heat until golden and cooked through, about 5 minutes per side. Remove chicken and set aside.

3   Add onions, garlic, and mushrooms to skillet. Cover and cook over medium heat until mushrooms are tender, stirring occasionally.

4   Pour nut milk into mushroom mixture, stir, and bring to a boil. Cook for about 2 minutes. Pour sauce over chicken breasts and serve over noodles, rice, or couscous. Sprinkle with parsley.

MAKES 4 SERVINGS

NUTRITIONAL ANALYSIS PER SERVING **378 calories** ▪ **60 percent fat (total fat 25 g, saturated fat 4 g)** ▪ **11 percent carbohydrate (3.3 g fiber)** ▪ **29 percent protein.**

Herb-Roasted Chicken

My family loves roast chicken, and it's so simple to make. The extra benefit is that leftovers can be used to make chicken salad for sandwiches and wraps the next day. Maple-Glazed Brussels Sprouts with Portabello Mushrooms and Walnuts (page 213), Roasted Gingered Vegetables (page 214), Glazed Carrots (page 215), and/or Cranberry Chutney (page 53) are all great accompaniments to this dish. (Notice the difference in calories, fat, and saturated fat between chicken breast and dark meat. If you are watching your weight or cholesterol, choose chicken breast.)

---

5 pound chicken, giblets removed, rinsed inside and outside, patted dry

½ teaspoon salt

½ teaspoon ground pepper

4 sprigs fresh rosemary

4 sprigs fresh sage

½ lemon, cut in half

3 cloves garlic

1 teaspoon olive oil

salt and pepper

Preheat oven to 425°.

1   Rub cavity of chicken with salt and pepper. Stuff with herbs, lemon, and garlic. Rub outside of bird with olive oil and generously salt and pepper. Tuck legs together (use string or tinfoil) to make bird as compact as possible.

2   Place bird on rack in covered roasting pan. Roast for 1 hour 15 minutes or until thigh meat is 170 degrees and juices run clear. Baste every 15 minutes after first half hour. If bird browns too quickly, lower oven temperature to 400°.

3   Let chicken rest for 5 to 10 minutes before carving.

MAKES 4 SERVINGS

NUTRITIONAL ANALYSIS PER 3-OUNCE SERVING OF BREAST MEAT **167 calories** ▪ **36 percent fat** (total fat 6.7 g, saturated fat 1.8 g) ▪ **0 percent carbohydrate (0 g fiber)** ▪ **64 percent protein.**

NUTRITIONAL ANALYSIS PER 3-OUNCE SERVING OF DARK MEAT **210 calories** ▪ **58 percent fat** (total fat 13.5 g, saturated fat 3.7 g) ▪ **0 percent carbohydrate (0 g fiber)** ▪ **42 percent protein.**

Stir-Fried Chicken Mu-Shu

Searching for that mu-shu recipe that tastes just like the one from your favorite Chinese restaurant? Here it is! We have taken shortcuts by using prepared coleslaw mix, purchased Asian plum sauce, and tortillas. Skip the chicken, and this recipe becomes vegetarian mu-shu.

2 teaspoons sesame oil

1 medium sweet yellow onion, peeled, thinly sliced, and chopped

¼ pound fresh shiitake mushrooms, thinly sliced

½ cup fat-free chicken broth

1 (16-ounce) package coleslaw mix

1 tablespoon cooking sherry

3 tablespoons Asian plum sauce or hoisin sauce

2 tablespoons soy sauce

2 teaspoons cornstarch

1 pound skinless, boneless chicken breasts, boiled and shredded

¼ cup green onion, thinly sliced

8 (6-inch) flour tortillas, warmed

¼ cup fresh cilantro, chopped

1. Heat sesame oil in a large nonstick wok or frying pan. When pan is hot, add onion and shiitake mushrooms. Cook until onion is tender, about 3 to 5 minutes. Add a little chicken broth if necessary to prevent from burning.

2. Add 1 package coleslaw mix, add remaining chicken broth, and stir-fry approximately 2 minutes until coleslaw is wilted but crisp. Do not overcook.

3. Mix together in a small bowl the sherry, plum or hoisin sauce, soy sauce, and cornstarch until smooth. Add to vegetables in pan, along with shredded chicken. Stir until sauce is thickened, approximately 1 minute.

4. Transfer to a large platter. Sprinkle with green onion.

5. Wrap tortillas in damp towel and warm in microwave for 1 minute.

6. To serve, spread each warmed tortilla with warmed plum or hoisin sauce. Add chicken mu-shu, sprinkle with cilantro, and roll up.

MAKES 8 SERVINGS

NUTRITIONAL ANALYSIS PER SERVING **260 calories** ▪ **21** percent fat (total fat 6 g, saturated fat 1 g) ▪ **43** percent carbohydrate (3 g fiber) ▪ **36 percent protein.**

Black Beans with Cumin and Chipotle Peppers

This hearty black bean recipe is a personal favorite at our house. It's quick, easy, not too saucy or messy, which adds versatility to creative recipe ideas. The smoky hot flavors from the chipotle peppers pair up perfectly with the sweet smooth taste of the onions. Serve with rice or warm tortillas, over soft polenta, with any of the tossed salads on pages 121 to 142, or in any of the following black bean recipes: Black Bean Chili with Chicken (page 95), Black Bean Burritos (page 64), or Black Bean Dip with Pita Wedges (page 38).

MOOD TIP

Beans are an excellent source of iron, supplying 3.6 milligrams for every cup. A deficiency of this mineral contributes to shortened attention span, lowered IQ and intelligence, lack of motivation, poor hand-eye coordination, lowered scores on vocabulary tests, inability to concentrate, and poor work performance.

2 tablespoons olive oil

1 large sweet yellow onion, chopped

1 medium green or red bell pepper, chopped

2 cloves garlic, minced

2 teaspoons ground cumin

1½ teaspoons ground coriander

1 (4-ounce) can diced green chilies

1 teaspoon canned chipotle pepper, rinsed, seeded, and minced (from a 7-ounce can of chipotle peppers in adobo sauce. 2 teaspoons minced chipotle pepper if you like it hot).

3 teaspoons canned chipotle adobo sauce (save rest of can for another use)

1 (14.5-ounce) can diced Mexican stewed tomatoes

2 (15-ounce) cans black beans, drained

½ cup fresh cilantro, chopped

⅓ cup fat-free sour cream (optional)

1   Warm oil in a heavy large pot or Dutch oven over medium-high heat. Add onion, pepper, and garlic. Sauté 5 minutes or until soft.

2   Add all remaining ingredients except cilantro and sour cream.

3   Simmer on medium heat for 20 minutes, then add cilantro.

4   Serve in a large bowl. Top with sour cream if desired.

5   Store leftover black beans in your freezer, or make a double batch for use in black bean recipes.

MAKES 10 SERVINGS

NUTRITIONAL ANALYSIS PER SERVING **142 calories** ▪ **19 percent fat (total fat 3 g, saturated fat < 0.5 g)** ▪ **63 percent carbohydrate (6.2 g fiber)** ▪ **18 percent protein.**

Crusty Cranberry Salmon

The sweet flavors of dried fruit go well with the fresh thyme and lemon in this flavorful dish. It's pretty, too! Serve with couscous and a green vegetable, such as green beans or sautéed spinach. Each serving supplies 2.5 grams of mood- and mind-boosting omega-3 fats.

MOOD TIP
The fats In salmon, called omega-3 fats, might help reduce depression, according to a study from Massachusetts General Hospital in Boston.

1½ pounds salmon or steelhead fillet

1 tablespoon fresh lemon juice

⅓ cup dried cranberries or cherries, diced

⅓ cup green onions, diced

½ cup bread crumbs

2 tablespoons fat-free mayonnaise

1 tablespoon fresh thyme leaves

pinch of red pepper flakes

salt, to taste

1 teaspoon lemon peel, grated

Preheat oven to 375°.

1. Place salmon on foil-lined cookie sheet and sprinkle with lemon juice.

2. Dice dried fruit in food processor. Remove and dice green onions in food processor. In medium bowl, combine bread crumbs, diced dried fruit, diced green onions, mayonnaise, thyme, red pepper flakes, salt, and lemon peel. Blend with fork until mixture is wet and can be pressed together in clumps.

3. Place dried fruit mixture on top of salmon and press together, covering entire top of fish. Bake until fish is flaky but not dry, approximately 20 minutes (time will vary depending on thickness of fish).

MAKES 4 SERVINGS

NUTRITIONAL ANALYSIS PER SERVING 406 calories ▪ 41 percent fat (total fat 18.5 g, saturated fat 4.5 g) ▪ 22 percent carbohydrate (1.6 g fiber) ▪ 37 percent protein.

Chicken 'n' Mushrooms in Sherry Cream Gravy

Serve over Creamy Comfort-Food Mashed Potatoes (page 186), noodles, or biscuits.

---

1 pound skinless, boneless chicken breast, cut into bite-size pieces

salt and pepper, to taste

¼ cup fat-free chicken broth

¾ cup fat-free half-and-half

5 tablespoons sherry

3 teaspoons olive oil

½ cup baby carrots, thinly sliced

1 pound mushrooms, washed, stemmed, and sliced

½ cup onion, chopped

⅔ cup green peas

1 tablespoon fresh thyme leaves

2 teaspoons cornstarch mixed with 2 tablespoons water

2 tablespoons fresh parsley, chopped

1   Season chicken with salt and pepper. Set aside.

2   In a small bowl, mix broth, half-and-half, and sherry. Set aside.

3   Warm 1 teaspoon oil in large nonstick skillet over medium heat. Add carrots and stir for 5 minutes. Add mushrooms and cook, stirring occasionally, until softened and golden brown, about 5 minutes. Transfer to medium bowl.

4   In the same skillet, add 1 teaspoon oil and chicken. Cook until underside of chicken is golden brown, then toss and continue to stir occasionally until almost cooked, about 8 minutes total. Add chicken to bowl of mushrooms and carrots.

5   Add last teaspoon of oil and onion to same skillet and cook until onion is translucent, about 3 minutes.

6   Add cream mixture and stir, including any browned bits from pan into sauce. Add peas, thyme, and cornstarch mixture, and simmer sauce for 5 minutes. Sauce should be slightly thickened.

7   Reduce heat to medium-low and stir in chicken, mushrooms, and carrots. Season with salt and pepper. Heat through, but do not boil. Remove from heat, sprinkle with parsley, and serve.

MAKES 6 SERVINGS

NUTRITIONAL ANALYSIS PER SERVING **190 calories** ▪ **30 percent fat (total fat 6.3 g, saturated fat 2.7 g)** ▪ **25 percent carbohydrate (2.4 g fiber)** ▪ **45 percent protein.**

C

Halibut with Tomatoes, Basil, and Capers

This dish goes especially well with Glazed Carrots (page 215) and Barley, Red Pepper, and Green Onion Pilaf (page 199).

FOOD TIP

Tomatoes are an excellent source of lycopene, a phytochemical that helps protect against cancer.

2 cups fresh tomatoes, chopped

4 tablespoons fresh basil, chopped

3 tablespoons capers, with 1 teaspoon caper juice

3 tablespoons fresh lemon juice

rind of 1 lemon, grated fine

½ teaspoon sugar

1 tablespoon olive oil

4 halibut steaks or 4 halibut fillets, 1¼ inches thick

lemon wedges and basil leaves

Preheat oven to 425° or preheat grill to high.

1   In a medium bowl, mix all ingredients, except halibut, lemon wedges, and basil.

2   Brush halibut with a small amount of the liquid from the tomato-caper mixture.

3   Arrange halibut on a baking sheet, roast until fish is opaque in center, about 4 to 5 minutes on each side, or grill over direct heat for 3 to 4 minutes per side or until opaque in center. Brush fish with more tomato-caper liquid if needed. Save remaining mixture for topping.

4   Remove from oven or grill. Serve with remaining sauce spooned over each halibut fillet or steak. (Tomato-caper sauce can be heated in microwave for 2 minutes or served at room temperature.) Garnish with lemon wedge and fresh basil.

MAKES 4 SERVINGS

NUTRITIONAL ANALYSIS PER SERVING **242 calories** ▪ **29 percent fat** (total fat 7.7 g, saturated fat 1 g) ▪ **10 percent carbohydrate** (1.4 g fiber) ▪ **61 percent protein.**

Grilled Pork Tenderloin with Rosemary-Orange Sauce

This pork is full of flavor and so tender, thanks to the quick-brine technique. There are so many rubs, marinades, and sauces from which to choose, so use your imagination. If you don't have orange marmalade, use any type of fruit jam. Serve with Fluffy Mashed Potatoes with Horseradish (page 187), Creamy Sweet Potatoes and Yams with Chipotle Peppers (page 217), and a green vegetable, such as broccoli or asparagus. Cranberry Chutney (page 53) also goes well with this dish.

8 cups water

½ cup coarse salt

½ cup sugar

2 pork tenderloins (about 1½ pounds each)

1 tablespoon fresh rosemary, minced

1 teaspoon thyme, dried

½ teaspoon ground cumin

¼ teaspoon ground cinnamon

1 tablespoon olive oil

SAUCE

1 teaspoon olive oil

1 shallot, peeled and minced

1 teaspoon fresh rosemary, minced

½ cup orange marmalade (reduced sugar)

1½ tablespoons balsamic vinegar

1   In a large bowl, prepare brine by mixing water, salt, and sugar until dissolved.

2   Trim excess fat from tenderloins and add them to brine. Submerge in brine for 30 minutes.

3   In a small bowl, mix ingredients for pork rub: rosemary, thyme, cumin, and cinnamon. Set aside.

4   Remove pork from brine, rinse with water, and pat dry. Rub each tenderloin with oil, then pat on pork rub, covering all sides evenly. Place in a shallow baking dish, cover, and refrigerate until ready to grill (up to 24 hours).

5   Heat gas grill to high (preheat for 5 to 10 minutes). Place pork over hot grate, insert a meat thermometer, and close lid. Grill for about 8 minutes, turn, and grill another 8 minutes on opposite side. Cook until meat reaches 145° to 150°. Remove pork from grill, cover with aluminum foil, and let rest for 5 minutes. (For perfect pork, remove it from the grill when it is slightly pink; while it rests, it completes the cooking process.)

6   To prepare the sauce: Warm oil in a small saucepan over medium heat. Add shallots and rosemary and cook for 2 minutes or until shallots are tender. Add marmalade and vinegar, and heat until mixture simmers. Add juices from resting pork tenderloin.

7   Slice pork into 3-inch rounds, place on a large serving platter, drizzle with sauce, and serve.

MAKES 8 SERVINGS OF APPROXIMATELY 4 OUNCES EACH

NUTRITIONAL ANALYSIS PER SERVING **335 calories** ▪ **44 percent fat (total fat 16 g, saturated fat 5 g)** ▪ **18 percent carbohydrate (0 g fiber)** ▪ **38 percent protein.**

Chilies Rellenos Casserole with Red Sauce

This is a family favorite. It's easy to make, and if you're lucky enough to have extra, the leftovers make a great lunch or second dinner later in the week.

CASSEROLE
cooking spray

3 cans whole chilies, drained, cut lengthwise, and seeded

8 ounces low-fat cheddar cheese, grated

1 (1 pound, 14 ounces) can fat-free refried beans

2 cups frozen corn, thawed

1/3 cup all-purpose flour

1/2 teaspoon salt

1 cup nonfat milk

dash of tabasco

1 cup liquid egg substitute (equivalent to 4 whole eggs)

3 egg whites, whipped until stiff

SAUCE
1 teaspoon olive oil

1 cup onions, diced

1 clove garlic, minced

2 tablespoons tomato paste

1 cup fresh tomatoes, chopped

1 cup fat-free chicken broth

1 teaspoon sugar

1/2 teaspoon salt

1/4 teaspoon ground cumin

1 teaspoon dried oregano

1/4 teaspoon freshly ground black pepper

1 teaspoon red wine vinegar

1 tablespoon all-purpose flour

CASSEROLE

Heat oven to 350°. Spray a 13-by-9-inch baking dish with cooking spray.

1   Spread half of chilies evenly on bottom of baking dish. Sprinkle half of the cheese (4 ounces) over top of chiles. Spread beans over top of cheese, then layer corn, rest of cheese, and second half of chilies.

2   In a small bowl, combine flour, salt, milk, tabasco, and egg substitute. Stir until thoroughly blended. Fold in whipped egg whites.

3   Pour milk-egg mixture over top of casserole, spreading evenly. Bake for 1 hour 20 minutes or until set. Let stand 5 minutes before serving.

MAKES 8 SERVINGS

SAUCE

1   Warm oil in small nonstick skillet over medium heat. Add onions and garlic and cook until transparent, approximately 4 minutes. Add tomato paste and chopped tomatoes. Simmer for 5 minutes. Add broth, sugar, salt, cumin, oregano, pepper, and vinegar. Continue to simmer until tomatoes begin to fall apart, approximately 5 minutes.

2   Pour tomato mixture into blender and whip until smooth. Add flour and blend for 30 seconds. Return to skillet and cook over medium-high heat until sauce bubbles and thickens slightly.

3   Serve in a small gravy boat or pitcher to pour over individual servings of casserole.

MAKES ABOUT 1⅔ CUPS SAUCE

NUTRITIONAL ANALYSIS PER SERVING **334 calories** ▪ **13 percent fat (total fat 4.8 g, saturated fat 1.9 g)** ▪ **59 percent carbohydrate (15 g fiber)** ▪ **28 percent protein.**

Individual Meat Loaves with Fresh Thyme

Meat loaf is a classic comfort food but is often very high in saturated fat and calories. Not this time! Shaped into individual loaves, this dish is lower in fat (by 47 percent), lower in cholesterol (by more than half), and lower in calories (by 25 percent) than traditional meat loaf yet is moist and tender, with a flavor punch from the fresh thyme and other classic ingredients. You can also shape the meat into one large traditional loaf, then use leftovers for sandwiches later in the week. Baking on a cookie sheet allows a crunchy coating to form all the way around the loaves.

MOOD TIP

Saturated fats and trans fats in commercial snack foods and processed vegetable oils, such as margarine or shortening, are not needed by the body, and at amounts greater than 5 to 10 percent of total calories contribute to memory loss, heart disease, and elevated blood cholesterol levels. That's why all the recipes in this cookbook use extra-lean meats, fat-free dairy products, and very little margarine.

cooking spray

1 teaspoon olive oil

1/2 cup onion, diced

1/2 cup red bell pepper, diced

2 cloves garlic, minced

1 pound extra-lean ground beef (7 percent or less fat by weight)

1/4 cup catsup

1 teaspoon Dijon mustard

1 teaspoon Worcestershire sauce

1/3 cup bread crumbs

1/3 cup liquid egg substitute (equivalent to 1 1/2 whole eggs)

1/2 teaspoon salt

1/4 teaspoon freshly ground black pepper

1 tablespoon fresh thyme leaves

1/4 cup fresh parsley, chopped

Preheat oven to 350°. Coat a cookie sheet with cooking spray.

1   In a medium nonstick skillet, warm oil over medium heat. Add onion, red pepper, and garlic and sauté for 4 minutes or until onion is transparent. Remove from heat and cool slightly.

2   In a large mixing bowl, combine all remaining ingredients and add onion mixture. Mix until ingredients are thoroughly combined. Don't overmash meat.

3   Divide loaf mixture into quarters and form into small, oval loaves. Place on sprayed cookie sheet and bake for 25 to 30 minutes or until meat thermometer reads 160°.

4   Remove from oven and let sit for 5 minutes to allow juices to redistribute.

MAKES 4 SERVINGS

NUTRITIONAL ANALYSIS PER SERVING **317 calories** ▪ **45 percent fat (total fat 16 g, saturated fat 5 g)** ▪ **18 percent carbohydrate (1.4 g fiber)** ▪ **37 percent protein.**

C

Shrimp Curry in a Hurry

This delicious dish takes only 15 minutes to prepare (not counting the rice). Use precooked shrimp when in a hurry, or peeled, raw shrimp when you have an extra 5 minutes. Experiment with other additions, such as sliced green onions or chopped apple, or substitute dried cranberries for the raisins.

FOOD TIP

A dollop of chutney—cranberry, mango, apricot, or other fruits—is a delicious complement to chicken, fish, lamb, or veal. Chutney has an intense flavor, so you don't need as much as you would with milder sauces.

2 teaspoons olive oil

2/3 cup onion, chopped

1/2 cup red bell pepper, chopped

1 1/2 tablespoons all-purpose flour

1 rounded tablespoon fresh ginger, peeled and minced

1 tablespoon curry powder

1 pound peeled medium-size shrimp, either precooked or raw

1 1/2 cups fat-free chicken broth

1/3 cup Major Grey chutney

2 rounded tablespoons raisins

salt, to taste

4 cups cooked jasmine rice

2 tablespoons dried coconut

1   Heat oil in a large nonstick skillet. Add onion and red pepper and cook over medium heat for 4 minutes or until onion is transparent.

2   Stir in flour, ginger, and curry. If adding raw shrimp, add them now and cook for 3 minutes, stirring frequently, until shrimp turn pink. If adding cooked shrimp, wait and add shrimp in step 3.

3   Add broth, bring to boil, and cook until sauce thickens, stirring constantly. Add cooked shrimp if you have not already added shrimp in step 2, and the chutney and raisins. Season with salt. Cook over medium heat for another 2 minutes to allow all ingredients to heat through.

4   Serve over jasmine rice and sprinkle with coconut.

MAKES 4 SERVINGS

NUTRITIONAL ANALYSIS PER SERVING **503 calories** ▪ **10 percent fat (total fat 5.8 g, saturated fat 2 g)** ▪ **63 percent carbohydrate (3 g fiber)** ▪ **27 percent protein.**

Classic Chicken Pot Pie

Low in fat, packed with nutrients, and providing all the flavor of the traditional comfort food, this chicken pot pie is a one-dish meal or can be served with a tossed salad. It also makes great leftovers later in the week.

CRUST/TOPPING

1 cup low-fat biscuit mix

¼ cup toasted wheat germ

½ cup plus 3 tablespoons nonfat milk

cooking spray

1 cup celery, diced (approximately 3½ stalks)

½ cup onion, diced

2 cups carrots, peeled and diced (approximately 3 carrots)

2 cloves garlic, minced

3½ cups fat-free chicken broth

1½ pounds skinless, boneless chicken breast

1 medium potato, peeled and diced

5 teaspoons cornstarch

1 cup fat-free half-and-half

1 cup frozen green peas

¼ cup fresh parsley, finely chopped

1 tablespoon fresh thyme leaves

salt and pepper, to taste

Preheat oven to 375°. Spray a 9-by-9-inch baking dish with cooking spray.

1 In a medium bowl, mix biscuit mix and wheat germ. Add milk and blend thoroughly. Set aside.

2 In a large nonstick skillet sprayed with cooking spray, cook celery, onion, carrots, and garlic over medium heat until onion is translucent, approximately 4 minutes.

3 Add 3 cups of the broth and the chicken. Bring to a boil, reduce heat to simmer, and cook uncovered until chicken is barely done, turning chicken once, approximately 8 minutes per side. Remove chicken and set aside.

4 Add potatoes to broth and cook uncovered until tender, approximately 10 minutes.

5 Blend cornstarch with remaining ½ cup chicken broth and half-and-half. Add to chicken broth and potato mixture, bring to a boil, stirring constantly, until mixture thickens. (If mixture is too thick, add 1 to 2 tablespoons of chicken broth.) Remove skillet from stove.

6 Cut chicken into bite-size pieces and add to skillet. Mix in peas, parsley, and thyme. Season with salt and pepper.

7 Pour mixture into baking dish, top evenly with biscuit mixture. Bake until golden brown and juices bubble, approximately 35 minutes.

MAKES 6 GENEROUS SERVINGS

NUTRITIONAL ANALYSIS PER SERVING **318 calories** ▪ **13 percent fat (total fat 4.5 g, saturated fat 1 g)** ▪ **42 percent carbohydrate (4.3 g fiber)** ▪ **45 percent protein.**

C

Grilled Asian Flank Steak with Wasabi Cream Sauce

Marinades add flavor while tenderizing meats. This slightly sweet marinated flank steak, which can be prepared in advance, is paired with the pungent wasabi cream sauce. Fresh Green Beans with Shallots, Red Onion, and Feta Cheese (page 219) or Roasted Beet Salad with Orange Vinaigrette (page 131) are especially good accompaniments to this dish.

FOOD TIP

Wasabi, often called Japanese horseradish, is found in the Asian foods section of the supermarket. Look for the powdered form of wasabi.

MARINADE

⅓ cup soy sauce

juice and zest of 1 orange

2 tablespoons molasses

1 teaspoon fresh ginger, peeled and minced

1 teaspoon minced garlic

1 teaspoon sesame oil

½ teaspoon red pepper flakes

1½ pounds flank steak, trim any surface fat

SAUCE

3 teaspoons wasabi powder mixed with 2 teaspoons water

¼ cup fat-free mayonnaise

¼ cup fat-free sour cream

1   In a medium bowl, whisk together all marinade ingredients, through red pepper flakes.

2   Place steak in a large resealable plastic bag and pour in the marinade. Press air out of bag and seal tightly. Turn the bag to distribute marinade. Place on a plate and refrigerate for at least 1 hour or up to 8 hours. Turn occasionally.

3   In a small bowl, mix together wasabi powder and water. Add mayonnaise and sour cream. Mix well. Cover and refrigerate until ready to use (up to 2 days).

4   Remove steak from plastic bag, discard remaining marinade. Allow steak to stand at room temperature for 20 to 30 minutes prior to grilling.

5   Grill over medium-high heat for 8 to 10 minutes or until internal temperature reaches 145° for medium-rare. Turn once halfway through grilling time. Remove from grill. Allow steak to rest for 5 to 10 minutes.

6   Cut steak across the grain into thin slices. Serve warm on a plate or platter. Pass wasabi cream sauce separately in a small bowl.

MAKES 4 SERVINGS

NUTRITIONAL ANALYSIS PER SERVING 269 calories ▪ 39 percent fat (total fat 11.6 g, saturated fat 5 g) ▪ 12 percent carbohydrate (0 g fiber) ▪ 49 percent protein.

Braised Chicken Parmesan

Chicken braised, then simmered in a savory well-seasoned tomato sauce is a complete meal when served with Creamy Comfort-Food Mashed Potatoes (page 186) and Green Beans and Toasted Slivered Almonds (page 216).

---

4 skinless, boneless chicken breasts (approximately 1 pound total)

½ cup liquid egg substitute (equivalent to 2 whole eggs)

⅓ cup low-fat Parmesan cheese, grated

½ cup bread crumbs

1 tablespoon olive oil

¼ cup shallots, chopped

2 carrots, peeled and chopped

2 cloves garlic, minced

1 (28-ounce) can tomatoes, chopped

2 tablespoons balsamic vinegar

2 tablespoons honey

1 teaspoon each: dried basil, marjoram, and oregano

½ cup low-fat mozzarella cheese, grated

1   Clean and pat dry chicken breasts. Lay chicken breasts between wax paper, flatten to 1 inch thick. (Use a rolling pin or mallet.) Set aside.

2   In a medium bowl, beat egg substitute. Set aside.

3   Mix together Parmesan cheese and bread crumbs. Place on a flat plate.

4   Dip chicken in eggs, then into Parmesan cheese mixture.

5   In a Dutch oven or heavy skillet, warm oil over medium-high heat. Add chicken breasts and cook until brown on each side, about 5 minutes per side. Remove chicken from skillet, keep warm.

6   In same skillet over medium-high heat, add shallots, carrots, and garlic. Cook for 5 minutes, stirring frequently. (Add water or a little chicken broth if vegetables stick.)

7   Add tomatoes, balsamic vinegar, honey, and seasonings. Cook for 10 minutes.

8   Return chicken to pan and cover. Simmer on medium-low heat for 30 minutes or until chicken is no longer pink in center. In the last few minutes of cooking, sprinkle with mozzarella cheese, cover skillet until cheese is melted, then serve hot.

MAKES 4 SERVINGS

NUTRITIONAL ANALYSIS PER SERVING 404 calories ▪ 26 percent fat (total fat 11.7 g, saturated fat 4.4 g) ▪ 33 percent carbohydrate (4.4 g fiber) ▪ 41 percent protein.

C

Southwest Fiesta Casserole with Corn Bread Topping

Sweet corn bread and spicy chipotle peppers pair up in this low-fat casserole, a great dish for Sunday night supper. Serve with a fresh green salad, tossed with fat-free ranch dressing.

cooking spray

1¼ pounds lean ground turkey breast

1 small yellow onion, diced

½ green bell pepper, stemmed, seeded, and diced

2 (14.5-ounce) cans Mexican-style stewed tomatoes, diced

¾ cup water

¼ cup orange juice (or water)

1 (4-ounce) can diced green chilies

1 tablespoon canned chipotle peppers in adobo sauce, minced

2 teaspoons ground cumin

1 teaspoon ground coriander

1 (14.5-ounce) can cut green beans, drained

1 (15.25-ounce) can yellow corn, drained

¼ cup fresh cilantro, minced

1 teaspoon Splenda

salt and pepper, to taste

1 box (14.5-ounce) fat-free corn bread mix

Heat oven to 350°. Spray a 3- to 4-quart casserole with cooking spray. Set aside.

1   In a large nonstick skillet or Dutch oven, place turkey, onion, and bell pepper. Sauté over medium-high heat for about 12 minutes, stirring frequently to break up turkey into small pieces. Drain any fat.

2   Add tomatoes, water, orange juice, chilies, chipotle peppers, cumin, and coriander. Cover and simmer for 20 minutes, stirring occasionally.

3   Add green beans, corn, cilantro, and Splenda. Stir to mix. Season with salt and bell pepper. Bring all ingredients to a gentle boil for 5 minutes. Pour into prepared casserole dish.

4   Prepare corn bread according to directions on package. Spread over meat mixture. Bake uncovered for 30 to 40 minutes or until corn bread is golden brown and cooked through. Serve hot.

MAKES 8 SERVINGS

NUTRITIONAL ANALYSIS PER SERVING **389 calories** ▪ **18 percent fat (total fat 7.8 g, saturated fat 1.9 g)** ▪ **58 percent carbohydrate (7.6 g fiber)** ▪ **24 percent protein.**

C

Baked Pork Florentine with Wild Rice

To make this a great-tasting low-fat vegetarian casserole, simply omit the pork and double the amount of chopped spinach.

MOOD TIP

Even though the pork is lean and this recipe has little added fat, the total percentage of fat calories and grams is high, as is the saturated fat. To keep this recipe within the Feeling Good Diet guidelines, keep the portion small and serve with lots of vegetables.

2 teaspoons olive oil

2 pounds boneless pork loin chops, trimmed

1 small yellow onion, diced

2 stalks celery, diced

2 carrots, peeled and diced

1 (10.75-ounce) can cream of mushroom soup (98 percent fat-free, low sodium)

½ cup fat-free chicken broth

1 cup fat-free half-and-half

⅓ cup cooking sherry

zest and juice of 1 small orange

1 teaspoon each of dried thyme, marjoram, and sage

cooking spray

1 (6-ounce) box long-grain wild rice mix

2 cups fresh spinach, chopped

¼ cup low-fat Parmesan cheese, grated

Preheat oven to 350°.

1   In a large skillet or Dutch oven, warm oil over medium-high heat. Add pork loin chops, brown on both sides (about 2 minutes per side). Remove from heat. Set pork aside.

2   In same skillet, add onion, celery, and carrots. Sauté until soft, about 5 to 7 minutes. (Add water or chicken broth if vegetables start to stick.) Set aside.

3   In a medium bowl, mix thoroughly cream of mushroom soup, chicken broth, half-and-half, sherry, orange zest and juice, and spices. Set aside.

4   Spray a 3- to 4-quart casserole pan with cooking spray. Add contents of wild rice mix (both rice and seasoning packet). Spread to cover bottom of casserole dish. Spoon sautéed vegetables over rice mixture. Pour half of soup mixture evenly over rice-vegetable mix. Cut each pork loin in half. Place pieces on top of soup mixture. Add remaining soup mixture to cover pork. Top with chopped spinach. Gently press spinach into soup mixture. Sprinkle with Parmesan cheese. Cover casserole and bake for 45 minutes (or until rice is tender).

5   Remove from oven. Let rest for 10 minutes to allow rice to completely soak up remaining juices, then serve.

MAKES 8 SERVINGS

NUTRITIONAL ANALYSIS PER SERVING **372 calories** ▪ **35 percent fat (total fat 14 g, saturated fat 4.1 g)** ▪ **31 percent carbohydrate (2 g fiber)** ▪ **34 percent protein.**

Fish Fajitas with Creamy Chipotle Coleslaw

The sliced mangos add a tropical twist to complement the warmth of the chipotle peppers. This is a great Friday night dinner!

4 (6-ounce) skinless, boneless fish fillets, about 1 inch thick (halibut, sea bass, cod, or red snapper)

2 tablespoons fresh lime juice

2 tablespoons fresh lemon juice

1 teaspoon Creole seasoning

1 tablespoon olive oil

COLESLAW

4 cups coleslaw mix

½ cup fat-free sour cream

¼ cup light mayonnaise

1 tablespoon canned chipotle peppers, minced in adobo sauce

2 teaspoons fresh lemon juice

¼ cup fresh cilantro, chopped

cooking spray

8 (10-inch) whole wheat tortillas, warmed

1 mango, peeled, pitted, and thinly sliced

1 Rinse, pat dry fish fillets. Set aside.

2 In a small bowl, whisk together lime juice, lemon juice, Creole seasoning, and oil. Spoon marinade on fish fillets to coat. Cover and place in refrigerator until ready to grill (up to 1 hour).

3 In a medium bowl, add coleslaw mix. Set aside.

4 In a small bowl, whisk together sour cream, mayonnaise, chipotle peppers, lemon juice, and cilantro. Pour over coleslaw mix. Toss well to combine. Cover and refrigerate until ready to use (up to 1 hour).

5 Spray grill with cooking spray. Heat grill to medium-high. Remove fish fillets from marinade. Place on grill. Cover lid and cook 3 minutes on each side or until no longer opaque in center. Remove from grill. Separate fish into 2-inch chunks with a fork. Cover to keep warm.

6 To assemble: Set up buffet style. Let everyone make their own fajitas. Place grilled fish on a plate, next to warm tortillas, coleslaw, and sliced mango. Spoon several pieces of grilled fish on bottom end of tortillas, cover with coleslaw, add mango slices. Fold over, roll up, and eat.

MAKES 8 FAJITAS

NUTRITIONAL ANALYSIS PER FAJITA **235 calories** ▪ **20 percent fat (total fat 5.2 g, saturated fat < 1 g)** ▪ **45 percent carbohydrate (3 g fiber)** ▪ **35 percent protein.**

Tandoori Chicken Made Simple

The Asian section of your supermarket is where you'll find great-tasting authentic Tandoori mixes. Not only is this recipe a snap, it has been tested against Jeanette's famous (well, at least locally) homemade Tandoori yogurt marinade. The Tandoori mix packed more authentic Indian flavor and took less time to prepare! Serve with Glazed Carrots (page 215) and Sunshine Rice with Basil and Parmesan (page 179) or wild rice.

½ cup Tandoori mix for chicken (comes in a 9.5-ounce jar)

¾ cup plain, nonfat yogurt

4 tablespoons fresh lemon juice

1 tablespoon fresh ginger, peeled and minced

4 skinless, boneless chicken breasts (approximately 4 ounces each)

lemon slices

1   In a large bowl, combine Tandoori mix, yogurt, lemon juice, and ginger.

2   Pierce chicken breasts several times each with a fork. Add chicken to marinade. Toss to coat well.

3   Place chicken and marinade in a large Ziploc plastic bag. Squeeze out any air. Turn to distribute marinade and place on a plate. Chill in the refrigerator for up to 24 hours.

4   Remove chicken from refrigerator 20 minutes before baking to allow meat to reach room temperature.

5   Preheat oven to 375°. Spread chicken on a large, flat baking sheet. Bake uncovered for 45 minutes or until chicken is no longer pink. Garnish with lemon slices.

MAKES 4 SERVINGS

NUTRITIONAL ANALYSIS PER SERVING **187 calories** ▪ **9 percent fat (total fat 1.9 g, saturated fat < 0.5 g)** ▪ **24 percent carbohydrate (1.5 g fiber)** ▪ **67 percent protein.**

Q

C —COMFORT FOOD

Q —QUICK FIX FOOD

A —ADVENTUROUS

S —SPECIAL OCCASION

Pasta, Rice, and Potato Dishes

Carbs for PMS, SAD, and Depression

WHAT DO A weepy young woman, a cranky old man at Thanksgiving, an insomniac, and someone who can't stop raiding the cookie jar have in common? They all might be suffering from low levels of a chemical called serotonin.

Serotonin turns on and off our cravings for carbohydrate-rich sweets and starches, helps regulate mood, and even determines whether we sleep well. Choose quality carbohydrates like those in this section, and you work in tune with serotonin to help sidestep many of the problems associated with premenstrual syndrome (PMS), seasonal affective disorder (SAD), and depression. Work against serotonin by snacking on sweets or skipping meals, and you only make matters worse.

Nerve Chemicals, Mood, and Cravings

What you eat and how you feel are determined by the nervous system, beginning with its tiniest functioning unit: the nerve cell. These cells "talk" to each other and to surrounding tissues by way of nerve chemicals called neurotransmitters. At least 70 neurotransmitters regulate nerve function, including memory, appetite and cravings, mental function, mood, and the wake-sleep cycle. What you eat has a direct and indirect effect on many of these neurotransmitters.

The interplay of serotonin levels and food choices, for example, is the classic chicken-and-egg scenario. The level of this neurotransmitter is dependent on what you eat, while what you choose to eat, in part, is dictated by the level of serotonin. This chemical is manufactured in the brain from a dietary amino acid called tryptophan, with the help of vitamins B_6, B_{12}, and folic acid. The omega-3 fats might also be involved in this process. When serotonin levels are low, you crave carbohydrates, such as sweets and starches, which are the very foods that raise levels of both tryptophan and serotonin and turn off the cravings. In short, cravers unconsciously turn to desserts, doughnuts, and other pastries, or pasta, cereals, and breads to relieve dwindling energy levels, grumpiness, and depression brought on by low serotonin levels. The snack works—it raises serotonin levels, curbs cravings, and boosts the craver's mood. Once serotonin levels are high, your sweet tooth subsides.

When a Craving Goes Bad

At one time or another, most of us have turned to food for solace, comfort, or relaxation. In most cases, the indulgence is harmless and comforting. However, some people, in an effort to soothe a bad mood, unknowingly choose foods that make them feel worse and set up a vicious cycle of feeling bad and overeating.

If you use food to treat depression, PMS, or SAD, you'd better choose the right stuff. Judith Wurtman, Ph.D., at Massachusetts Institute of Technology and an expert on the serotonin-mood link, acknowledges that "women with [PMS], those with seasonal weight gain, and individuals going through smoking withdrawal may need frequent 'doses' of carbohydrate." However, routinely turning to a highly processed sweet or salty carbohydrate, such as cookies or chips, is only a temporary mood fix that is likely to cause weight problems. Eating a sugar-rich diet leads to nutrient shortages that keep you from feeling your best. In short, depending on processed and junk food doesn't work over the long term and, in fact, aggravates the problem. On the other hand, choosing the right carbs will always help you feel better and, in some cases, might be the answer to depression, PMS, and SAD.

The Common Thread in PMS, SAD, and Depression

PMS is the moodiness, anxiety, depression, food cravings, weight gain, and bloated feelings many women experience in the 7 to 10 days before their periods. People with SAD—a more severe case of the winter blues—dread the autumn and winter, when they feel crabby and battle out-of-control appetites, weight gain, lethargy, and an insatiable need to sleep. General depression also typically leads to food cravings, weight gain, and sleep problems.

People who suffer from PMS, SAD, or depression have a lot in common, and much of it is linked to serotonin.

- All three conditions are associated with food cravings, especially for carbohydrates. For example, people who are depressed or battle SAD, as well as women during the premenstrual phase, are most likely to turn to chocolate and other sweets, with sugar intake increasing by up to 20 teaspoons daily above normal intake.

- Serotonin levels are low in all three conditions, so people understandably experience cravings for foods that help elevate levels of this appetite-control chemical.

  1. The link between serotonin and depression is so strong that many of the antidepressant medications, such as Prozac, are effective because they increase the activity of this chemical.

  2. During the winter months, serotonin levels are low and levels of melatonin (a derivative of serotonin) are high, especially in people who suffer from SAD.

  3. The most frequently reported symptoms of PMS, including cravings for carbohydrate-rich foods, sleep disturbances, and moodiness, coincide with dwindling serotonin levels, according to researchers at Massachusetts Institute of Technology. Snacking on carbohydrate-rich foods provides some relief from depression, tension, anger, confusion, sadness, and fatigue, leaving women feeling more alert and calm. The researchers state that premenstrual women overeat carbohydrates in an attempt to raise serotonin levels and improve their bad moods.

While working with serotonin by eating high-quality carbohydrate-rich foods can help solve these problems, using sugar to feel better is a temporary fix. The bad feelings always return, leaving only one option: to reach, once again, for another sugar fix. This creates a vicious cycle and magnifies PMS or SAD symptoms. The secret is to use the right kind of quality carbs to raise serotonin levels, without causing a spike in blood sugar levels, and get your mood back on track.

The Carb Solution

You get the same mood boost from quality carbohydrates, such as many of the whole grain, pasta, sweet potato, and other starchy vegetable dishes in this section, as you do from sugar, but the effect is sustained. With quality carbs, you are less likely to gain weight, more likely to consume all the nutrients needed to improve mood, and you will avoid the blood sugar roller coaster associated with sweets. For example, PMS sufferers report they are less tense, angry, confused, and tired after they eat a bowl of cereal than when they snack on a candy bar. They also feel more alert.

When it comes to grains, whole grains are the best, because they also help you manage weight, keep blood sugar at moderate levels, and lower the risk for heart disease, diabetes, hypertension, and possibly cancer. Unprocessed refined grains, such as egg noodles, jasmine rice, or pearl barley, are in-between choices, since they are better than sweetened grains in doughnuts or desserts and much better than sugar, but not as healthful as whole grains. Because not everyone is hooked on whole grains, you'll find recipes for both whole grain and some processed grains in this section. All are low in calories and saturated fat.

To boost your mood without jeopardizing your waistline and your health, limit sugar to no more than 10 percent of calories (that means about 10 teaspoons for someone on a 2,000-calorie diet). People battling depression who eliminate sugar (or caffeine) from their diets often feel much better within a few weeks. "Compared to the temporary high people get from sugar, eliminating sugar and/or caffeine from the diet is a permanent solution to depression for some people," says Larry Christensen, Ph.D., the chairman of the department of psychology at the University of South Alabama and an expert on sugar and depression.

The recipes in the "Desserts" section of this book are low in sugar but should still be consumed in moderation. Limit soda to one or two servings per week (8 to 10 teaspoons of sugar in one can), candy to an occasional treat (another 5 to 8 teaspoons per candy bar), and cookies to a few small ones each week. Read labels, since sugar is added to most processed foods, from baked beans to fruited yogurt. (Hint: 4 grams = 1 teaspoon of sugar.)

12 QUICK-FIX CARB DISHES

1. **COUSCOUS:** To 4 cups of cooked couscous, add (1) 1 cup green peas and 1 tablespoon chopped fresh tarragon, (2) ¼ cup grated low-fat Parmesan and 1 tablespoon chopped fresh basil or oregano, or (3) ⅔ cup diced green onions and 4 tablespoons chopped pecans.

2. **DILLED CORN:** Coat ears of corn-on-the-cob with butter-flavored cooking spray, sprinkle with chopped fresh dill and salt. Wrap in tinfoil and bake at 325° until done, approximately 20 minutes.

3. **ASIAN-STYLE NOODLES:** Cook Japanese noodles according to package directions. Drain and combine with $2/3$ cup diced green onions, 3 tablespoons soy sauce, and 1 teaspoon dark sesame oil.

4. **CITRUS RICE:** Prepare rice according to package directions. Remove from heat and toss with ground ginger and grated orange rind.

5. **CURRIED RICE:** Prepare rice according to package directions. Remove from heat and toss with curry powder, salt, chopped green onions, and thawed green peas.

6. **HERBED RICE:** Cook instant brown rice according to package directions, using chicken broth instead of water and adding fresh or dried herbs, such as rosemary, thyme, garlic powder, and marjoram.

7. **HERBED BAKED POTATO:** Slice a baker in half, lay fresh herbs or bay leaves, salt, and pepper in middle, then tie baker together with string. Microwave until tender, approximately 10 to 13 minutes on high. Remove herbs before eating.

8. **TOMATO 'N' HERB PASTA:** Mix 2 chopped tomatoes, 1 tablespoon fresh chopped basil, 1 minced garlic, and salt and pepper in a small bowl. Set aside for 1 hour for flavors to blend. Cook 6 ounces of pasta according to package directions, drain, and add tomato mixture.

9. **LINGUINE AND PESTO:** Cook 12 ounces of linguine according to package directions. Mix with 4 tablespoons pesto sauce and sprinkle with low-fat Parmesan cheese. Serve with a steamed vegetable and tossed salad.

10. **FETTUCCINE ALFREDO:** Cook 9 ounces of fettuccine according to package directions. Heat cooked pasta with $3/4$ cup fat-free half-and-half, 1 tablespoon butter, and $1/4$ teaspoon ground nutmeg until a creamy consistency forms, approximately 3 to 5 minutes. Sprinkle with $1/2$ cup low-fat Parmesan cheese and freshly ground pepper. Serve with a tossed salad and steamed vegetables.

11. **PLENTY OF POLENTA:** Simmer 4 cups chicken broth with 1 cup cornmeal polenta for 10 minutes, stir in $1/2$ cup chopped roasted red peppers and 1 tablespoon fresh thyme leaves. Use as a bed for any meat dish that has gravy or sauce, such as Chicken 'n' Mushrooms in Sherry Cream Gravy (page 156) or Chicken with Mushrooms in Creamy Garlic-Pecan Sauce (page 151).

12. **OVEN-FRIED POTATO WEDGES:** Rub potato wedges with paprika, ground black pepper, salt, and garlic powder. Spray potato wedges and cookie sheet with cooking spray and bake at 450° for 15 minutes or until golden brown and crisp.

To satisfy a craving and raise serotonin levels turn to minimally processed, wholesome carbohydrates, such as the grain and starchy vegetable dishes in this section. Or snack on a whole grain English muffin drizzled with honey or a toasted cinnamon bagel with jam, and you'll get the same serotonin boost that you'd get with candy but without the drop in blood sugar. Also, be patient. You can't expect pasta to work like Prozac, at least not immediately. It will take two to three weeks of eating well before you notice an improvement in your mood and cravings. In addition, the following tips should prove helpful.

- *Work with a craving.* Make sure every meal contains reasonable portions of carbohydrate-rich foods, such as the Baked Apple–Cinnamon Pancake (page 13) or the Ginger-Pumpkin Muffins (page 14) for breakfast, the Black Bean Burritos (page 64) for lunch, and any of the recipes in this section as an accompaniment to dinner. Plan a complex carbohydrate–rich snack during that time of the day when you are most vulnerable to snack attacks. (See the "Appetizers" section for ideas.)

- *Identify your craving.* Is it for something crunchy or chewy? Cold, sweet, or creamy? Once you pinpoint exactly what you want, find a low-calorie food that satisfies that craving. Luckily, the better you eat, the more likely your cravings for fatty or overly sweet foods will dwindle.

- *Eat breakfast.* I don't care if you're not hungry, eat something nutritious anyway. Breakfast replenishes dwindling energy reserves and fuels the body during the first half of the day. The protein and carbohydrates in a morning meal also help regulate the nerve chemicals and hormones that help curb the symptoms of PMS, SAD, and depression.

- *Make changes gradually.* Any dramatic change in normal eating patterns can alter brain chemistry. Binge on sweets, skip meals, or eat erratically, and you tinker with your neurotransmitter levels and mood. You can ward off a chocolate chip cookie binge by consuming several small meals or snacks throughout the day, which maintains steady blood sugar and neurotransmitter levels.

- *Exercise.* Daily movement, especially aerobic activity, such as walking, jogging, swimming, or bicycling, helps regulate blood sugar levels and other nerve chemicals, and provides an energy boost without the calories. This is not an option—you *must* exercise if you want to control or even prevent symptoms of PMS, SAD, and depression.

- *Try light therapy.* Lights that provide the full spectrum of ultraviolet rays have worked wonders for many SAD sufferers!

Habit, Not Chemistry

Sometimes we simply eat out of habit, not because our body's chemistry is dictating our mood. If a midafternoon sweet snack tastes good, you are likely to have it again. Repeating the snack over and over, day after day, results in a habit or even a craving. In these cases, you can take charge by substituting a more nutritious snack, replace the midmorning doughnut with a whole wheat bagel or exchange the afternoon candy bar with an almond stuffed into a date. Or develop a new habit to replace the old one, such as taking a walk at the time of day when cravings are most intense or riding an exercise bicycle instead of snacking while watching television.

Some people suffer from serious PMS, SAD, or clinical depression. In all cases, eating well helps these situations, but it may not be the sole answer. Always discuss your health concerns with a physician, especially if they persist after making healthy changes in your life, exercise schedule, and diet.

Low-Fat Potato Latkes

This low-fat version of latkes uses an egg substitute and bakes the pancakes. They taste great and are almost fat- and cholesterol-free.

FOOD TIP
Potato pancakes, or latkes, are a traditional food served at Hanukkah. They typically are fried in oil or other fats.

cooking spray

9 cups (about 1½ pounds) frozen, shredded hash browns, thawed

1¼ cups onions, diced

3 tablespoons matzo meal

½ teaspoon salt or salt substitute (omit if hash browns are salted)

½ teaspoon freshly ground pepper

½ cup fat-free egg substitute

1 teaspoon dill weed

Heat oven to 425°. Spray 2 nonstick cookie sheets with cooking spray.

1   Place remaining ingredients (everything except cooking spray) in a large bowl and blend well.

2   Form mixture into small pancakes about 3 to 4 inches wide (approximately ⅓ cup each) and place on cookie sheets. Spray top of pancakes with more cooking spray.

3   Bake pancakes for 10 minutes, flip with a spatula, bake for another 10 minutes or until golden brown.

4   Spray with a light coating of cooking spray and top with fat-free sour cream, apple-sauce, or topping of your choice.

MAKES 16 PANCAKES

NUTRITIONAL ANALYSIS PER PANCAKE **52 calories** ▪ **10 percent fat (total fat < 1 g, saturated fat 0 g)** ▪ **74 percent carbohydrate (< 0.5 g fiber)** ▪ **16 percent protein.**

C

Sunshine Rice with Basil and Parmesan

This light side dish is fresh and flavorful without being overpowering. Serve with Grilled Halibut with Ginger-Mango Chutney (page 149) or Crusty Cranberry Salmon (page 155).

(page 149) ... (page 155)

FOOD TIP

Citrus juice and zest give lots of recipes an added boost. For example:

- *use lemon or lime juice to liven up a soup or stew*
- *squeeze lemon juice on roasted or grilled vegetables*
- *enhance salad dressing with a little lemon or lime zest*
- *accompany any Mexican or southwest dish with a side of lemon wedges*
- *add a little zing to fruit salads and desserts with lime or lemon juice or zest.*

2 quarts water

1 cup arborio rice

½ cup yellow onion, chopped

½ cup fresh parsley, finely chopped

1 tablespoon butter

2 tablespoons fresh basil, finely chopped

1 tablespoon fresh lemon juice

1 teaspoon grated lemon peel

1 teaspoon salt

¼ cup low-fat Parmesan cheese, grated

fresh basil sprigs or lemon slices

1   Bring water to a boil in medium saucepan. Add rice and onion and continue to boil until rice is tender, approximately 20 minutes. Drain.

2   Mix parsley, butter, basil, lemon juice, lemon peel, and salt in a medium bowl. Add rice mixture and stir until thoroughly mixed and butter has melted. Add Parmesan and toss. Garnish with basil sprigs or lemon slices.

MAKES 6 SERVINGS OF ½ CUP EACH

NUTRITIONAL ANALYSIS PER SERVING **157 calories** ▪ **19 percent fat (total fat 3.3 g, saturated fat 1.3 g)** ▪ **73 percent carbohydrate (0.8 g fiber)** ▪ **8 percent protein.**

Grandma's Homemade Chicken 'n' Noodles

Dad made this dish when I was a kid, but it's really my grandmother's recipe. She made it for the family in the early 1900s when they lived on a dairy farm west of Portland, Oregon. My sister Gayle taught me how to make it. You can cut back on the cholesterol (each serving has 119 milligrams of cholesterol) by using egg substitute instead of whole eggs, but the noodles will be a bit chewier. If you want to double or triple the batch of noodles, add one extra egg to the entire batch. Serve with steamed vegetables, such as green beans or peas and carrots, and a salad, and you have an all-American comfort meal.

FOOD TIP

The biggest mistake people make when preparing homemade noodles is not sprinkling enough flour over the dough as they are rolling out and cutting the noodles. Err on the side of excess, and you'll do fine.

1¼ cups all-purpose flour, plus a sprinkle can filled with flour (I use an old jam jar with nail holes punched in the top)

pinch of salt

2 jumbo whole eggs (or 3 medium eggs) (or ½ cup egg substitute), beaten

9 cups fat-free chicken broth

2 pounds chicken breast, skinned, defatted, and deboned

1 tablespoon "Better Than Bouillon" Chicken Base (optional)

1   In a large bowl, blend flour and salt. Make a well in the middle and add beaten eggs. With a fork blend flour-egg mixture until it is thoroughly mixed. Dough should hold together but be slightly moist.

2   Sprinkle flour heavily over a working surface, divide flour-egg dough in half, form into a ball, and place on floured surface. With a rolling pin and generous sprinklings of flour, roll dough until it is ¼ inch thick. Frequently sprinkle more flour over and under the dough as you are rolling.

3   When dough is the desired thickness, sprinkle more flour over entire surface. Starting at one end, flip about 1 inch of dough over and sprinkle with flour. Roll the dough over again and sprinkle more. Repeat until entire dough is rolled into a 1-inch-wide roll. Sprinkle with more flour. Cut roll into ½-inch slices with a steady chop of the knife. Don't saw the noodles off the roll. Unroll each slice to make a long noodle and place in the bowl. Sprinkle with more flour and toss lightly to completely cover noodles with flour. Repeat the above process with second half of dough. Don't overtoss, since this will compact noodles, leaving them thicker and more starchy. Cover bowl with

a damp towel and place in refrigerator for 1 hour or more. (You can leave it there overnight and finish making the dish the next day.)

4   While noodles are chilling, place chicken broth in large saucepan. Bring broth to a boil and add chicken breasts. Cook until breasts are cooked through, about 30 minutes. (Time will vary depending on thickness of breasts.) Remove breasts and add bouillon. Bring liquid to a boil and add noodles, being careful to gently pull them apart so they don't clump. Return to a boil and reduce heat to simmer.

5   While noodles are cooking, tear chicken apart into small, bite-size pieces. Add to noodles, cover, and cook until noodles are done, about 45 minutes.

MAKES 10 CUPS

NUTRITIONAL ANALYSIS PER CUP **217 calories** ▪ **15 percent fat (total fat 3.6 g, saturated fat 1 g)** ▪ **30 percent carbohydrate (0.5 g fiber)** ▪ **55 percent protein.**

C

Creamy Mashed Potatoes, Parsnips, and Carrots

With the same comfort-food texture as mashed potatoes, this dish is sweeter and more colorful. It's a great accompaniment to pork or roast chicken. A serving provides almost three times your daily minimum requirement for beta-carotene and hefty amounts of vitamin C, manganese, and potassium.

FOOD TIP

Any mashed potato dish is creamier if you warm the additions, such as milk or half-and-half, before adding. Butter should be soft, but not liquid, when added.

2 cups yellow potatoes, peeled and chopped (about 3 medium potatoes)

4 parsnips, peeled and chopped (about 3½ cups)

4 carrots, peeled and chopped (about 3½ cups)

2 tablespoons butter, at room temperature

¾ cup low-fat (1 percent) milk

½ cup fat-free half-and-half

1 teaspoon salt

½ teaspoon ground black pepper

dash of cayenne pepper

2 tablespoons fresh parsley, finely chopped

1   Place potatoes, parsnips, and carrots in a steamer over medium-high heat and steam until very tender, approximately 25 minutes.

2   Transfer vegetables to a large bowl. Whip potato mixture with an electric mixer, then slowly add butter, milk, and half-and-half, salt, pepper, and cayenne and whip with an electric mixer until smooth and creamy. Add parsley and continue to whip until thoroughly blended.

MAKES 6 SERVINGS OF 1 CUP EACH

NUTRITIONAL ANALYSIS PER CUP **205 calories** ▪ **20 percent fat (total fat 4.5 g, saturated fat 2.7 g)** ▪ **71 percent carbohydrate (7.3 g fiber)** ▪ **9 percent protein.**

Southwest Corn-Potato Cakes

This flavorful alternative to regular potato pancakes goes well with salsa and fat-free sour cream as a side to any Mexican dish or as a lunch or snack accompanied by a tossed salad. My kids love these cakes as leftovers, topped with grated low-fat cheese and heated for one minute in the microwave.

4 quarts water

5 cups russet potatoes, peeled and cubed

1 (16-ounce) package frozen corn

½ cup sharp cheddar cheese, grated

½ cup fat-free cottage cheese

¾ cup egg substitute (equivalent to 3 large eggs)

½ cup green onion, minced (white and green portions)

3 tablespoons red bell pepper, minced

½ cup firmly packed fresh cilantro, chopped

2 tablespoons canned diced green chilies

3 tablespoons yellow cornmeal

2 teaspoons ground cumin

1 teaspoon salt

½ teaspoon ground black pepper

cooking spray

1   In a large saucepan, bring water to a boil over high heat. Add potatoes, return to a boil, reduce heat, and simmer until tender, approximately 20 minutes. Drain and mash until smooth.

2   While potatoes are cooking, mix well all other ingredients (except cooking spray) in a large bowl. Add mashed potatoes and blend well.

3   In a nonstick skillet or griddle sprayed with cooking spray over medium heat, place ⅓ cup of potato-corn mixture. Pat down to form a 3-inch patty and cook until golden brown. Flip and cook other side until golden brown, approximately 6 minutes per side. Place in a warming oven while cooking remaining cakes. (Batter keeps in refrigerator for 2 days.)

MAKES APPROXIMATELY 20 CAKES

NUTRITIONAL ANALYSIS PER CAKE **86 calories** ▪ **16 percent fat (total fat 1.5 g, saturated fat ‹ 1 g)** ▪ **66 percent carbohydrate (2 g fiber)** ▪ **18 percent protein.**

Thai Fettuccine with Chicken

Serve this pasta dish hot or warm for dinner with steamed broccoli or Chinese pea pods or for lunch with a tossed salad. Replace chicken with jumbo shrimp for another great combo. This dish is especially rich in vitamin C, B vitamins, trace minerals, and the antioxidant selenium.

FOOD TIP

Red peppers are especially rich in vitamin C and other antioxidants. They can be added raw to salads or cooked in soups, stews, and stir-fries. Peppers are also good roasted and marinated, or they can be stuffed and baked or microwaved.

8 ounces fettuccine

cooking spray

1 pound skinless, boneless chicken breasts

1 teaspoon sesame oil

3 cloves garlic, minced

4 teaspoons fresh ginger, peeled and minced

2 cups red bell pepper, stemmed, seeded, and sliced into thin strips

⅔ cup fat-free chicken broth

⅓ cup peanut butter

⅓ cup hoisin sauce

½ teaspoon salt

1 tablespoon rice wine vinegar

1 teaspoon chili-garlic sauce

⅔ cup green onion, thinly sliced

⅔ cup fresh cilantro, chopped

1   Cook pasta according to directions on package, omitting fat. Drain.

2   Spray a medium nonstick frying pan with cooking spray and place over medium heat. Sauté chicken breasts until cooked through, approximately 10 minutes on each side depending on thickness of breasts. Remove from pan and set aside to cool. Cut into ½-inch cubes.

3   In pan used for chicken, add oil, garlic, and ginger and sauté over medium heat for 3 minutes, stirring frequently. Add red pepper and cook an additional 2 minutes. Add chicken broth, peanut butter, hoisin sauce, salt, vinegar, and chili-garlic sauce. Blend well over medium heat for 3 minutes.

4   In a large serving bowl, toss hot pasta, chicken, and sauce to coat. Sprinkle with onion and cilantro and toss gently.

MAKES 8 CUPS

NUTRITIONAL ANALYSIS PER CUP **258 calories** ▪ **26 percent fat (total fat 7.4 g, saturated fat 1 g)** ▪ **43 percent carbohydrate (3.4 g fiber)** ▪ **31 percent protein.**

Spicy Couscous and Chickpeas

A simple side dish that blends the delicate flavor and texture of couscous with a slight hint of pizzazz from the chili sauce. A great accompaniment to any chicken dish.

FOOD TIP
Chickpeas were first domesticated in the Middle East but are now harvested primarily in India. Also called garbanzo beans and when mashed called hummus, this legume is especially rich in magnesium and fiber.

¼ cup slivered almonds

2 cups fat-free chicken broth

1 box (approximately 2 cups) plain couscous

2 teaspoons olive oil

1 cup red bell pepper, stemmed, seeded, and diced

1 (14-ounce) can chickpeas (approximately 1½ cups)

3 teaspoons commercial chili-garlic sauce

salt, to taste

2 teaspoons fresh parsley, chopped

Heat oven to 325°.

1 Toast almonds until golden brown, about 12 minutes.

2 In medium pan, bring broth to a boil, pour in couscous, stir to wet, turn off heat, and set aside 5 minutes.

3 While couscous is cooking, in small sauté pan, heat olive oil and sauté red pepper until slightly soft, 5 minutes.

4 Add red pepper, almonds, chickpeas, and chili-garlic sauce to couscous. Salt if desired. Toss gently with fork. Sprinkle with parsley and serve.

MAKES 0 SERVINGS

NUTRITIONAL ANALYSIS PER SERVING **213 calories** ▪ **18 percent fat (total fat 4.3 g, saturated fat ‹ 0.5 g)** ▪ **67 percent carbohydrate (5.7 g fiber)** ▪ **15 percent protein.**

Creamy Comfort-Food Mashed Potatoes

Simple but mouthwatering, these potatoes are low in fat and full of flavor. (Traditional mashed potatoes contain more than three times the fat and have 42 percent more calories!) Serve with any fish, chicken, or meat dish. The potatoes are especially good with Chicken 'n' Mushrooms in Sherry Cream Gravy (page 156).

2½ **pounds Yukon Gold or any medium-starch potato, peeled and cut into large pieces**

2 **teaspoons salt**

1 **cup fat-free half-and-half**

2 **tablespoons butter**

salt and pepper, to taste

1   Place potatoes in large pot, cover with cold water, and add salt. Bring water to a gentle boil and cook potatoes until they are very soft and fall apart, approximately 30 minutes.

2   Drain potatoes well, return to pot, and mash with electric mixer or potato masher, adding half-and-half and butter a little at a time. Make potatoes as lumpy or creamy as you want, but don't overwhip, since this can make them too sticky. Season with salt and pepper.

MAKES 6 SERVINGS

NUTRITIONAL ANALYSIS PER SERVING **223 calories** ▪ 16 percent fat (total fat 4 g, saturated fat 2 g) ▪ 75 percent carbohydrate (2.8 g fiber) ▪ 9 percent protein.

Fluffy Mashed Potatoes with Horseradish

To minimize calories and fat, replace some or all of the fat with the following: low-fat buttermilk, fat-free half-and-half, chicken broth, fat-free sour cream, and fat-free cream cheese. The horseradish gives this traditional side dish a spark of flavor, making it an excellent side for Grilled Pork Tenderloin with Rosemary-Orange Sauce (page 158), Herb-Roasted Chicken (page 152), or any other meat dish.

FOOD TIP
Yukon Golds make the creamiest mashed potatoes, but brown russets are preferred for fluffiness.

2½ pounds russet potatoes, peeled (leaving some skin on) and cubed

⅓ cup fat-free chicken broth

⅓ cup low-fat buttermilk

⅓ cup fat-free sour cream

1 tablespoon butter

2 tablespoons prepared creamy horseradish

¾ teaspoon salt

½ teaspoon freshly ground black pepper

1   Place potatoes in large pot of cold water, bring to a boil, reduce heat, and simmer until tender, about 15 to 20 minutes. Drain and return potatoes to pan.

2   Add all remaining ingredients. Mash to desired consistency. Add more chicken broth or buttermilk if too thick.

MAKES 8 SERVINGS OF APPROXIMATELY ⅔ CUP EACH

NUTRITIONAL ANALYSIS PER SERVING **158 calories** ▪ **10 percent fat (total fat 1.7 g, saturated fat 1 g)** ▪ **80 percent carbohydrate (2 g fiber)** ▪ **10 percent protein.**

South-of-the-Border Rice

This rice is just spicy enough to make it interesting—and a great side to Chilies Rellenos Casserole with Red Sauce (page 160), tacos, or burritos—but mild enough that even your kids will like it. Use it in Mexican wraps by adding black beans and extra cilantro and rolling into a tortilla. It's easy to prepare, too.

---

1 teaspoon olive oil

1 medium onion, chopped fine (approximately 1½ cups)

4 cloves garlic, minced

1½ cups fat-free chicken broth

1 (10-ounce) can diced tomatoes with green chilies (undrained)

1 cup uncooked long-grain brown rice

⅓ cup fresh cilantro, chopped

1   Heat oil in a 10-inch nonstick skillet. Add onion and garlic and sauté over medium heat until transparent, approximately 4 minutes.

2   Add broth and tomatoes, stir, and bring to a boil. Add rice and return to a boil, cover, reduce heat, and simmer until rice is tender, approximately 45 minutes.

3   Just before serving, fluff rice with a fork to mix well. Top with cilantro.

MAKES 6 SERVINGS OF APPROXIMATELY ½ CUP EACH

NUTRITIONAL ANALYSIS PER SERVING **121 calories** ▪ **12 percent fat (total fat 1.6 g, saturated fat ‹ 0.5 g)** ▪ **76 percent carbohydrate (2 g fiber)** ▪ **12 percent protein.**

Spicy Linguine with Red Clam Sauce

Serve this pasta dish with a crisp salad of assorted greens tossed with a balsamic vinaigrette dressing. A loaf of rustic Italian bread or Crusty French Bread (page 18) completes the meal.

2 quarts water

salt

8 ounces linguine

2 tablespoons olive oil

2 cloves garlic, minced

2 tablespoons tomato paste

1 teaspoon sugar

1 (8-ounce) bottle clam juice

1 (28-ounce) can Italian tomatoes, chopped

½ to 1 teaspoon crushed red pepper flakes

2 (6.5-ounce) cans chopped clams (undrained)

2 tablespoons fresh parsley, chopped

2 tablespoons fresh basil, chopped

1 pound littleneck clams, cleaned

parsley and basil leaves

1   Bring salted water to a boil and cook linguine according to package directions. (Water should be salty enough to taste like ocean water.) Drain and set aside.

2   Warm oil in a heavy skillet or Dutch oven over medium heat. Add garlic and sauté for 30 seconds. Don't let it brown.

3   Add tomato paste and sugar, cook for 1 minute. Add clam juice, tomatoes, and red pepper flakes (amount depends on personal taste). Simmer for 20 minutes or until sauce begins to thicken.

4   Add chopped clams, parsley, and basil. Simmer for 5 minutes.

5   Meanwhile in another pot, steam littleneck clams until shells open, about 3 to 5 minutes.

6   In a large pasta bowl, pour sauce over freshly cooked linguine. Arrange littleneck clams on top of pasta. Garnish with parsley and basil.

MAKES 6 SERVINGS

NUTRITIONAL ANALYSIS PER SERVING 345 calories ▪ 18 percent fat (total fat 6.9 g, saturated fat < 1 g) ▪ 54 percent carbohydrate (4.1 g fiber) ▪ 28 percent protein.

Linguine with Tomatoes and Fresh Basil

This recipe is easy to make and a staple at my house. Vary it by adding sliced green onions, slivered orange or yellow peppers, chopped sun-dried tomatoes, or any other vegetable in your refrigerator! It requires only the time to cook the pasta yet feeds eight people as a main dish. Even the leftovers serve as a quick lunch or dinner.

4 quarts water

salt

1 pound linguine

2¼ pounds fresh tomatoes, chopped (approximately 4 cups)

2 bundles fresh basil leaves, chopped (approximately 1 cup)

2 cloves garlic, minced

⅓ cup fresh parsley, minced

4 ounces Gorgonzola cheese, crumbled

4 ounces feta cheese, crumbled

⅓ cup slivered almonds, toasted (optional)

1 Bring a large pot of salted water to a boil, add linguine, and cook according to directions on package (approximately 10 to 12 minutes). Remove from heat and drain.

2 In a large bowl, toss the tomatoes, basil, garlic, parsley, Gorgonzola, and feta cheese. Add pasta and toss until Gorgonzola begins to melt. If desired, sprinkle with toasted almonds and serve.

MAKES 8 GENEROUS SERVINGS OF APPROXIMATELY 1½ CUPS EACH

NUTRITIONAL ANALYSIS PER SERVING WITHOUT ALMONDS **326 calories** ▪ **25 percent fat (total fat 9 g, saturated fat 5 g)** ▪ **58 percent carbohydrate (4.6 g fiber)** ▪ **17 percent protein.**

NUTRITIONAL ANALYSIS PER SERVING WITH ALMONDS **359 calories** ▪ **29 percent fat (total fat 11.6 g, saturated fat 5 g)** ▪ **55 percent carbohydrate (5 g fiber)** ▪ **16 percent protein.**

Sautéed Scallops with a Creamy Pink Sauce over Fettuccine

Delicate sweet scallops are tender and glamorous when draped in this creamy pink sauce. The unusual hue is a combination of balsamic-sweetened tomatoes and cream (fat-free, of course!).

2 quarts water

8 ounces fettuccine

1 pound fresh sea scallops, cleaned and patted dry

1 tablespoon all-purpose flour

1 tablespoon olive oil

2 cloves garlic, minced

2 cups canned Italian tomatoes, chopped

1 tablespoon balsamic vinegar

1 teaspoon Splenda or regular sugar

½ cup fat-free half-and-half

¼ cup freshly grated Parmesan cheese

2 tablespoons fresh basil leaves, chopped

1 tablespoon chopped basil leaves (garnish)

1 In a large saucepan, boil water and cook fettuccine according to package directions. Drain.

2 In a medium bowl, dust scallops with flour.

3 Warm oil in a large Dutch oven or deep skillet over medium heat. Add scallops, sauté until brown on both sides, about 2 minutes on each side, or until opaque in center. Remove scallops from skillet (keep warm).

4 Add garlic to same skillet, cook for 30 seconds, add tomatoes, balsamic vinegar, and sugar. Boil over medium-high heat for 5 minutes.

5 Turn heat to low, add half-and-half and Parmesan cheese. Stir until cheese is melted. Add basil and scallops. Stir to combine.

6 Serve scallops and sauce over fresh, hot fettuccine. Garnish with leftover chopped basil.

MAKES 6 SERVINGS

NUTRITIONAL ANALYSIS PER SERVING 423 calories ▪ 16 percent fat (total fat 7.5 g, saturated fat 2 g) ▪ 54 percent carbohydrate (5.6 g fiber) ▪ 30 percent protein.

S

Ginger-Teriyaki Rice Bowls

This dish uses leftover rice and vegetables for a quick, healthy rice bowl. Keep teriyaki sauce on hand so you can make this meal when in a time crunch.

3 skinless, boneless chicken breasts, rinsed and patted dry

1½ cups commercial teriyaki sauce (ginger-teriyaki sauce works best)

1 tablespoon fresh ginger, peeled and minced

1 teaspoon hot pepper flakes

4 cups cooked, cold rice, mixed with 1 teaspoon sesame oil

⅓ cup fat-free chicken broth

4 cups coleslaw mix

1 cup cooked broccoli, chopped

1 cup clean bean sprouts (optional)

½ cup carrots, peeled and shredded

½ cup green onions, thinly sliced

½ cup fresh cilantro, chopped

cooking spray

1   Place chicken in a large plastic Ziploc bag, seal, and set aside.

2   In a small bowl, mix teriyaki sauce, ginger, and pepper flakes. Pour ½ cup teriyaki sauce mixture into Ziploc bag with chicken. (Save remaining 1 cup teriyaki mixture.) Seal. Turn to distribute marinade. Place in refrigerator until ready to grill (up to 24 hours).

3   In a large bowl, add cold rice mixed with sesame oil. Set aside.

4   In a large skillet over medium-high heat, add chicken broth. Bring to a simmer, add coleslaw mix, and cook quickly, until tender-crisp, approximately 2 minutes. Remove from heat. Add to bowl of rice, toss well. Add remaining ingredients (except cooking spray) and reserved 1 cup of teriyaki mixture. Mix well. Set aside.

5   Spray grill with cooking spray and heat to medium-high. Remove chicken from marinade (discard marinade). Place chicken on grill, close lid. Cook for about 5 minutes on each side or until juices run clear. Remove from grill. Slice into thin strips.

6   Spoon rice mixture into 6 bowls, top with several slices of chicken, and serve. Store leftovers in refrigerator.

MAKES 6 SERVINGS

NUTRITIONAL ANALYSIS PER SERVING **343 calories** ▪ **6 percent fat (total fat 2.2 g, saturated fat < 0.5 g)** ▪ **66 percent carbohydrate (3 g fiber)** ▪ **28 percent protein.**

Soba Noodles with Spicy Peanut Sauce

Earthy-flavored Soba noodles pair up nicely with peanut sauce, crisp cucumbers, cilantro, and mint. Clean tasting and packed with vegetables and complex carbohydrates, this dish is designed to keep you feeling upbeat and energized.

FOOD TIP

Soba noodles are thin, brownish noodles made from wheat and buckwheat flours. They have a nutty flavor and are traditionally served cold in Japanese dishes.

1 (16-ounce) package Soba noodles or whole wheat pasta

1 teaspoon sesame oil

⅓ cup fat-free chicken broth

3 cups coleslaw mix

½ cup peanut sauce (commercial brand)

2 tablespoons soy sauce

1 large cucumber, peeled and diced

½ cup fresh cilantro, minced

1 tablespoon fresh mint leaves, minced

2 teaspoons toasted sesame seeds (optional)

1   Cook Soba noodles or pasta according to package directions. Rinse with cold water, drain. In a large salad bowl, toss noodles with sesame oil. Set aside.

2   In a large skillet or Dutch oven over medium high-heat, add chicken broth and coleslaw mix. Stir-fry quickly for 1 to 2 minutes, until tender crisp. Remove from heat. Add peanut sauce and soy sauce and mix well. Pour mixture over Soba noodles.

3   Add cucumber, cilantro, and mint and mix well. Sprinkle with sesame seeds, if desired, and serve. Or cover the dish and chill in refrigerator for up to 24 hours, then mix well before serving.

MAKES 6 SERVINGS OF APPROXIMATELY 1 CUP EACH

NUTRITIONAL ANALYSIS PER SERVINGS **195 calories** ▪ **22 percent fat (total fat 4.7 g, saturated fat ‹ 1 g)** ▪ **60 percent carbohydrate (3 g fiber)** ▪ **18 percent protein.**

Coconut Rice with Ginger and Cardamom

Jasmine rice has a light perfumed aroma when cooking, and it is simply delicious if prepared with a little extra attention. Rice should be rinsed thoroughly several times to remove excess starch, which otherwise makes rice mushy. This side dish goes well with any Indian or Asian entrée, such as Grilled Asian Flank Steak with Wasabi Cream Sauce (page 165).

FOOD TIP

Coconut milk is often mistaken for the fluid inside a coconut, but it is actually a combination of water and shredded coconut meat that is simmered and strained. Coconut milk is a common ingredient in curries in Thailand and in satays in Malaysia. The light version used in this recipe contains less fat and calories than regular coconut milk, 132 versus 447 calories per cup.

2 cups water

1 tablespoon fresh ginger, peeled and minced

1 tablespoon toasted shredded coconut

½ teaspoon salt

¼ cup golden raisins

⅛ teaspoon ground cardamom

1 cup jasmine rice

2 tablespoons slivered almonds

3 tablespoons "light" coconut milk or fat-free half-and-half

2 tablespoons fresh cilantro, minced

1   In a medium heavy pot, place water, ginger, shredded coconut, salt, raisins, and cardamom. Bring water to a boil. Wash rice in cold water 3 times and drain well. (If you have time, soak rice for 10 minutes.) Add rice to pot and cook uncovered over medium heat, stirring once, until water is almost absorbed, approximately 15 minutes.

2   Reduce heat to low simmer, cover tightly, and steam until rice is tender, about 10 minutes. Remove from heat, let rest with cover on for another 10 minutes. Fluff with a fork.

3   Spoon rice into a serving bowl, add slivered almonds, coconut milk, and cilantro. Mix well. Serve immediately.

MAKES 5 SERVINGS OF APPROXIMATELY ½ CUP EACH

NUTRITIONAL ANALYSIS PER SERVING **190 calories** ▪ **13 percent fat (total fat 2.7 g, saturated fat ‹ 1 g)** ▪ **79 percent carbohydrate (1.4 g fiber)** ▪ **8 percent protein.**

Thai Curry Pasta with Fresh Crab and Basil

Intensely flavored, this dish is not for the lighthearted. Thai red curry paste is pungent and hot; when it is combined with sweet flavors from ingredients such as apples and cinnamon, the flavor is irresistible.

FOOD TIP

Fish sauce is also called nam pla in Thailand. It is made by packing fish with a brine in crocks and allowing them to ferment. The brown liquid that forms provides a distinctive flavor to Thai dishes.

½ cup fat-free chicken broth

1 cup light coconut milk

1 large apple, peeled, seeded, and diced (any variety)

½ cup sweet yellow onion, diced

1½ teaspoons curry powder

1 teaspoon fish sauce (in the Asian section of the grocery store)

¼ teaspoon Thai red curry paste (in the Asian section of the grocery store)

¼ teaspoon ground cinnamon

1 pound penne pasta

½ pound fresh crabmeat, cleaned and picked over (remove any shells)

2 tablespoons fresh basil, minced

1   In a medium saucepan over high heat, add chicken broth, ½ cup coconut milk, apple, onion, curry, fish sauce, curry paste, and cinnamon. Stir well. Bring ingredients to a boil, reduce heat to low, cover, and simmer for 10 minutes or until apples are soft. Remove from heat. Set aside.

2   Cook penne according to package directions. Drain.

3   Pour Thai sauce ingredients into a food processor or blender. Blend until smooth. Pour back into saucepan, add remaining ½ cup coconut milk, and stir to mix. Simmer on low heat until pasta is cooked.

4   Transfer cooked, drained penne to a large pasta bowl. Pour simmering Thai sauce over penne, toss to coat well. Gently fold in fresh crab. Sprinkle with fresh basil and serve hot.

MAKES 6 SERVINGS

NUTRITIONAL ANALYSIS PER SERVING **178 calories** ▪ **19 percent fat (total fat 3.7 g, saturated fat 2 g)** ▪ **57 percent carbohydrate (3.8 g fiber)** ▪ **24 percent protein.**

Creamy Risotto with Wild Mushrooms and Fresh Thyme

Creating a creamy risotto needn't be intimidating. Commercially prepared boxed risotto is a welcome addition to the kitchen for the informed cook looking for a shortcut. Feel free to add your favorite vegetable, herb, or seafood.

FOOD TIP
Risotto is Italy's version of rice and is as much a technique as it is a grain. Chefs refer to risotto as a dish that is built, not cooked.

1 (5.5-ounce) box risotto (garlic flavored works well)

2 cups mushrooms, chopped (shiitake, oyster, or button)

1 tablespoon cooking sherry

2 tablespoons fat-free half-and-half

2 teaspoons fresh thyme or sage, minced

1   Prepare risotto according to package instructions but make the following change: add mushrooms to the risotto mixture after you add the water. Continue to cook and stir according to directions.

2   Just before serving, remove cooked risotto mixture from heat and add sherry, half-and-half, and fresh thyme. Stir well to combine. Serve immediately.

MAKES 4 SERVINGS

NUTRITIONAL ANALYSIS PER SERVING **160 calories** ▪ **3 percent fat (total fat 0.5 g, saturated fat 0 g)** ▪ **85 percent carbohydrate (1 g fiber)** ▪ **12 percent protein.**

Old-Fashioned (Low-Fat) Macaroni and Cheese

Mac 'n' cheese is a classic comfort food. This recipe has been adjusted to reduce the overall fat content by half. You will be surprised by the creamy-rich cheese texture. Add a cup of fresh chopped spinach, peas, or cooked asparagus for more color and nutrients.

FOOD TIP

Hardly a dish you would serve at a formal dinner, yet this classic comfort food is said to have been served by President Thomas Jefferson at the White House in 1802. Kraft Foods turned a once-in-a-while dish into an all-time American favorite when it packaged this dinner in 1937.

cooking spray

1 tablespoon reduced-fat margarine

2 tablespoons all-purpose flour

2⅓ cups fat-free half-and-half

4 ounces Velveeta light cheese, cubed

½ cup reduced-fat cheddar or jack cheese

½ teaspoon salt

¼ teaspoon pepper

pinch of cayenne

4 cups hot cooked Rotelle pasta (spiral) or any other favorite pasta

1 slice whole wheat bread

1 tablespoon Parmesan cheese, grated

Preheat oven to 425°. Coat 2-quart baking dish with cooking spray and set aside.

1   Melt margarine in a large nonstick saucepan over medium heat. Add flour, cook for 30 seconds, stirring constantly. Gradually add half-and-half and whisk until well blended. Bring to a boil; cook until thick, approximately 1 to 2 minutes. Add Velveeta and cheddar cheese. Cook until melted, stirring frequently. Add salt, pepper, and cayenne, stirring to mix.

2   Add cooked pasta to sauce, stir gently to mix. Spoon pasta into baking dish. Set aside.

3   Place whole wheat bread and Parmesan in a food processor and pulse until coarse bread crumbs are produced. Sprinkle over casserole. Bake for 20 minutes or until bubbly.

MAKES 4 SERVINGS

NUTRITIONAL ANALYSIS PER SERVING **426 calories** ▪ **16 percent fat (total fat 7.5 g, saturated fat 2.6 g)** ▪ **61 percent carbohydrate (3 g fiber)** ▪ **23 percent protein.**

C

East Coast Goulash

Wednesday at noon the lunch bell would ring. The most popular lunch was waiting: goulash, green beans, a salad, and a roll. Jeanette's memory collaborated with her taste buds to re-create this childhood favorite.

FOOD TIP
The secret to a good goulash is the paprika. If you can find fresh Hungarian paprika, it will add a hot and sweet taste to this dish.

1 pound ground sirloin beef (7 percent fat by weight)

1½ cups celery, diced

1 cup sweet yellow onion, diced

½ cup green bell pepper, diced

2 (14.5-ounce) cans stewed tomatoes, chopped (Italian-style stewed tomatoes are especially good)

2 teaspoons dried basil

1 teaspoon dried marjoram

1 teaspoon paprika

1 tablespoon brown sugar

1 tablespoon Worcestershire sauce

½ teaspoon salt

¼ teaspoon pepper

2½ cups Elbo-Roni pasta, uncooked

1   In a large Dutch oven or saucepan over medium-high heat, brown beef, celery, onion, and green pepper. Sauté for about 8 minutes, breaking up meat into small pieces. Drain any fat.

2   Stir in the remaining ingredients, except pasta. Reduce heat to medium and simmer for 20 minutes. (The longer you simmer the ingredients, the more tender the meat becomes.)

3   Cook the pasta according to package directions. Rinse, drain, and set aside. When sauce is done simmering, add pasta to sauce. Mix well. Serve hot.

MAKES 6 SERVINGS

NUTRITIONAL ANALYSIS PER SERVING **266 calories** ▪ **19 percent fat (total fat 5.6 g, saturated fat 2 g)** ▪ **46 percent carbohydrate (4.5 g fiber)** ▪ **35 percent protein.**

Barley, Red Pepper, and Green Onion Pilaf

A simple yet flavorful dish that goes well with chicken, fish, or meat.

2 teaspoons olive oil	1 cup pearl barley	salt, to taste
1 cup onion, diced	2 cups fat-free chicken broth	¼ cup green onion, chopped
¾ cup red bell pepper, stemmed, seeded, and diced	1 cup water	2 tablespoons slivered almonds or chopped pecans

1   In a large nonstick skillet, warm oil over medium heat. Add onion and red pepper and sauté, stirring frequently, for 5 minutes. Add barley and stir for 3 minutes.

2   Add broth, water, and salt to taste, bring to a boil, reduce heat, cover, and simmer for 40 minutes or until liquid is absorbed and barley is tender. Five minutes before barley is done, sprinkle green onions on top, return cover, and continue to simmer remaining 5 minutes.

3   Transfer to serving bowl and sprinkle with nuts. Serve hot.

MAKES APPROXIMATELY 8 SERVINGS OF ½ CUP EACH

NUTRITIONAL ANALYSIS PER SERVING 131 calories ▪ 20 percent fat (total fat 2.9 g, saturated fat < 0.5 g) ▪ 67 percent carbohydrate (4.7 g fiber) ▪ 13 percent protein.

Q

Potato Gratin with Light Boursin Cheese

Serve with comfort foods, such as Individual Meat Loaves with Fresh Thyme (page 162) and Petite Peas with Shiitake Mushrooms (page 226).

1½ cups plus 1 tablespoon fat-free half-and-half

1½ pounds small red potatoes, thinly sliced (baby reds are good, leave skins on)

2 leeks (white part only), thinly sliced

½ teaspoon salt

¼ teaspoon fresh cracked pepper

1 teaspoon dried thyme

2 teaspoons all-purpose flour

3 tablespoons light Boursin cheese spread

1 tablespoon Parmesan cheese, grated

Preheat oven to 425°.

1   In a medium saucepan, combine 1½ cups half-and-half, potatoes, leeks, salt, pepper, and thyme. Bring to a simmer over medium heat. Cook for about 12 minutes or until potatoes are tender. Stir frequently. Use a slotted spoon to transfer potatoes to a round 1-quart dish or a quiche dish. Set potatoes aside.

2   In a small cup, whisk together 1 tablespoon half-and-half and flour. Add flour mixture to hot saucepan and whisk to blend thoroughly. Cook over medium heat until thick, about 1 minute. Remove saucepan from heat. Whisk in Boursin cheese. Add more half-and-half if mixture is too thick.

3   Pour sauce over potatoes, sprinkle with Parmesan cheese, and bake for 20 minutes or until bubbly hot. Cool for 5 minutes before serving.

MAKES 4 SERVINGS

NUTRITIONAL ANALYSIS PER SERVING **277 calories** ▪ **16 percent fat** (total fat 4.9 g, saturated fat 3 g) ▪ **69 percent carbohydrate** (3.5 g fiber) ▪ **15 percent protein**.

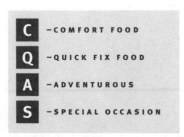

C —COMFORT FOOD

Q —QUICK FIX FOOD

A —ADVENTUROUS

S —SPECIAL OCCASION

Vegetables

Antiaging Mind Boosters

I WHIMPER A bit when I notice an extra pound on the scale, another wrinkle, or a few more gray hairs, but when I forget what I was about to say or where I put my glasses, I get downright worried. Reshape my girlish figure, even add a few years to my looks, but don't rob me of my mind!

As early as our middle 30s, most of us notice a slow, steady drop in mental sharpness. It's called age-related memory loss, cognitive decline, generalized slowing, and even—heaven forbid—a senior moment. Is it inevitable? Does forgetting a name lead ultimately to forgetting your loved ones?

The answer is a definite "no!" Granted, the average 75-year-old is a little slower at Jeopardy than people in their 20s, but the minor short-term memory loss that begins in a person's 40s is a nuisance, not a mental death sentence. Even then, the difference has more to do with diet and lifestyle than with age. And although scientists used to say the brain was one of the few tissues that did not repair itself, we now know the brain can generate new cells in the hippocampus—a portion of the brain important for memory—throughout life. That means the sooner you start caring for your mind, the better. It's always easier to keep the brain humming in good order than to get it started again once the pipes are clogged . . . but it's never too late. You can supply the brain at any age with the building blocks it needs to protect itself from damage, slow the aging process, and function at its best.

The Three Tenets of Brain Smarts

Fatigue, lack of sleep, stress, and depression can undermine your short-term memory. These topics are addressed in other sections of this book. The three basic tenets to stay mentally sharp are: (1) challenge your mind, (2) keep moving, and (3) eat the right foods. (It's a given that you shouldn't smoke!) Follow these tenets, and at any age you can

- hone your ability to concentrate,

- tune your sensory-motor nerves,

- keep motivated (by staying energized),

- amp up your memory,

- speed your reaction times,

- diffuse stress, and

- slow or even prevent brain aging.

Exercise Your Mind and Body

Give your mind and body a daily workout, and they will repay you with sharper thinking and better health throughout life. People who stay mentally challenged, whether it is by working crossword puzzles or taking college courses, compensate for the changes caused by aging in the brain that lead to memory loss. Mental planning, organization, and problem solving remain strong when people turn off the television and pick up a book, play chess, learn new skills, or engage in stimulating conversations.

The same goes for staying physically active. Even moderate exercise stimulates blood flow to the brain and nerve growth. Study after study show that people who stay physically fit also stay mentally fit. Combine daily exercise and mental stimulation with a great diet, and you stack the deck in favor of thinking clearly throughout life.

Brain Food

What you eat affects your mental health long before it affects your physical health. What you eat for breakfast could affect how fast you react, how well you concentrate, and how clever your ideas are midmorning and into the afternoon. Skipping meals, not eating enough, adopting a low-carbohydrate diet, forgetting to take your vitamins, or even not drinking enough water are all linked to slowed reaction times, poor memory, and hit-or-miss recall. In contrast, people who eat well think more clearly and have longer attention spans.

In a nutshell, a good diet protects your mind by providing nutrients that

- are building blocks for nerve and brain cells,

- serve as assembly-line workers to maintain optimal brain function, and

- act as warriors and ammunition to protect delicate brain tissue from damage.

Many vitamins and minerals, such as the B vitamins, iron, and zinc, are essential for the proper function of cells, their components, and nerve chemicals. For example, by lowering a compound in the blood called homocysteine, vitamins B_6, B_{12}, and folic acid protect against injury to small blood vessels that supply oxygen to brain cells, prevent the formation of scar tissue that interferes with nerve function, and help maintain well-functioning brain cells. Compounds in soy might also help ward off age-related memory loss.

On the other hand, poor diets not only fail to provide these essential brain protectors but add insult to injury by flooding the brain with harmful substances. For example, saturated fat clogs blood vessels, which are then less able to transport oxygen to the brain. High-saturated-fat diets also cause tiny brain lesions and blood clots that lead to depression, reduced reaction times, and poor memory. Add sugar to that high fat diet, and you further compromise memory and the ability to learn new information. It's no wonder that people who shun vegetables and eat lots of meat, fast foods, and fatty dairy products are most prone to depression, memory loss, and poor concentration, whereas people with the sharpest minds typically eat diets low in saturated fat and cholesterol but feast on fruits, vegetables, and the nutrients in these foods, such as vitamin C, beta-carotene, and folic acid.

Don't get me wrong. Your brain needs fat—but the right kind. While saturated fats in red meats and fatty dairy products, and *trans* fats in processed foods made with hydrogenated oils muddle your mind, the omega-3 fats in fish and moderate amounts of the monounsaturated fats in nuts, avocados, seeds, and olive and canola oils are essential building blocks for brain cell membranes. They allow electrical messages to pass from one cell to another, thus speeding thought processes. They also help protect the brain from damage and heal damage when it occurs. Fish oils are so important to brain function that preliminary research shows that people who include the most fish in their weekly diets have the lowest risk for memory loss, dementia, and even Alzheimer's disease. The old adage "fish is brain food" is really true!

Avoid the Rust

You don't have to worry about growing old,
you have to worry about rusting.
—GEORGE BURNS, COMEDIAN

Like the bumper on a car, your body "rusts" when exposed to oxygen. Free radicals are oxygen fragments inhaled in air pollution and tobacco smoke, consumed in fatty foods, and manufactured within the body during normal metabolic processes. Left unchecked, these oxygen fragments, or oxidants, attack cell membranes and the genetic code—a process called oxidation. While the bumper on an old jalopy turns crusty red and the Statue of Liberty's copper turned green when oxidized, a human cell either dies or mutates to form a potential cancer cell when exposed to oxidants. Free radicals contribute to all age-related diseases, from heart disease and cancer to cataracts and possibly osteoporosis. The same oxidative processes that clog your arteries and cause cancerous changes in body cells also damage the delicate communication pathways in your brain.

Oxygen is a double-edge sword. It is the most important nutrient to life, yet it also contains tissue-damaging free radicals. The brain consumes more oxygen than any other tissue, so it is the most vulnerable to free-radical exposure. Minute by minute, day by day, year after year, decade upon decade, free radicals are attacking and damaging one brain cell after another until the cumulative damage results in memory loss, slowed reaction times, and reduced alertness.

Why Your Brain Needs Antioxidants

The good news is that your body has an anti–free radical arsenal, called the antioxidants, which sweep up, deactivate, and prevent oxidants from damaging cells. Antioxidants also help keep the heart beating strong and protect the tiny blood vessels that transport nutrients to brain cells, keeping them elastic and free of "debris." Since 20 percent of the heart's output goes to the brain, all of these benefits mean improved blood flow and better thinking. The trick is to maintain an antioxidant arsenal equal to or better than the onslaught of free radicals.

Stockpiling antioxidants is essential throughout life, especially when we are stressed and as we age. Stress is a death sentence for brain cells, especially as we get older. As mentioned on pages 29 to 31, stress sets off a cascade of events, releasing chemicals and hormones, including cortisol, that generate a free-radical flood that is toxic to brain cells. A study at McGill University in Montreal found that people with high blood levels of cortisol scored lower on short-term memory tests than did people who were relatively stress-free. As we get older, oxidative damage to tissues, including the brain, intensifies, so that a 30-year-old woman needs more antioxidant-rich foods than a 12-year-old girl, and the required dose increases even more with every decade.

12 QUICK-FIX VEGETABLES

1. **BROCCOLI:** Cut a large head into 2-inch pieces and steam until crisp-tender. Briefly sauté in a medium skillet with 2 teaspoons olive oil along with 2 sliced garlic cloves, 1 teaspoon red pepper flakes, or 1 tablespoon pecans.

2. **CARROTS:** Peel 5 carrots and cut into 2-inch pieces. Place in a roasting pan or on a baking sheet and toss with 1 tablespoon olive oil and salt to taste. Add fresh thyme leaves, freshly ground black pepper, curry powder, or strips of fresh ginger and roast for 30 minutes or until tender-firm.

3. **GREENS:** Steam your favorite greens, including spinach, chard, or kale. Chop and blend with mashed potatoes.

4. **ZUCCHINI:** Slice zucchini lengthwise into 4 strips, approximately 1/4 inch thick. Spray a hot barbecue grill with cooking spray, place zucchini on grill, and sprinkle with Italian seasoning. Close hood and cook for 7 minutes on each side or until zucchini is cooked through but not translucent.

5. **ROASTED VEGETABLES:** Toss a 1-pound bag of frozen stew vegetables (thawed) with 3 whole garlic cloves, 1 tablespoon olive oil, 1 tablespoon fresh rosemary, and salt and pepper to taste. Roast at 475° for 25 minutes or until vegetables are tender.

6. **CAJUN SWEET POTATOES:** Cut sweet potatoes into 1-inch-thick slices. Toss with olive oil, prepared Cajun seasoning, and freshly ground pepper. Bake at 375° for 40 minutes or until lightly brown and cooked through.

7. **BROILED TOMATOES:** Mix bread crumbs, low-fat Parmesan cheese, and salt and pepper to taste. Cut tomatoes in half and sprinkle with crumb mixture. Broil until brown and crispy, approximately 4 minutes.

8. **SNOW PEAS:** Microwave (on high power) 2 (6-ounce) packages of frozen snow peas for 3 to 4 minutes or until heated through and crisp. Toss with 1 tablespoon yogurt-based spread and 1 teaspoon lemon zest.

9. **SWEET POTATO WITH MAPLE SYRUP:** Mash 1 small cooked sweet potato with 2 tablespoons reduced-calorie maple syrup. Salt and pepper to taste.

10. **STUFFED RED BELL PEPPERS:** Stem, seed, and blanch whole red peppers. Fill with cooked instant rice, minced onions, minced garlic, chopped steamed spinach, salt and pepper, and herbs. Microwave on high power for 5 minutes or until heated through.

11. **GREEN BEANS:** Trim and steam green beans until tender but crisp, approximately 8 minutes. Toss with lemon zest, lemon juice, parsley, minced garlic, and salt and pepper.

12. **BRUSSELS SPROUTS:** Steam sprouts until tender but still green, approximately 5 minutes. Toss with a little butter, fresh dill, and fresh chives.

Vegetables and Fruits=Total Recall

Vegetables and fruit are the number one supplier of brain-protecting antioxidants. Plants are your best source of antioxidant vitamins, such as vitamin C and beta-carotene. In addition, they contain most of the 12,000 plant compounds, called phytochemicals, that are also antioxidants, such as the flavonoids in citrus, anthocyanins in red cabbage and cherries, lycopene in tomatoes and watermelon, lutein in spinach, sulphorophane in broccoli, ellagic acid in berries, and sulfur compounds in garlic, to name only a few. The darker the plant's color, the greater the antioxidant punch.

The research overwhelmingly shows that the more color-rich produce you eat, the better you think. At Tufts University in Boston, animals fed diets enriched with extra produce, such as blueberries and spinach, performed best on memory tests throughout life. The same holds true for people. Folks who eat the most broccoli, sweet potatoes, spinach, and other deep-colored produce maintain the highest blood levels of antioxidants. They also score highest on memory tests, exhibit the best judgment and reasoning, maintain a youthful ability to learn new tasks, and react quickly.

How Many Vegetables Do You Need?

You should limit your intake of sugar, saturated fat, salt, and processed foods, but when it comes to vegetables—*the more you eat, the better*. Aim for 8 to 10 servings each day for starters. That recommendation is not as unreasonable as it might sound. All you need to do is:

- Include two fruits and/or vegetables at every meal and one at every snack.

- Double a serving size of any bright-colored vegetable, such as any vegetable dish in this section or any salad in the "Salads" section, and you have two servings! (See page 147 for guidelines on serving size.)

THE BEST ANTIOXIDANT-RICH FOODS
(Hint: The higher the value, the better)

Fruit or Vegetable (3½ ounces)	Antioxidant Value	Fruit or Vegetable (3½ ounces)	Antioxidant Value
Kale	1,770	Orange	750
Strawberries	1,540	Grapes	739
Raspberries	1,220	Red bell pepper	710
Spinach	1,260	Cherries	670
Brussels sprouts	980	Onion	450
Plums	949	Corn	400
Broccoli	890	Eggplant	390
Beets	840		

The recipes in this section are designed to fuel your mind as well as satisfy your taste buds. Double a recipe and use the leftovers for lunch the next day. Enjoy!

Pan-Seared Asparagus with Gingered Onions

Pan-searing seals in flavor and gives this vegetable an exotic personality it doesn't have when steamed. One serving supplies half your daily requirement for folic acid, a B vitamin that helps regulate mood and thinking, and whopping doses of vitamin C, iron, and selenium, which also protect your brain from age-related memory loss. This dish is especially delicious with Chicken with Mushrooms in Creamy Garlic-Pecan Sauce (page 151), Crusty Cranberry Salmon (page 155), or Baked Pork Florentine with Wild Rice (page 168).

---

1 tablespoon orange peel, thinly sliced

⅓ cup fat-free chicken broth

4 cups onions, thinly sliced into rounds

1 teaspoon fresh ginger, peeled and grated

1 teaspoon brown sugar

salt, to taste

1 teaspoon olive oil

1½ pounds fresh asparagus, washed and ends snapped off

orange slices (optional)

1   Soak orange peel in chicken broth for 5 minutes.

2   Warm 1 tablespoon of the chicken broth in a medium nonstick skillet over medium heat. Add onions and orange peel. Cook, turning frequently, for 10 minutes or until onions are translucent and peel is tender. Add additional chicken broth, 1 tablespoon at a time, to keep onions moist but not wet. Add ginger, brown sugar, and salt to taste. Continue to stir until onions are golden and limp, approximately 10 minutes. Set aside.

3   During the last 10 minutes while onions are cooking, pour olive oil in a large skillet over medium-high heat. Add asparagus and salt to taste. Stir gently and frequently until asparagus turns bright green and is cooked through but still crunchy, approximately 12 minutes. Add 1 tablespoon of chicken broth if pan is too dry.

4   Arrange asparagus spears on a platter and top with gingered onions. Garnish with orange slices.

MAKES 4 SERVINGS

NUTRITIONAL ANALYSIS PER SERVING **103 calories** ▪ **14 percent fat (total fat 1.7 g, saturated fat 0 g)** ▪ **66 percent carbohydrate (5 g fiber)** ▪ **20 percent protein.**

Ginger Squash

This butternut squash is a great accompaniment to both Asian dishes and less spicy fare. For example, serve it with grilled halibut and steamed broccoli or with Tandoori Chicken Made Simple (page 170) or Grilled Asian Flank Steak with Wasabi Cream Sauce (page 165). It is also packed with antioxidants, such as beta-carotene, which protect delicate brain cells from damage, and is a good source of iron, which helps carry oxygen to your memory banks.

1½ pounds butternut squash, peeled, seeded, and cut into strips or cubes (approximately 4 cups raw)

2 tablespoons orange juice concentrate

3 tablespoons maple syrup

½ teaspoon ground ginger

¼ teaspoon ground nutmeg

salt and pepper, to taste

⅓ cup crystalline ginger

1   Steam squash until tender, approximately 10 minutes.

2   Stir in orange juice, maple syrup, ginger, and nutmeg. Stir until thoroughly blended and squash is partially mashed. Season with salt and pepper.

3   Transfer to a serving bowl and sprinkle with crystalline ginger. Serve hot.

MAKES 4 SERVINGS OF ½ CUP EACH

NUTRITIONAL ANALYSIS PER ½ CUP **110 calories** ▪ 1 percent fat (total fat < 0.5 g, saturated fat 0 g) ▪ 95 percent carbohydrate (3 g fiber) ▪ 4 percent protein.

Zucchini-Tomato Lasagna with Fresh Thyme and Caramelized Onions

This easy-to-make au gratin is a great way to use up those garden vegetables in the summertime. It also makes a tasty accompaniment to any Italian dish in the winter. Prepare the zucchini and squash while the onions are sautéeing, and you'll save time.

1 tablespoon olive oil

2 large yellow onions (about 6 cups), peeled and thinly sliced

5 cloves garlic, minced

2 tablespoons fresh thyme leaves

3 large tomatoes, halved and cut into ¼-inch slices

1½ pounds zucchini, cut into ¼-inch diagonal slices

1½ pounds yellow squash, cut into ¼-inch diagonal slices

2 tablespoons olive oil

⅓ cup fresh thyme leaves

salt and pepper, to taste

1½ cups low-fat Parmesan cheese, grated

salt, to taste

Heat oven to 375°.

1   Warm 1 tablespoon oil in large skillet over medium heat. Add onions and sauté for 10 minutes, stirring frequently. Add garlic and continue to stir and sauté for another 10 minutes or until onions are limp and golden. Spread onion-garlic mixture evenly in bottom of a 13-by-9-by-2-inch glass baking dish. Sprinkle with 2 tablespoons thyme. Set aside.

2   Place tomatoes on paper towel to remove any excess liquid.

3   Toss zucchini, yellow squash, 2 tablespoons olive oil, ⅓ cup thyme, and salt and pepper in a large bowl.

4   Set aside half of cheese to use as topping. Start at one end of the baking dish, press an overlapping layer of tomato slices, laid upright across end of dish. Sprinkle lightly with cheese. Overlap with a dense layer of zucchini, again positioned upright, followed by a dense layer of yellow squash. Repeat tomato, cheese, zucchini, and yellow squash and finish with a layer of tomatoes. Push the rows back to make more room

for additional rows and to firmly pack the vegetables. Any remaining pieces can be fit into the layers so that the red, green, and yellow layers are packed firmly. Sprinkle remaining half of cheese evenly over top.

5   Bake for 75 minutes or until top is golden brown and a fork easily moves through squash. Liquid should be bubbling and have reduced considerably. Let stand for a few minutes before serving.

MAKES 10 SERVINGS AS A SIDE DISH AND 6 TO 8 SERVINGS AS A MAIN DISH

NUTRITIONAL ANALYSIS PER SIDE DISH SERVING **183 calories** ▪ **39 percent fat (total fat 8 g, saturated fat < 1 g)** ▪ **49 percent carbohydrate (4 g fiber)** ▪ **12 percent protein.**

S

Veggie Stir-Fry with Ginger and Black Bean Sauce

Not just another stir-fry, this Japanese-inspired dish can be served alone, as a side dish, or over buckwheat Soba noodles, rice, or any favorite grain. Be creative and add your favorite vegetables.

2 tablespoons olive oil

1 green zucchini, coarsely chopped

1 yellow zucchini, coarsely chopped

3 Japanese eggplants, coarsely chopped (do not peel)

1 large sweet onion, peeled and thinly sliced

1 large carrot, peeled and thinly sliced

2 cloves garlic, minced

1 tablespoon fresh ginger, peeled and grated

12 mushrooms of choice (button, oyster, shiitake, or a combination), sliced

3 tablespoons black bean sauce

1 tablespoon soy sauce

¼ teaspoon crushed red pepper flakes

2 tablespoons fresh cilantro, chopped

1 Warm oil in a large skillet over medium-high heat.

2 Add zucchinis, eggplants, onion, carrot, garlic, ginger, and mushrooms. Stir-fry until vegetables are tender but still crisp, about 2 to 3 minutes.

3 Stir in remaining ingredients, mixing well to combine.

4 Transfer to your favorite serving plate or serve over noodles or rice. Garnish with a fresh cilantro sprig or two.

MAKES 6 SERVINGS OF APPROXIMATELY ⅔ CUP EACH

NUTRITIONAL ANALYSIS PER SERVING **93 calories** ▪ **47 percent fat (total fat 5 g, saturated fat < 1 g)** ▪ **43 percent carbohydrate (3 g fiber)** ▪ **10 percent protein.**

Portabello Mushrooms and Walnuts

The rich flavors in this dish are likely to win over even those who are unsure about Brussels sprouts. Serve with Chicken with Mushrooms in Creamy Garlic-Pecan Sauce (page 151), Grilled Pork Tenderloin with Rosemary-Orange Sauce (page 158), or any holiday meal.

MOOD TIP

Mushrooms contain a variety of phytochemicals, such as lentinan, which have antiviral and possibly antitumor properties.

2 pounds Brussels sprouts, washed and trimmed

2 teaspoons olive oil

½ yellow onion, chopped (approximately ¾ cup)

1 medium portabello mushroom, stemmed and chopped

⅓ cup walnuts, chopped

¼ cup maple syrup

1   Steam Brussels sprouts until crisp, approximately 10 minutes. Set aside.

2   In a large nonstick skillet, warm oil over medium heat. Add onion and mushroom and sauté until onion is transparent, approximately 5 minutes. Stir in Brussels sprouts.

3   Remove from heat and toss with walnuts and maple syrup. Serve immediately.

MAKES 6 SERVINGS

NUTRITIONAL ANALYSIS PER SERVING **169 calories** ▪ **29 percent fat (total fat 5.4 g, saturated fat < 1 g)** ▪ **56 percent carbohydrate (7.6 g fiber)** ▪ **15 percent protein.**

Roasted Gingered Vegetables

The extra ginger added at the end gives these vegetables a fresh flavor. Better yet, this dish provides an entire day's requirement for vitamin C and three-quarters of that for beta-carotene, antioxidants that protect the mind from age-related damage! Serve with Herb-Roasted Chicken (page 152) or Individual Meat Loaves with Fresh Thyme (page 162).

cooking spray

2 large parsnips, peeled and cut into 2-inch slices

1 medium red onion, peeled and quartered, then halved

1 pound baby carrots

3 medium red potatoes, washed and cut into eighths

½ pound Brussels sprouts, stems trimmed and wilted leaves removed

1 medium red sweet potato, peeled and cut into large chunks

⅓ cup fresh ginger, peeled and cut into 3-inch toothpick slices

2 tablespoons olive oil

salt and pepper, to taste

2 teaspoons fresh ginger, peeled and grated

2½ tablespoons maple syrup

Heat oven to 425°. Spray a large baking dish (13 inches by 9 inches by 2 inches) with cooking spray and set aside.

1   In a large bowl, toss first 9 ingredients (from parsnips through salt and pepper) to thoroughly coat vegetables with oil. Spread evenly in baking dish. Roast for 45 minutes, tossing twice, or until vegetables are tender, but not mushy, and golden brown in spots.

2   While vegetables are roasting, mix grated ginger and maple syrup and set aside.

3   Remove vegetables from oven and pour ginger-syrup mixture over top. Mix well to coat thoroughly. Serve warm.

MAKES 6 SERVINGS OF APPROXIMATELY 1 CUP EACH

NUTRITIONAL ANALYSIS PER SERVING **213 calories** ▪ **21 percent fat (total fat 5 g, saturated fat ‹ 1 g)** ▪ **72 percent carbohydrate (7.8 g fiber)** ▪ **7 percent protein.**

Glazed Carrots

A fresh twist on traditional glazed carrots, this dish is simple to make and goes well with any chicken, fish, or pork entrée.

2 pounds carrots, peeled

²/₃ cup fat-free chicken broth

1 tablespoon butter

1 teaspoon sugar

salt, to taste

1 tablespoon fresh ginger, peeled and minced

2 tablespoons fresh cilantro, chopped

1   Cut carrots lengthwise, then diagonally, to form 2-inch-long chunks.

2   Place carrots and broth in large sauté pan (almost single layer). Add butter, sugar, and salt, and bring to a boil. Cover and reduce heat to medium. Simmer until carrots are slightly tender but still firm, about 5 minutes.

3   Uncover carrots and add ginger, return to a gentle boil, and cook until broth is reduced to syrup, approximately 10 minutes. Stir occasionally to prevent burning.

4   Toss with cilantro and serve.

MAKES 8 SERVINGS

NUTRITIONAL ANALYSIS PER SERVING 75 calories ▪ 21 percent fat (total fat 1.7 g, saturated fat < 1 g) ▪ 69 percent carbohydrate (3.8 g fiber) ▪ 10 percent protein.

Q

Green Beans and Toasted Slivered Almonds

So simple, yet so flavorful, the toasted almonds bring this dish to life! Especially good with Chicken 'n' Mushrooms in Sherry Cream Gravy (page 156).

cooking spray

⅓ cup almonds

1 tablespoon butter

2 pounds green beans, trimmed and washed

4 cloves garlic, minced

½ teaspoon salt

1¼ cups fat-free chicken broth

salt and pepper, to taste

Heat oven to 325°. Spray a cookie sheet with cooking spray.

1   Place almonds on cookie sheet and bake for 10 minutes or until almonds are toasty brown. Remove and set aside.

2   Melt butter in a large pan over medium heat. Add green beans, garlic, and salt. Toss to coat beans. Add chicken broth and simmer gently, stirring occasionally, until beans are tender but still firm, approximately 25 minutes. The liquid should be reduced to less than ¼ cup.

3   Season with salt and pepper. Transfer to a serving platter and sprinkle with almonds.

MAKES 6 SERVINGS

NUTRITIONAL ANALYSIS PER SERVING **112 calories** ▪ **44 percent fat (total fat 5.4 g, saturated fat 1.6 g)** ▪ **41 percent carbohydrate (5.7 g fiber)** ▪ **15 percent protein.**

Creamy Sweet Potatoes and Yams with Chipotle Peppers

You will make this recipe time and again. The chipotle chilies combine with coconut milk to give the subtle hint of heat and sweetness. Few can guess the secret ingredients! These potatoes pair nicely with Grilled Pork Tenderloin with Rosemary-Orange Sauce (page 158).

FOOD TIP

What are called yams in the United States are really just a pale version of the redder sweet potatoes. True yams are much drier in texture, starchier, and scalier in appearance and are found only in ethnic or specialty markets. The deeper the color, the higher the nutrient and phytochemical content, so reach for the reddest sweet potato at the grocery store, which has six times your daily requirement for beta-carotene (yams have next to none) and much more vitamin C and trace minerals.

2 yams (approximately 1½ pounds), peeled and cubed

2 sweet potatoes (approximately 1½ pounds), peeled and cubed

1 chipotle pepper and 2 tablespoons of adobo sauce (from a 7-ounce can chipotle peppers in adobo sauce)

½ cup light coconut milk

½ cup fat-free chicken broth

2 tablespoons butter

¾ teaspoon salt

pinch of cinnamon

1   Steam yams and potatoes until tender, about 15 to 20 minutes.

2   Rinse chipotle pepper with water. Remove most of seeds and finely chop. Add to sauce. Set aside.

3   Drain and return potatoes to pan. Add chipotle mixture plus all remaining ingredients. Mash to desired consistency. If too thick, add more coconut milk or chicken broth.

MAKES 10 SERVINGS OF APPROXIMATELY ½ CUP EACH

NUTRITIONAL ANALYSIS PER SERVING **155 calories** ▪ **18 percent fat (total fat 3 g, saturated fat 2 g)** ▪ **76 percent carbohydrate (3.4 g fiber)** ▪ **6 percent protein.**

Swiss Chard with Garlic and Oregano

Packed with folic acid, vitamin C, beta-carotene, iron, and fiber, Swiss chard is one of the most nutritious vegetables. This recipe is simple and goes well with any Italian dish. Leftovers can be whipped into mashed potatoes for a great accompaniment to any chicken, beef, or pork recipe. Try this recipe using spinach or any dark green leafy vegetable. Sprinkle with low-fat Parmesan cheese for a different taste.

2 teaspoons olive oil

4 cloves garlic, minced

16 cups Swiss chard, washed, drained, and chopped

1 tablespoon fresh oregano leaves

¼ teaspoon salt

dash of black pepper

pinch of red pepper flakes

1 tablespoon red wine vinegar

1   In a large nonstick skillet, warm oil over medium heat. Add garlic and sauté for 2 minutes, stirring frequently.

2   Add chard, toss to mix with garlic, cover, and cook for 3 minutes or until chard begins to wilt.

3   Stir in oregano, salt, black pepper, and red pepper flakes. Cover and cook 5 minutes or until chard is tender but still bright green.

4   Remove from heat, add vinegar, toss, and serve.

MAKES 3 CUPS OR 6 SERVINGS OF ½ CUP EACH

NUTRITIONAL ANALYSIS PER SERVING **35 calories** ▪ **38 percent fat (total fat 1.5 g, saturated fat 0 g)** ▪ **44 percent carbohydrate (1.7 g fiber)** ▪ **18 percent protein.**

Q

Fresh Green Beans with Shallots, Red Onion, and Feta Cheese

Serve beans hot as a side dish to Grilled Asian Flank Steak with Wasabi Cream Sauce (page 165) or cold as a salad.

FOOD TIP

Are fresh vegetables more nutritious than canned or frozen? It depends on how fresh is fresh. Fresh tastes best, but if your produce was picked before ripening, held in storage, transported over long distances, and displayed at the store for days prior to purchase, then you might get more nutrients from frozen plain vegetables that were processed immediately after picking. Canned is better than not eating vegetables at all; just make sure you drink the liquids in the can, since many vitamins have migrated from the vegetables into this juice.

4 cups water

1 pound fresh green beans, washed and trimmed

1 tablespoon olive oil

1 tablespoon balsamic vinegar

2 shallots, minced (approximately 2 tablespoons)

2 cloves garlic, minced

2 tablespoons red onion, minced

2 tablespoons feta cheese, crumbled

salt and pepper, to taste

1   In a large heavy skillet, bring water to a boil over high heat. Add beans and cook covered, until tender-crisp, about 15 to 20 minutes. Drain and pour into a bowl of ice water to stop the cooking process. Drain and set aside.

2   In the same skillet over medium-high heat, add oil, balsamic vinegar, shallots, and garlic. Sauté for 2 to 3 minutes or until shallots are tender.

3   Add green beans to skillet and toss to coat with shallot mixture. Simmer for 1 minute to reheat beans.

4   Place green beans on a platter, sprinkle with red onion and feta cheese. Season with salt and pepper. Serve hot or at room temperature.

MAKES 4 SERVINGS

NUTRITIONAL ANALYSIS PER SERVING **97 calories** ▪ **44 percent fat (total fat 4.7 g, saturated fat 1.6 g)** ▪ **43 percent carbohydrate (3.8 g fiber)** ▪ **13 percent protein.**

A

Baked Sweet Potatoes Topped with Apples, Cranberries, and Nuts

Creamy, sweet, and crunchy, all rolled into one, these potatoes can be made the day before and reheated without losing a bit of flavor. They go well with turkey, chicken, or pork. They pack a hefty antioxidant punch, supplying three times the minimum requirement for beta-carotene, almost three-quarters of the daily requirement for vitamin E, and half the day's need for vitamin C.

4 medium sweet potatoes, scrubbed

½ cup dried cranberries

1 tablespoon butter

1 large Granny Smith apple, peeled, seeded, and diced

¼ cup pecans or walnuts, chopped

6 teaspoons brown sugar

⅛ teaspoon ground cinnamon

dash of ground nutmeg

salt, to taste

Preheat oven to 350°. Line a cookie sheet with tinfoil.

1 Pierce potatoes with a fork, place on cookie sheet, and bake for 1 hour or until tender when pierced with a fork. Set aside until warm and easy to handle.

2 Place cranberries in a small bowl and cover with hot water. Set aside for 10 minutes. Drain.

3 Melt butter in a medium nonstick skillet over medium-high heat. Add apples and sauté until slightly soft and golden, approximately 5 minutes. Stir in cranberries, nuts, and 2 teaspoons brown sugar, and continue to sauté for 1 minute. Remove from heat and add cinnamon, nutmeg, and salt.

4 With a sharp knife, remove an oval of skin off the top of each potato, large enough to allow you to mash the pulp without disturbing the remaining skin. Sprinkle pulp with salt to taste and 1 teaspoon brown sugar per potato. Gently mash the pulp with a fork until smooth and sugar is completely blended.

5 Divide the apple mixture evenly and mound on top of each potato. Serve immediately or cool and cover with plastic wrap, store in refrigerator, and reheat uncovered in oven at 350° for approximately 20 minutes or until heated through.

MAKES 4 SERVINGS

NUTRITIONAL ANALYSIS PER SERVING **302 calories** ▪ **23 percent fat (total fat 7.7 g, saturated fat 2.3 g)** ▪ **72 percent carbohydrate (6 g fiber)** ▪ **5 percent protein.**

Slow-Roasted Tomatoes
with Garlic and Herbs

If you can imagine tomatoes as candy, then this dish is it! Roast these tomatoes long and slow for the most delicious accompaniment to any fish or chicken dish. Leftovers can be used for the appetizer Slow-Roasted Tomatoes and Pesto on Polenta Pizzas (page 51).

cooking spray	3 cloves garlic, minced	salt and pepper, to taste
10 large plum tomatoes, washed, dried, trimmed, and cut in half lengthwise	1 tablespoon fresh thyme leaves	Parmesan cheese, grated (optional)

Heat oven to 350°. Cover a cookie sheet with tinfoil and spray with cooking spray.

1   Place tomatoes, cut side up, on lined cookie sheet. Sprinkle garlic and thyme evenly over each tomato half. Season with salt and pepper, then spray with more cooking spray.

2   Place in oven and bake for 1 hour 20 minutes or until tomatoes are wrinkled and starting to blacken. Turn once during baking.

3   Serve while hot. Sprinkle with Parmesan cheese if desired.

MAKES 4 SERVINGS

NUTRITIONAL ANALYSIS PER SERVING 68 calories ▪ 12 percent fat (total fat 1 g, saturated fat 0 g) ▪ 75 percent carbohydrate (4.2 g fiber) ▪ 13 percent protein.

Quick-Baked Cherry Tomatoes with Olive Oil, Balsamic Vinegar, and Basil

If you're in a hurry, skip the roasting step! Serve tomatoes as a side dish at room temperature or chilled.

---

1 pound cherry tomatoes
(20 to 30), rinsed and patted dry

1 tablespoon olive oil

1 tablespoon balsamic vinegar

1 teaspoon dried basil

1 teaspoon Splenda

salt and pepper, to taste

Preheat oven to 400°.

1   In a medium bowl, place all ingredients. Mix gently to coat tomatoes.

2   Pour into a small round baking pan. Bake for 7 minutes or until tomatoes are heated through. Remove from oven and serve hot.

MAKES 4 SERVINGS

NUTRITIONAL ANALYSIS PER SERVING **55 calories** ▪ **56 percent fat (total fat 3.4 g, saturated fat < 1 g)** ▪ **37 percent carbohydrate (1.6 g fiber)** ▪ **7 percent protein.**

Q

Baked Lima and Butter Beans in a Thick BBQ Sauce

For those who shy away from lima beans, try this recipe, a delicious blend of beans in a spicy BBQ sauce. Horseradish and molasses pair up as spicy and sweet flavors. Serve with grilled chicken, hamburgers, or Turkey Burgers with Caramelized Onions (page 74).

1 cup commercial barbecue sauce

1 tablespoon horseradish sauce

1 tablespoon dark or light molasses

2 tablespoons brown sugar

2 (15-ounce) cans pork and beans

1 (15.25-ounce) can lima beans, drained

1 (15-ounce) can butter beans, drained

1 small sweet onion, finely chopped

½ small green bell pepper, finely chopped

Preheat oven to 350°.

1   In a large 2-quart casserole dish, blend barbecue sauce, horseradish, molasses, and brown sugar.

2   Add the remaining ingredients to the barbecue mixture and blend well. Bake uncovered for 45 minutes or until onions and peppers are tender.

MAKES 10 SERVINGS OF APPROXIMATELY ⅔ CUP EACH

NUTRITIONAL ANALYSIS PER SERVING **279 calories** ▪ **7 percent fat (total fat 2.2 g, saturated fat ‹ 1 g)** ▪ **73 percent carbohydrate (18 g fiber)** ▪ **20 percent protein.**

Polenta-Crusted Eggplant Parmesan

A delicious, crusty vegetable side dish or vegetarian entrée. Serve with your favorite pasta and Low-Fat Caesar Salad (page 142) for a complete meal.

cooking spray

½ cup dry polenta

¼ cup low-fat Parmesan cheese, grated

1 teaspoon dried basil

½ teaspoon salt

½ cup liquid egg substitute (equivalent to 2 whole eggs)

1 medium eggplant (about 1 pound), peeled and cut into 1½-inch-thick slices

3 cups tomato sauce (a commercial brand with added basil and garlic or herbs and garlic)

1 cup part-skim mozzarella cheese

Preheat oven to 350°. Spray a large flat cookie sheet with cooking spray. Set aside.

1 Place dry polenta, Parmesan cheese, basil, and salt on a large plate, mix well to combine. Set aside.

2 Place egg substitute in a shallow bowl. Set aside.

3 Dip eggplant slices into egg substitute, then roll in polenta mixture to coat both sides. Place on cooking sheet and bake for 25 minutes or until crust of eggplant is crispy brown. Remove from oven. Set aside.

4 Spray a 9-by-5-by-3-inch loaf pan with cooking spray. Add enough tomato sauce to cover bottom of pan. Add 1 layer of crusty eggplant (may need to cut, to fit) on top of tomato sauce. Pour about ⅓ cup tomato sauce over eggplant and sprinkle with ⅓ cup mozzarella cheese. Continue to layer eggplant slices, sauce, and cheese. Save enough sauce to cover top of casserole. Bake for 30 minutes or until bubbly and cheese has melted. Remove from oven and serve hot.

MAKES 8 SERVINGS

NUTRITIONAL ANALYSIS PER SERVING **133 calories** ▪ **27 percent fat (total fat 4 g, saturated fat 2 g)** ▪ **47 percent carbohydrate (4 g fiber)** ▪ **26 percent protein.**

Creamy Cauliflower Puree

Cauliflower is available year round, yet some of us push our grocery carts past these cream-colored heads. Cauliflower is a member of the cabbage family and is packed with a phytochemical called indole, which lowers cancer risk.

---

1 head (1½ pounds) cauliflower, broken into small florets

1½ cups fat-free chicken broth

2 teaspoons reduced-fat margarine

2 tablespoons reserved chicken broth (from steaming cauliflower)

4 tablespoons fat-free sour cream

1 teaspoon prepared horseradish

¼ cup green onions, thinly sliced

salt and pepper, to taste

paprika

1   In a medium saucepan, combine cauliflower and chicken broth. Bring to a boil. Reduce heat to low, cover pan, and simmer until cauliflower is very tender, approximately 15 minutes.

2   With a slotted spoon, place cauliflower in a food processor or blender, add margarine and 2 tablespoons of reserved chicken broth, and process until smooth. Add sour cream and horseradish, process until blended.

3   Pour cauliflower puree into a medium bowl, stir in green onions, and season with salt and pepper. If puree is too thick, add more chicken broth or sour cream. Sprinkle with paprika. Serve hot.

MAKES 4 SERVINGS OF APPROXIMATELY ¼ CUP EACH

NUTRITIONAL ANALYSIS PER SERVING 46 calories ▪ 47 percent fat (total fat 2.4 g, saturated fat 0 g) ▪ 26 percent carbohydrate (0.4 g fiber) ▪ 27 percent protein.

Petite Peas with Shiitake Mushrooms

Experiment with various types of mushrooms for this quick-fix side dish; just about any mushroom will taste great. These peas go especially well with Braised Chicken Parmesan (page 166).

---

1 (16-ounce) bag frozen petite peas

⅓ cup fat-free chicken broth

6 medium shiitake mushrooms, thinly sliced

½ teaspoon dried marjoram

1 tablespoon diced pimentos

1   Place peas in a steamer and steam over high heat for 5 minutes or until just heated through.

2   In a nonstick skillet, warm chicken broth over medium-high heat. Add mushrooms and stir-fry quickly for 3 minutes. Add more chicken broth if mushrooms start to stick.

3   Add peas to skillet with mushrooms, sprinkle with marjoram, and toss to coat peas and mushrooms in remaining chicken broth. Spoon into a serving bowl, garnish with pimentos. Serve hot.

MAKES 4 SERVINGS

NUTRITIONAL ANALYSIS PER SERVING **108 calories** ▪ **5 percent fat (total fat ‹ 1 g, saturated fat 0 g)** ▪ **71 percent carbohydrate (6.4 g fiber)** ▪ **24 percent protein.**

Q

Grilled Vegetables with Garlic and Balsamic Vinaigrette

Simple and delicious, these vegetables go well with grilled chicken or salmon. Feel free to replace one of the listed vegetables with another, such as zucchini, sweet potato, asparagus, or carrot strips. Keep in mind that grilling time may be longer or shorter depending on the vegetable.

cooking spray

1 small eggplant, skin intact

1 large portabello mushroom

1 medium-size green or red bell pepper

VINAIGRETTE

1 tablespoon olive oil

2 tablespoon balsamic vinegar

2 cloves garlic, minced

1 teaspoon dried basil

1 teaspoon Splenda

salt and pepper, to taste

Spray grill with cooking spray and preheat to medium.

1　Slice eggplant lengthwise into 4 (½-inch-thick) pieces, then slice each piece in half. Clean mushroom, remove stem, and slice into 1-inch-thick pieces. Slice pepper into 1-inch-thick pieces.

2　Place vegetables in a single layer on a large rectangular baking pan or cookie sheet. Set aside.

3　In a small bowl, whisk together the vinaigrette ingredients.

4　Brush vinaigrette mixture on both sides of vegetables. Grill until vegetables are tender, turning occasionally, about 6 minutes for eggplant and mushrooms, 5 minutes for peppers. Serve on a large plate.

MAKES 4 SERVINGS

NUTRITIONAL ANALYSIS PER SERVING **87 calories** ▪ **36 percent fat** (total fat 3.5 g, saturated fat ‹ 1 g) ▪ **54 percent carbohydrate** (5.3 g fiber) ▪ **10 percent protein**.

Quick Steamed Broccoli
with Parmesan Cheese

An easy way to prepare and serve a much loved vegetable.

FOOD TIP
If you should overcook the broccoli by mistake, just make it a pureed side dish. Place the broccoli in your food processor, add some fat-free half-and-half, and blend until smooth. Sprinkle with reduced-fat Parmesan cheese.

1 cup fat-free chicken broth

1 pound fresh broccoli florets

2 tablespoons reduced-fat Parmesan cheese, grated

1   Place chicken broth in a medium saucepan and bring to a boil. Add broccoli, reduce heat to medium, cover pan, and cook broccoli until tender-crisp, about 3 minutes. Remove from heat and drain broccoli.

2   Spoon broccoli into a bowl and sprinkle with Parmesan cheese. Serve hot.

MAKES 4 SERVINGS

NUTRITIONAL ANALYSIS PER SERVING **197 calories** ▪ **19 percent fat (total fat 4.2 g, saturated fat 0.5 g)** ▪ **52 percent carbohydrate (12.7 g fiber)** ▪ **29 percent protein.**

Q

C –COMFORT FOOD

Q –QUICK FIX FOOD

A –ADVENTUROUS

S –SPECIAL OCCASION

Desserts, Chocolate, and Other Sweets

Curbing Sweet Cravings

IT'S AMAZING WHAT we do to soothe a sweet tooth:

- It's late at night and you're driving to the ice cream parlor in your ratty pj's to satisfy a craving for a scoop of mocha almond fudge ice cream.

- You tear up the kitchen, opening drawers, rifling through cabinets, frantically searching for that last chocolate mint granola bar.

- You've driven all the way to your in-laws focused on one thought, that homemade cheesecake your mother-in-law will be serving for dessert.

- You ache for a chocolate chip cookie but snack instead on a tub of yogurt, a bag of chips, a can of soda, and a few bites of last night's casserole. You're stuffed and still craving the cookie.

Almost all women, most dieters, and 7 out of 10 men admit they give in to cravings on occasion. Most cravings are for sweets, typically sweet and creamy foods, such as ice cream, chocolate, cookies, or pastries. In many cases, the yearning is just a need to reward ourselves or relieve boredom. In other cases, daily cravings can undermine our best intentions to eat well.

Why do we crave chocolate when our bodies need vegetables? As my daughter says, "It's a no-brainer; chocolate tastes better!" That statement appears straightforward at face value, but the chemistry that drives us to indulge is so complex it has most experts baffled. According to recent research, sugar might even be addicting.

Your Sweet Origins

It is difficult to imagine in this era of gluttony, but for 99.9 percent of the millions of years our ancestors walked the earth, finding food was a challenge. To survive, our Stone Age ancestors needed concentrated calories—the sweet and greasy foods that pack the greatest calorie punch per bite. These foods were rare and limited to fruit or honey in season, wild game, and a few nuts, seeds, and avocados. As a result, the human body evolved complex appetite-control systems to ensure we eat enough when these foods are around and to drive us to look for them when they're not.

The elaborate control center for cravings is located in the brain, where such chemicals as neuropeptide Y (NPY) and serotonin increase our yearnings for carbohydrate-rich foods. Today, those chemicals create a strong desire for any starch or sweet, from cereal, pasta, and rice to cakes, cookies, and pies. Other chemicals in the brain, such as galanin and the endorphins, drive our modern desires for fatty foods, such as pizza, hamburgers, chocolate, fries, and chips. There appears to be no chemistry driving us to crave low-calorie, fiber-rich broccoli, chard, or lima beans, so we depend on our highly evolved rational minds to make these food choices!

In addition to these internal controls, many sweets tickle our brain chemistry from the outside in. Chocolate contains theobromine and caffeine, both central nervous system stimulants that pack an energy kick; phenylethylamine (PEA), a nerve chemical that produces warm-fuzzy feelings; and cannabinoids such as anandamide that produce the "high" as well as the food munchies associated with marijuana. You must eat a lot of chocolate, say 50 pounds, to get an anandamide "high" or a PEA rush, but the complex chemistry of this sweet helps explain why it's the number one food that people crave. (Of course, there is also that irresistible melt-in-your-mouth creamy texture, but that's another story!)

Are You a Sugar Addict?

People have confided in me for years about their addictions to sugar. They say they must have something sweet every day. They get irritable, have headaches, and even start to sweat or shake when they avoid sweets. The cravings subside after a few weeks of abstinence, only to return if sugar even graces their lips. I always sympathized (I have a bit of a chocolate addiction, too), but there was no research to support this phenomenon.

12 QUICK-FIX DESSERTS

1. **BERRY PARFAIT:** Layer fresh raspberries and lemon low-fat yogurt in parfait glasses. Top with a dollop of nonfat dairy topping.

2. **CHOCOLATE CHIP FROZEN YOGURT:** Mix chocolate chips into softened nonfat vanilla or coffee-flavored frozen yogurt.

3. **FRUIT DUNK:** Dip fresh strawberries in fat-free dark-chocolate syrup.

4. **ICE CREAM COOKIES:** Spread softened fat-free ice cream (vanilla, chocolate, coffee, or your favorite flavor) onto the flat side of chocolate wafer cookies. Top each with another wafer cookie. Wrap in Saran Wrap and freeze until ready to serve.

5. **FROZEN YOGURT PIE:** Fill a commercial graham cracker crust with softened fat-free frozen yogurt (any flavor). Freeze. When ready to serve, cut into individual servings and top with fresh fruit and fat-free dairy topping.

6. **RASPBERRY BROWNIE SUNDAE:** Top a low-fat commercial brownie with a scoop of fat-free vanilla yogurt and warmed raspberry all-fruit jam.

7. **STRAWBERRY SHORTCAKE:** Top a thin slice of commercial fat-free pound cake, angel food cake, or leftover cake from the Mixed Berry Trifle (page 244) with fresh strawberries and fat-free whipped topping.

8. **BLUEBERRY FROZEN YOGURT:** Mix fresh blueberries and a little honey into softened fat-free vanilla yogurt.

9. **HAVE YOUR CAKE:** Top store-bought angel food cake with fresh raspberries.

10. **STRAWBERRY CUSTARD SUNDAE:** Layer instant sugar-free vanilla pudding, fresh strawberries, and crushed low-fat vanilla wafers in a tall glass and top with fat-free dessert topping.

11. **CHOCOLATE FONDUE:** Melt semisweet chocolate, and add fat-free dark-chocolate syrup, fat-free half-and-half, a touch of orange liqueur, and a splash of rum or rum extract. Dip banana slices and fresh strawberries.

12. **ORANGES WITH A ZING:** Top canned mandarin oranges with crystallized ginger.

Granted, research from Johns Hopkins and Cornell Universities had shown that the very taste of sugar on the tongue has a calming effect in infants and raises levels of endorphins in the brains of animals. These endorphins are morphinelike chemicals that produce a pleasurable feeling, so it was theorized that perhaps people become addicted to an endorphin "high" brought on by sugar. Withdrawal symptoms may result when the brain doesn't get its "fix" of endorphins, just as a drug addict goes through withdrawals when the drug is withheld. All of this was speculation—until recently.

Preliminary research on animals at Princeton University has added credibility to the suspicion that sugar is addicting. Animals fed high-sugar diets exhibit all the symptoms of withdrawal, including agitation and nervousness, when sugar is taken away; reintroduce sugar to their diets, and the animals binge—all of which are classic symptoms of substance abuse. Changes in the animals' brains also resemble changes seen in morphine and heroin addiction. The researchers theorize that the sweet taste releases endorphins in the brain, making the snack pleasurable. Another neurotransmitter called dopamine permanently stamps the experience into our memory banks to entice us to seek this yummy taste again. The response is so powerful that even the sight of the food, let alone the smell, at a later date will release dopamine and a craving for another taste.

Sugar Binge

Obviously, addiction to drugs is a much more serious issue than sugar dependency. Besides, all the studies on sugar dependency have been on animals, not people. We are much more socially and intellectually complex in our food choices than a lab rat. However, drug addicts, alcoholics, and smokers all crave sugar during recovery, which suggests that sugar dependency might also be a problem for people.

In the United States, our love affair with sugar has grown to obsessive proportions. My father, growing up on a farm in Oregon in the early 1900s, consumed about 4 teaspoons of added sugar a day, which Grandma used in her homemade pies, jams, and breads. Fast-forward to 2002, when each American averaged 31 teaspoons of added sugar every day, an almost eightfold increase in the past 100 years, and three times the recommended upper limit of 10 teaspoons. If you are that average person, you ate almost 100 pounds of added sugar last year! Never in the history of the human species or the planet has any animal ever eaten so much refined sugar. There appears to be no limit to our sugar cravings.

Our bodies weren't designed to eat this much sugar. Our Stone Age ancestors only had mangos, figs, honey, apples, and other fruits to satisfy their sweet teeth. The natural sugar in fruits comes packaged with fiber, water, vitamins, minerals, and thousands of health-enhancing phytochemicals. In contrast, the vast majority of the sugar most people eat today is refined sugar added to nutrient-depleted, processed foods. You don't even benefit from the sweetness, since much of that sugar is hidden in regular foods like tomato soup, flavored hot cereals, baked beans, hot dogs, catsup, and other processed foods, which average three to nine teaspoons of sugar per serving. Hey, if I'm going to squander my sugar allowance, at least let it be on something deliciously sweet!

Granted, the body doesn't care whether glucose comes from a date or a doughnut. But, ounce for ounce, the doughnut has seven times more calories, lots more fat, and none of the phytochemicals in fruit. We currently average 500 calories from refined sugar every day. In a study at the University of Minnesota, researchers found that the more refined foods a person eats, the higher the calorie intake and the lower the intake of vitamins, minerals, and other health-enhancing compounds. According to another study from the Harvard School of Public Health, children's weight problems are directly proportional to how many soft drinks (the number one source of sugar) they drink. Granted, people gain weight when they eat too many calories, regardless of which kind, but we obviously have a major problem with sugar!

The 12-Step Program

Wouldn't it be great if cravings were simple signals from our bodies to restock necessary nutrients? If that was the case, young women would crave iron-rich spinach and kidney beans, middle-age women would crave calcium-rich nonfat milk, and everyone would yearn for more kale, tofu, and Brussels sprouts. Instead, our ancient brain chemistry compels us to seek sweets, which typically are some of the highest fat and calorie items on the menu.

Never fear. You can have your cake and eat it, too. Just follow the 12 simple steps in the box below—many of which are used in the recipes in this section—for taming your sweet tooth.

1.   **EAT SMALL PORTIONS.** Don't deprive yourself of your favorite treats—it will only backfire and lead to bingeing. Instead, make room in your diet for a thin slice of Lemon Cheesecake Piled High with Blueberries (page 236) or a small bowl of The Ultimate Bittersweet Chocolate Pudding (page 242), and enjoy every bite. Remember, the first two bites will satisfy your brain chemistry; anything after that is pure indulgence. We have focused on highly flavorful, small portions in the dessert recipes that follow.

2. STICK TO THE GOOD STUFF. Just because it's there, doesn't mean you have to eat it. Skip the boxed cookies, the commercial doughnuts, and the cheap candy bars; instead, focus on small amounts of the best desserts, which are the most satisfying.

3. SKIP OR SPLIT DESSERTS. Drink a cup of coffee instead of having a dessert or share a dessert with two other people.

4. PLAN AHEAD. Bring healthful foods with you so you're not caught short midafternoon when sweet cravings are at an all-time high.

5. GET STRUCTURED. People who eat regularly throughout the day, starting with breakfast, are less prone to out-of-control cravings for sweets.

6. SET GROUND RULES. Establish rules about when and how you will indulge, such as not eating at the kitchen counter, out of the pie pan, off someone else's dessert plate, or while doing anything else.

7. PAMPER YOURSELF. Find nonfood ways to feel good, such as a bubble bath, quiet time to read the newspaper, or a romp with the dog.

8. TAKE INVENTORY. Cravers often report they feel tired, depressed, anxious, or bored just before they dive for the sweets. Before you grab a couple of Chocolate Chip Granola Cookies (page 254), ask yourself if you're really hungry or if you're trying to soothe a mood with food. Have the cookies if you're hungry; find another alternative if you're not.

9. GO FOR THE GOLD. If you really want Creamy, Low-Fat Fudge (page 235), chances are a bowl of fruit won't do. Listen to your cravings and satisfy them with a small amount of the desired food.

10. READ LABELS. Added sugars are not distinguished from natural sugars on labels, so go directly to the ingredients list. High-sugar items are those with sugar or any of its nicknames (glucose, sucrose, high-fructose corn syrup, dextrose, corn syrup, brown sugar, honey) as the top three ingredients or with several mentions of sugar. (Remember, 4 grams of sugar equals 1 teaspoon.) Switch to unsweetened foods, such as applesauce, plain yogurt, and instant oatmeal, and flavor them at home.

11. CUT BACK. Limit sweetened soft drinks to one or two servings a week. In the recipes that follow, we cut back on sugar by using sugar substitutes, such as Splenda, and fat by using fat substitutes, such as baby food prunes, which cut calories without sacrificing taste and texture.

12. SPICE IT UP. In the following recipes we use sweet-tasting (calorie-free) spices, such as vanilla, cinnamon, mint, and nutmeg, to offset the reduced sugar content.

Creamy, Low-Fat Fudge

Fudge is notoriously high in fat, sugar, and calories. But, hey, what are the holidays without it? This yummy fudge takes some of the guilt out of indulgence. By using fat-free instead of whole evaporated milk, prunes instead of fat, and Splenda to replace much of the sugar, this fudge tastes just like the original but packs a much lower calorie, fat, and sugar punch.

---

2 tablespoons salted butter

1½ cups sugar

1 cup Splenda

⅔ cup fat-free evaporated milk

16 ounces semisweet chocolate chips

1 (2.5-ounce) jar of baby prunes

1 (7-ounce) jar of marshmallow creme

⅓ cup walnuts, chopped

2 teaspoons vanilla extract

1 Line a 13-by-9-by-2-inch baking pan with wax or parchment paper, extending the paper over the edges of the pan. Set aside.

2 In a large saucepan, melt butter over medium heat. Stir in sugar, Splenda, and milk. Bring mixture to a boil, stirring constantly. Boil gently for 5 minutes, stirring constantly.

3 Remove saucepan from heat and slowly stir in chocolate chips. Stir until chocolate melts. Then stir in prunes, marshmallow creme, walnuts, and vanilla until well combined.

4 Spread mixture in the prepared pan. Chill in refrigerator until firm (overnight or at least 3 hours). To serve, use the wax or parchment paper to lift fudge from pan. Cut into pieces. Keep extra pieces refrigerated.

MAKES 48 PIECES

NUTRITIONAL ANALYSIS PER PIECE **94 calories** ▪ **34 percent fat (total fat 3.5 g, saturated fat 2 g)** ▪ **64 percent carbohydrate (0.8 g fiber)** ▪ **2 percent protein.**

Lemon Cheesecake
Piled High with Blueberries

This dessert is creamy and flavorful yet derives only a fraction of its calories from fat. It's easy to make, too.

CHEESECAKE

cooking spray

$\frac{1}{3}$ cup graham cracker crumbs

24 ounces fat-free cream cheese, at room temperature

8 ounces low-fat cream cheese, at room temperature

$1\frac{3}{4}$ cups white sugar

$\frac{3}{4}$ cup fat-free half-and-half

$\frac{1}{4}$ cup fresh lemon juice

2 tablespoons lemon peel, finely grated

2 teaspoons vanilla extract

$1\frac{1}{2}$ cups liquid egg substitute (equivalent to 6 eggs)

TOPPING

4 cups blueberries (fresh or frozen)

$\frac{2}{3}$ cup white sugar

3 tablespoons fresh lemon juice

1 tablespoon cornstarch

Preheat oven to 350°.

1   Spray the bottom and sides of a 9-inch-diameter springform pan with 3-inch sides. Sprinkle graham cracker crumbs in pan and tilt pan to spread evenly over bottom and sides, leaving extra crumbs on bottom.

2   Beat cream cheese and sugar with an electric beater until creamy and well blended. Slowly add half-and-half, lemon juice, lemon peel, and vanilla and continue to beat. Add egg substitute until mixture is thoroughly blended and creamy. Pour into crumb-lined pan.

3   Place springform pan in large roasting pan. Pour enough water into roasting pan to come halfway up sides of springform pan (no higher, or water will bubble into cheese-cake during baking). Bake cheesecake until firm, slightly golden, and sides crack, about 1 hour 25 minutes. Remove springform pan from water and refrigerate, uncovered, until cold (about 3 hours or overnight).

4   To prepare topping: Place blueberries, sugar, and lemon juice in a nonstick saucepan over medium heat and stir gently until sugar dissolves and juices form. Continue heating for 5 minutes. Remove $\frac{1}{2}$ cup of juice, add cornstarch, and stir until cornstarch is completely dissolved. Pour juice-cornstarch mixture into blueberries and stir over high heat until mixture boils and thickens slightly. Remove from heat, cool completely, then refrigerate for at least 1 hour or until ready to serve cheesecake.

5   To serve cheesecake: Run knife around sides of cheesecake and remove springform pan sides. Top each slice with a generous helping of the blueberry sauce.

MAKES 12 SERVINGS

NUTRITIONAL ANALYSIS PER SERVING **343 calories** ▪ **14 percent fat (total fat 5.24 g, saturated fat 2.47 g)** ▪ **67 percent carbohydrate (1.3 g fiber)** ▪ **19 percent protein.**

Citrus-Scented Caramel Flan

This homemade creamy, yet light, custard has a hint of orange. It is the queen of simple, with only four ingredients and no baking. Chill thoroughly before serving.

FOOD TIP

Flan is the dessert of Spain and Latin America, although also a favorite in France, where it is called crème caramel. Flan is a stiff egg custard baked in a mold with caramel sauce on the bottom. When served, it is turned upside down so the caramel sauce drizzles from the top and down the sides.

2 (3-ounce) packages Jell-O Flan (Spanish-style custard)

zest of 1 orange

3 cups fat-free half-and-half

1 cup fat-free condensed milk

light whipped cream

1   Pour both packets of caramel sauce (from Jell-O Flan) into a 9-inch nonstick cake pan. Rotate pan to help evenly distribute sauce to cover pan bottom. (Sauce will not completely cover pan at this point.) Sprinkle orange zest evenly over sauce. Set aside.

2   In a medium saucepan, whisk together 2 packages of dry flan ingredients, half-and-half, and condensed milk. Bring mixture to a boil over medium heat, stirring constantly. (Liquid will be thin.) Remove from heat. Pour hot mixture carefully over sauce. Refrigerate overnight.

3   To serve, run a knife between flan and pan edge. Invert cake pan on a flat cake dish. Hold tightly together. Flan will slip off onto dish. Cut into 8 wedges and use a pie server to transfer to plates. Garnish each slice with light whipped cream if desired.

MAKES 8 SERVINGS

NUTRITIONAL ANALYSIS PER SERVING **245 calories** ▪ **< 1 percent fat (total fat < 0.5 g, saturated fat 0 g)** ▪ **90 percent carbohydrate (0 g fiber)** ▪ **10 percent protein.**

Individual Bread Puddings with Brandy White Sauce

Who doesn't love old-fashioned bread pudding! These wonderful treasures are served hot from muffin pans. A fun and easy way to impress family and friends, and ideal for portion control.

BREAD PUDDING

cooking spray

1 cup fat-free half-and-half

½ cup nonfat milk

1 tablespoon butter

½ cup liquid egg substitute (equivalent to 2 eggs)

½ cup sugar

1 teaspoon ground cinnamon

1 teaspoon vanilla extract

6 cups dry bread cubes (8 slices bread of your choice)

¼ cup dried currants

2 tablespoons brandy or bourbon

SAUCE

1 cup plus 2 teaspoons fat-free half-and-half

2 teaspoons cornstarch

1 tablespoon Splenda

1 tablespoon brandy or bourbon

Preheat oven to 400°. Coat a 12-cup muffin pan with cooking spray.

1 In a medium saucepan, add half-and-half, milk, and butter. Cook over medium heat until butter is melted and milk is hot. Set aside.

2 In a large bowl, mix egg substitute, sugar, cinnamon, and vanilla. Stir in bread cubes. Add warm milk mixture and blend thoroughly.

3 In a small bowl, place currants and brandy. Heat in the microwave for 1 minute. Add to bread mixture and stir well.

4 Scoop about ¼ cup of bread pudding mixture into each cup and bake for 30 minutes, or until golden brown.

5 To prepare sauce: Place 1 cup half-and-half in a small saucepan, and simmer over medium heat. In a small cup, mix cornstarch and 2 remaining teaspoons of the half-and-half. Add to saucepan, increase heat to medium-high, and let mixture boil for 1 to 2 minutes, stirring frequently until thickened. Remove from heat, add Splenda and brandy. Mix well.

6 Serve bread puddings on dessert plates. Drizzle with warm sauce.

MAKES 12 SERVINGS

NUTRITIONAL ANALYSIS PER BREAD PUDDING **160 calories** ▪ **13 percent fat (total fat 2.3 g, saturated fat 1 g)** ▪ **70 percent carbohydrate (3 percent alcohol; 1 g fiber)** ▪ **14 percent protein.**

C

Low-Fat Panna Cotta with Fresh Raspberry Sauce

This delicate, smooth cream is so delicious you won't believe that it's almost fat-free (traditional panna cotta is 69 percent fat calories!) and has a third of the calories of the original version. Cool this cream in custard cups or ramekins as described below (this is the best presentation when drizzling sauces over the dessert), or pour liquid mixture into parfait or wineglasses, chill, and serve with chunks of fresh fruit, such as mango, apricots, berries, or kiwi. The raspberry sauce is also a delicious topping for ice cream or chunks of mango.

FOOD TIP
Panna cotta is a delicate "cooked cream" pudding from Italy. It can be flavored with a variety of ingredients, including cinnamon, lemon or orange zest, or rum extract.

PANNA COTTA
3 tablespoons water
2½ teaspoons unflavored gelatin
1 cup fat-free half-and-half
4 tablespoons sugar
3 tablespoons Splenda
1½ cups low-fat buttermilk

1 teaspoon vanilla extract

SAUCE
2 cups fresh raspberries (if necessary, substitute frozen raspberries or any other berry)
2½ tablespoons sugar
1 teaspoon fresh lemon juice

1   Pour water into a small bowl and sprinkle with gelatin. Stir and let stand for 5 minutes until gelatin softens and forms a stiff gel.

2   Combine half-and-half, sugar, and Splenda in medium saucepan and warm over medium-high heat until just about to boil. Remove from heat, add gelatin mixture, and stir until gelatin is completely dissolved and mixture is smooth. Set aside and cool, approximately 45 minutes.

3   Stir buttermilk and vanilla into cream mixture. Pour into 6 custard cups or ramekins. Refrigerate for 3 hours or until panna cotta is completely set.

4   Run thin sharp knife around edges and set each ramekin in hot water for 1 minute to loosen gel. Place plate on top of ramekin and invert to allow panna cotta to settle onto plate.

5   To prepare sauce: Blend berries in food processor or blender. Pass liquified berries through a fine sieve, pressing with spatula, to remove all seeds. Whisk sugar and lemon juice into berry liquid.

6   Pour sauce over panna cotta and serve. Sauce can be stored in a well-sealed container in the refrigerator for up to 1 week.

MAKES 6 SERVINGS OF PANNA COTTA AND ABOUT 1 CUP OF SAUCE

NUTRITIONAL ANALYSIS PER SERVING OF PANNA COTTA **90 calories ▪ 6 percent fat (total fat 0.5 g, saturated fat 0 g) ▪ 73 percent carbohydrate (0 g fiber) ▪ 21 percent protein.**

NUTRITIONAL ANALYSIS PER 1-OUNCE SERVING OF SAUCE **38 calories ▪ 4 percent fat (total fat < 0.5 g, saturated fat 0 g) ▪ 93 percent carbohydrate (1 g fiber) ▪ 3 percent protein.**

S

The Ultimate Bittersweet Chocolate Pudding

This bittersweet chocolate pudding is so rich and thick, you'll be satisfied with less. It's also low in fat and sugar. Top with low-fat whipped topping, just eat it plain, or pour into a graham cracker crust for an ultra-rich chocolate cream pie.

MOOD TIP

Sugar substitutes do not promote hunger or cause people to eat more food later in the day, according to a study from the University of Michigan.

2½ cups nonfat milk

1 cup Dutch processed cocoa powder

1½ tablespoons cornstarch

dash of salt

1 cup fat-free half-and-half

½ cup sugar

½ cup Splenda

¼ cup liquid egg substitute (equivalent to 1 whole egg)

1 large egg yolk, lightly beaten

1 ounce bittersweet chocolate, broken into small chunks

2 teaspoons vanilla extract

1   In a large bowl, combine 1 cup milk, cocoa, cornstarch, and salt. Mix thoroughly. Set aside.

2   In a medium saucepan, place remaining 1½ cups milk and half-and-half. Cook over medium heat, stirring constantly, until hot but not boiling. Remove from heat and add sugar and Splenda. Stir with a whisk until smooth and sugar has dissolved. Add cocoa mixture and stir until thoroughly blended. Return to heat and bring to boil. Cook for 1 minute, stirring constantly with a whisk. Remove from heat and set aside.

3   In a medium bowl, combine egg substitute and egg yolk. Gradually add hot milk–cocoa mixture, stirring constantly with a whisk. Return to saucepan and cook over medium heat until pudding thickens and bubbles, approximately 3 minutes.

4   Remove pudding from heat, add bittersweet chocolate shavings and vanilla. Stir until chocolate dissolves. Spoon into pudding cups, cover with plastic wrap, and refrigerate until firm.

MAKES 8 SERVINGS OF ½ CUP EACH

NUTRITIONAL ANALYSIS PER ½ CUP **157 calories** ▪ **22 percent fat (total fat 3.8 g** ▪ **saturated fat 2 g)** ▪ **62 percent carbohydrate (3.8 g fiber)** ▪ **16 percent protein.**

C

Ricotta Tart with Strawberry Coulis

Although ricotta is typically used in traditional Italian dishes like lasagna and stuffed manicotti, its slightly sweet and creamy flavor and consistency work well in desserts. Read labels carefully, since some ricotta contains up to 4 grams of fat per ounce. Nonfat ricotta is what you want. Both the ricotta tart and coulis in this recipe can be prepared a day ahead and refrigerated.

MOOD TIP

Lemons are a great source of vitamin C, and the peel (also called zest) is rich in limonene and coumarin, phytochemicals that help the body eliminate toxins.

COULIS

2 cups fresh strawberries, cleaned, hulled, and coarsely chopped (or use frozen strawberries)

¼ cup water

3 tablespoons Splenda

2 teaspoons fresh lemon juice

TART

cooking spray

1 Pillsbury pie crust (unfold, fill, and bake)

1 (15-ounce) container fat-free ricotta cheese, drained

⅓ cup sugar

⅓ cup Splenda

¼ cup liquid egg substitute (equivalent to 1 whole egg)

2 tablespoons cornstarch

1 teaspoon vanilla extract

¼ teaspoon almond extract

zest of 1 small orange

zest of 1 small lemon

powdered sugar

1   To prepare coulis: Combine strawberries, water, Splenda, and lemon juice in blender. Puree until smooth. Cover and refrigerate until well chilled, at least 2 hours.

2   Preheat oven to 350°. Spray a 10-inch tart pan with cooking spray.

3   Unfold pie crust and position in tart pan. Gently press dough to cover bottom and sides of pan. Set aside.

4   In a medium bowl, combine drained ricotta cheese and remaining ingredients, except for powdered sugar. Mix well. Pour into prepared tart pan and bake for 45 to 50 minutes or until filling is set in center.

5   When ready to serve, remove side of tart pan and cut tart into 12 servings. Place each slice on a dessert plate. Spoon strawberry coulis over top and sprinkle with powdered sugar.

MAKES 12 SERVINGS

NUTRITIONAL ANALYSIS PER SERVING **216 calories** ▪ **31 percent fat (total fat 7.4 g, saturated fat 3 g)** ▪ **53 percent carbohydrate (1 g fiber)** ▪ **16 percent protein.**

S

Mixed Berry Trifle

Make the pudding and cake ahead of time, assemble in the evening, and let this dessert blend its flavors overnight or through the day and you have a delicious dessert for company or family with no last-minute preparation. If you want to splurge, use real whipped cream instead of the dessert topping (this adds 24 more calories and 2 grams of saturated fat per serving). Bake the leftover cake mix and freeze to use for strawberry shortcake at a later date. An extra bonus, this dessert supplies a third of your daily requirement for vitamin C and 25 percent of that for calcium and vitamin B_2.

FOOD TIP

Stock up on fresh berries when they are in season and less expensive. Spread them unwashed on a cookie sheet and freeze. Once frozen, you can transfer them to freezer bags. In the winter, they are a refreshing addition to desserts, salads, and smoothies. They also make a great garnish for roast chicken, pork tenderloin, and duck or Cornish game hens.

cooking spray

1 box commercial white or yellow cake mix (French vanilla works especially well)

¼ cup canola oil

¾ cup liquid egg substitute (equivalent to 3 whole eggs)

⅔ cup water

1 (4.6-ounce) box vanilla pudding

2 cups fat-free evaporated milk

1 cup nonfat milk

2 (16-ounce) bags frozen mixed berries (strawberries, blackberries, raspberries, blueberries), thawed

1 (50-ml) bottle Grand Marnier

2 tablespoons sugar

1½ teaspoons lemon zest, finely grated

1 cup fat-free whipped topping

1 tablespoon sliced almonds

Coat a loaf pan with cooking spray. Preheat oven to 350°.

1   Place cake mix, oil, egg substitute, and water in a large bowl and beat with an electric mixer for 2 minutes (or stir by hand for 3 minutes). Don't overbeat. Pour enough batter into loaf pan to fill pan halfway up the sides. (You will have about a third of the batter left over, which you can bake in a separate pan for later use.) Bake for 35 minutes or until toothpick inserted in center comes out clean. Remove cake from pan and cool completely. Cut 7 slices of cake, each ⅔ inch thick. (Freeze the remaining quarter of cake.)

2   Make pudding according to directions on box, except use evaporated milk and nonfat milk. Pour into bowl, cover with plastic wrap so that top does not form a skin, and refrigerate until completely cool.

3   Place berries in a colander and drain some of the excess juice. Transfer berries to a large bowl and mix with Grand Marnier, sugar, and lemon juice. Set aside.

4   Assemble the trifle in a 2½-quart glass serving bowl. Arrange half the cake pieces snugly in the bottom of the bowl (break them into pieces if needed). Spoon half the berries with their juices over the cake slices. Spoon half the pudding over the berries and spread evenly to coat top. Repeat, ending with pudding. Cover with plastic wrap and refrigerate for at least 4 hours and up to 1 day.

5   Just before serving, top trifle with dollops of dessert topping and sprinkle with almonds.

MAKES 12 SERVINGS

NUTRITIONAL ANALYSIS PER SERVING **330 calories** ▪ **22 percent fat (total fat 8 g, saturated fat 1 g)**
▪ **67 percent carbohydrate (3.3 g fiber)** ▪ **11 percent protein.**

S

Carrot Cake with Coconut Cream Frosting

Traditional carrot cake has up to one and a half cups of salad oil, two to three whole eggs, and two cups of sugar. And that's not including the cream cheese frosting. This carrot cake has one-fifth the fat, half the sugar, and no cholesterol, yet it is light, moist, and rich with traditional carrot cake flavor. Top the cake with fluffy coconut cream frosting, and you can have your cake and eat it, too! The flavors improve with time, so make the cake and frost it the day before and store in the refrigerator.

CAKE

cooking spray

2 cups all-purpose flour

1 teaspoon baking powder

½ teaspoon baking soda

¼ teaspoon salt

2 teaspoons ground cinnamon

½ teaspoon ground nutmeg

⅛ teaspoon ground allspice

½ cup sugar

½ cup Splenda

⅓ cup light coconut milk

2 tablespoons canola oil

½ cup liquid egg substitute
(equivalent to 2 whole eggs)

1 teaspoon vanilla extract

2 cups carrots, peeled and shredded

1 (8-ounce) can crushed pineapple
in juice, undrained

⅓ cup low-fat buttermilk

FROSTING

1 envelope dessert topping dry mix
(such as Dream Whip)

½ cup nonfat milk

½ teaspoon vanilla extract

3 tablespoons nonfat cream cheese

1 tablespoon Splenda

½ teaspoon coconut flavoring or
extract

2 tablespoons flaked coconut

Preheat oven to 325°. Spray 2 (8-inch) round cake pans with cooking spray. Set aside.

1   In a medium bowl, stir together flour, baking powder, baking soda, salt, cinnamon, nutmeg, allspice, sugar, and Splenda.

2   In a large bowl, beat coconut milk, oil, and egg substitute. Add vanilla, shredded carrots, pineapple, and buttermilk. Mix well.

3   Add liquid ingredients to flour mix. Stir until evenly moistened. Pour mixture into prepared pans and bake for 20 to 25 minutes or until center of cake springs back when touched.

4   To prepare frosting: In a deep bowl, place dessert topping dry mix, milk, and vanilla. With an electric mixer, beat on low speed for 30 seconds, then on high speed for 4 minutes or until topping thickens. Add cream cheese, Splenda, coconut flavoring, and flaked coconut and beat until smooth. Cover and chill frosting for at least 1 hour. Best if chilled overnight.

5   Once cake is cool, top with chilled frosting and keep refrigerated.

MAKES 10 SERVINGS

NUTRITIONAL ANALYSIS PER SERVING **235 calories** ▪ **22 percent fat (total fat 5.7 g, saturated fat 2.5 g)** ▪ **67 percent carbohydrate (1.7 g fiber)** ▪ **11 percent protein.**

C S

Lemon Bundt Cake with Raspberry Filling

This cake is incredibly moist with lots of lemony flavor, yet low in fat and calories. It's also quick and easy to prepare.

cooking spray

1 (1 pound, 2.25-ounce) box reduced-fat lemon cake mix

1¼ cups water

⅓ cup fat-free sour cream

½ cup liquid egg substitute (equivalent to 2 whole eggs)

zest of 1 lemon

⅔ cup red raspberry filling (Solo brand comes in 12-ounce cans)

1 tablespoon powered sugar

Preheat oven to 350°. Coat a 12-cup bundt cake pan with cooking spray. Set aside.

1   In a large bowl, place cake mix, water, sour cream, egg substitute, and lemon zest. Beat on low speed of mixer for 30 seconds, then on medium speed for 2 minutes.

2   Pour a third of the batter into a prepared bundt cake pan. Dollop raspberry filling in center of batter. Pour the remaining batter over the raspberry filling. Spread evenly.

3   Bake for 40 to 45 minutes or until toothpick inserted in center comes out clean. Don't overbake.

4   Cool cake for 20 minutes in pan. Invert cake onto a serving plate. When cool, sprinkle with powered sugar.

MAKES 16 SERVINGS

NUTRITIONAL ANALYSIS PER SERVING 186 calories ▪ 18 percent fat (total fat 3.7 g, saturated fat < 1 g) ▪ 76 percent carbohydrate (0.5 g fiber) ▪ 6 percent protein.

Q

Mixed Berries with Custard Sauce

This light-custard sauce enhances the sweet natural flavors of fresh berries.

---

1 cup nonfat milk

1 cup fat-free half-and-half

2 tablespoons cornstarch

½ cup liquid egg substitute (equivalent to 2 whole eggs)

¼ cup Splenda

1 teaspoon vanilla extract

1 tablespoon bourbon, brandy, or Grand Marnier (or substitute brandy-flavored extract)

2 cups fresh strawberries, cleaned and hulled

2 cups fresh blueberries, cleaned and dried

ground nutmeg

1   In a heavy saucepan over medium-high heat, place milk, half-and-half, and cornstarch. Whisk constantly until mixture boils and thickens, about 3 minutes.

2   Remove from heat and add egg substitute and Splenda. Return to medium-high heat and whisk until mixture comes to a boil. Continue to cook for 1 minute, stirring constantly.

3   Remove from heat and mix in vanilla and bourbon. Cool to room temperature. (This sauce can be made a day ahead, covered, and kept refrigerated. When ready to serve, whisk in additional milk to thin.)

4   Divide berries among 4 dessert bowls or cups. Spoon custard sauce over the top. Sprinkle with nutmeg and serve. Serve cold or reheat in microwave until warm.

MAKES 4 SERVINGS

NUTRITIONAL ANALYSIS PER SERVING **173 calories** ▪ **9 percent fat (total fat 1.7 g,** saturated fat < 0.5 g) ▪ 66 percent carbohydrate (3.6 g fiber) ▪ 21 percent protein, 4 percent alcohol.

Busy-Day Brownies

These moist, cakelike brownies are quick and easy to prepare yet have no added fat.

---

cooking spray

1 (1 pound, 3.8-ounce) box of fudge brownie mix

¼ cup prune-plum filling or baby prunes

⅓ cup warm water

¼ cup fat-free sour cream

½ cup liquid egg substitute (equivalent to 2 whole eggs)

cooking spray

Heat oven to 350°. Spray an 8-by-8-inch baking pan with cooking spray. Set aside.

1   Place brownie mix in a medium bowl and set aside.

2   In a small bowl, combine prune filling, water, and sour cream. Mix well.

3   Add prune mixture and egg substitute to brownie mix. Stir until well blended and smooth.

4   Spread brownie mixture evenly in prepared pan and bake for 20 to 25 minutes or until top is soft but not firm. Don't overbake.

5   Cool for 5 minutes, cut into 20 equal-sized portions, and remove from pan.

MAKES 20 BROWNIES

NUTRITIONAL ANALYSIS PER BROWNIE 129 calories ▪ 25 percent fat (total fat 3.6 g, saturated fat 1.7 g) ▪ 70 percent carbohydrate (0 g fiber) ▪ 5 percent protein.

Poached Pears with Chocolate-Orange Sauce

This elegant, low-fat dessert is perfect for special occasions.

2 cups water

⅓ cup honey

½ teaspoon ground cinnamon

¼ teaspoon ground nutmeg

2 strips orange peel from 1 medium orange (zest the remaining peel for chocolate sauce)

3 large fresh, firm pears (Anjou, Bartlett, or Comice), peeled, halved, and seeded

2 tablespoons Dutch processed cocoa powder

½ teaspoon vanilla extract

½ to 1 teaspoon Grand Marnier

pinch of ground nutmeg

1   Combine water, honey, cinnamon, nutmeg, and orange peel in a large saucepan or skillet. Mix well. Bring to a boil over medium-high heat.

2   Add pears. Reduce heat to medium-low and simmer, covered, until pears are just tender but still firm, about 10 to 15 minutes. Using a slotted spoon, transfer pears to a large bowl.

3   Boil poaching liquid until reduced to half, about 2 to 3 minutes, stirring frequently. Remove from heat. Pour 2 tablespoons poaching liquid over pears in bowl.

4   To remaining poaching liquid, add cocoa powder and remaining orange zest. Whisk well until chocolate melts and sauce is smooth.

5   Return chocolate sauce to medium-high heat. Whisk chocolate sauce to a gentle boil for 1 minute. Remove from heat, add vanilla and Grand Marnier, stir well.

6   Place 1 pear half on each plate. Sprinkle with nutmeg and drizzle with warm chocolate-orange sauce. (You can cover pears and sauce separately and refrigerate for up to 2 days. In this case, serve pears cold but reheat sauce in the microwave for 1 minute on high power.)

MAKES 6 SERVINGS OF ½ PEAR EACH

NUTRITIONAL ANALYSIS PER SERVING **124 calories** ▪ **4 percent fat (total fat < 1 g, saturated fat 0 g)** ▪ **93 percent carbohydrate (3.7 g fiber)** ▪ **2 percent protein, 1 percent alcohol.**

Baked Stuffed Apples with Toasted Walnuts, Currants, and Maple Syrup

Toasting walnuts intensifies the flavor, so you use less in recipes. Toasted wheat germ has a natural nutty flavor; the addition of currants gives it a sweet, rich taste.

2 tablespoons walnuts, chopped

2 tablespoons toasted wheat germ

4 large baking apples (Golden Delicious, Rome, or Granny Smith)

$\frac{1}{3}$ cup dried currants

1 tablespoon brown sugar

2 teaspoons reduced-fat margarine

$\frac{1}{2}$ teaspoon ground cinnamon

4 teaspoons light maple syrup

$1\frac{1}{2}$ cups apple juice

1 tablespoon honey

$\frac{1}{2}$ teaspoon ground nutmeg

$\frac{1}{2}$ cup fat-free half-and-half

Preheat oven to 350°.

1 In a small bowl, combine walnuts and wheat germ. Place together on tinfoil in a single layer and bake for 5 to 6 minutes or until golden brown. Set aside.

2 Using a melon baller, scoop out core of apple. Leave bottom intact. Peel a strip off top quarter of each apple or middle of apple (for decoration). Stand apples in an 8-by-8-inch baking pan. Set aside.

3 In a small bowl, combine walnut–wheat germ mixture, currants, brown sugar, margarine, and cinnamon. Mix into a paste.

4 Fill apple core with about 1 heaping tablespoon of walnut filling. Spoon 1 teaspoon maple syrup into each apple core, drizzling it on top of filling.

5 In a medium bowl, mix apple juice, honey, and nutmeg. Pour into baking pan with apples. Bake apples, uncovered, for about 50 to 60 minutes or until apples are soft when pierced with a fork. Baste several times with apple juice mixture while baking.

6 Cool for 5 minutes. To serve, slice each apple in half lengthwise. Press any loose filling back into each half. Place on individual dessert plates. Drizzle with warm fat-free half-and-half and serve immediately.

MAKES 8 SERVINGS OF $\frac{1}{2}$ APPLE EACH

NUTRITIONAL ANALYSIS PER SERVING **140 calories** ▪ **14 percent fat** (total fat 2.2 g, saturated fat 0 g) ▪ **81 percent carbohydrate** (3 g fiber) ▪ **5 percent protein**.

Strawberry-Blueberry Cobbler

Fruit cobbler is an easy and flexible dish. You can substitute just about any fruit or use a favorite combination. Serve alone or with fat-free vanilla frozen yogurt or fat-free half-and-half.

cooking spray

4 cups strawberries, sliced in half, or 1 (16-ounce) frozen bag

1 cup blueberries, fresh or frozen

⅓ cup Splenda

⅓ cup sugar

2 tablespoons cornstarch

¼ teaspoon ground nutmeg

1 tablespoon fresh lemon juice

½ teaspoon orange peel, dried

TOPPING

1½ cups reduced-fat Bisquick mix

½ cup plus 2 tablespoons nonfat milk

2 tablespoons Splenda

⅛ teaspoon ground nutmeg

Preheat oven to 350°. Spray a 2-quart baking dish with cooking spray and set aside.

1   In a large bowl, gently toss berries with Splenda, sugar, cornstarch, nutmeg, lemon juice, and orange peel. Pour into baking dish.

2   In a medium bowl, blend topping ingredients until well combined. Dollop mixture over berries. (It will not completely cover them.)

3   Bake for 30 to 40 minutes or until topping is golden brown and filling is bubbly.

MAKES 8 SERVINGS

NUTRITIONAL ANALYSIS PER SERVING **150 calories** ▪ **12 percent fat (total fat 2 g, saturated fat 0 g)** ▪ **81 percent carbohydrate (2.6 g fiber)** ▪ **7 percent protein.**

Rum-Scented Pear Clafouti

Although clafouti traditionally resembles a thin pancake, this low-fat recipe is a deep-dish version laced with a bit of rum flavoring. It is also good with sliced apples or pitted cherries. You can cut an additional 40 calories by using Splenda instead of sugar.

FOOD TIP
A custardlike dessert with French origins, clafouti is a simple dessert that combines an easy batter with fresh fruit.

cooking spray

1 tablespoon butter

4 large Anjou pears, peeled, seeded, and sliced thin

1 cup liquid egg substitute (equivalent to 4 whole eggs)

½ cup nonfat milk

½ cup fat-free half-and-half

½ cup sugar (or Splenda)

3 tablespoons all-purpose flour

1 teaspoon lemon peel, finely grated

1 teaspoon vanilla extract

1½ teaspoons rum extract

¼ teaspoon salt

Preheat oven to 325°. Spray a 9-inch deep-dish pie pan with cooking spray.

1   In a large nonstick skillet, melt butter over medium-high heat. Add pears and sauté until somewhat tender and slightly golden, approximately 10 minutes. Set aside to cool slightly.

2   In a blender, place remaining ingredients and blend until smooth.

3   Arrange pears evenly in pie pan. Pour batter over the top. Place pan on a cookie sheet to catch any spills and bake for 1 hour or until clafouti has set and begun to brown on top. Serve warm or at room temperature, or freeze in individual servings and warm quickly in the microwave for a quick treat later in the week.

MAKES 10 SERVINGS

NUTRITIONAL ANALYSIS PER SERVING **140 calories ▪ 15 percent fat (total fat 2.3 g, saturated fat ‹ 1 g) ▪ 73 percent carbohydrate (2.6 g fiber) ▪ 12 percent protein.**

Chocolate Chip Granola Cookies

I adapted this recipe from one created by my favorite granola company (Oat Cuisine),* giving it a low-fat face-lift. By exchanging butter for baby prunes, substituting most of the brown sugar with Splenda, and using egg substitute instead of whole egg, this recipe is about 30 percent lower in calories and almost 50 percent lower in saturated fat, with no loss of taste or texture.

cooking spray

3 tablespoons butter

1 jar baby prunes

¼ cup brown sugar

1 cup Splenda

¼ cup liquid egg substitute (equivalent to 1 large egg)

2 teaspoons vanilla extract

¾ cup whole wheat flour

½ teaspoon baking soda

¼ teaspoon salt

½ teaspoon ground cinnamon

⅛ teaspoon ground nutmeg

pinch of ground cloves

⅔ cup chocolate chips

3 cups granola (no raisins)

Heat oven to 350 °. Coat cookies sheets with cooking spray.

1   In a medium bowl, blend butter, prunes, brown sugar, Splenda, egg substitute, and vanilla. Set aside.

2   In a large bowl, thoroughly mix flour, soda, salt, cinnamon, nutmeg, and cloves.

3   Pour liquid mixture into flour mixture and stir until blended. Add chocolate chips and granola and stir until mixed.

4   Drop tablespoon-size dollops onto greased cookie sheets, press lightly to flatten, and bake for 12 minutes for crispy or 10 minutes if you like your cookies soft in the middle.

MAKES 3 DOZEN COOKIES

NUTRITIONAL ANALYSIS PER COOKIE **87 calories** ▪ **45 percent fat (total fat 4.3 g, saturated fat 1.6 g)** ▪ **47 percent carbohydrate (1.7 g fiber)** ▪ **8 percent protein.**

C

*Oat Cuisine, P.O. Box 1066, Alameda, CA 94501, (510) 562-8448.

Peach 'n' Blueberry Crisp with a Hint of Orange

Comfort just came home to roost with this dessert. Serve alone or top with fat-free vanilla frozen yogurt. This crisp can also double as breakfast if served with warm almond milk.

¾ cup sugar

¼ cup Splenda

⅓ cup all-purpose flour

¼ teaspoon ground cinnamon

⅛ teaspoon ground cardamom

⅛ teaspoon ground nutmeg

5 pounds fresh peaches, peeled, pitted, and sliced, or 3 (1-pound) bags frozen peach slices

1 cup blueberries, fresh or thawed

CRISP

⅔ cup whole wheat flour

1 cup old-fashioned rolled oats (not instant)

½ cup brown sugar

¼ cup Splenda

1 teaspoon ground cinnamon

pinch of salt

1½ tablespoons butter, cut into tiny pieces

1 tablespoon canola oil

3 tablespoons frozen orange juice concentrate

Preheat oven to 400°.

1   In a large bowl, blend sugar, Splenda, flour, cinnamon, cardamom, and nutmeg until thoroughly mixed. Add peaches and toss until all dry ingredients are wet and mixed with fruit. Gently fold in blueberries. Pour into a 13-by-9-by-2-inch baking dish and evenly spread over bottom of pan. Place in oven for 1 hour.

2   Make crisp during first 15 minutes of fruit baking. In a medium bowl, blend whole wheat flour, oats, brown sugar, Splenda, cinnamon, and salt. Add butter and oil and blend with a pastry knife or fingertips. Add orange juice concentrate and blend with fingertips until all ingredients are moistened and mixture is crumbly.

3   After fruit has been baking for 30 minutes, remove from oven and sprinkle flour-oat crisp mixture evenly over top. Return to oven and finish baking for remaining 30 minutes or until fruit is bubbling and mixture is golden brown.

MAKES 12 SERVINGS

NUTRITIONAL ANALYSIS PER SERVING **250 calories** ▪ **12 percent fat (total fat 3.3 g, saturated fat 1 g)** ▪ **82 percent carbohydrate (5 g fiber)** ▪ **6 percent protein.**

C

Pumpkin Pie with Rum Whipped Cream

For the rich flavor of this pie, there is no substitute for real whipped cream. The trick is to pack a small amount of whipped cream with extra flavor so a little goes a long way. For variation, add finely minced crystallized ginger or toasted chopped pecans to the filling. This pie is 35 percent lower in calories and has half the fat of traditional pumpkin pie.

MOOD TIP

Pumpkin pie is more than just a tasty dessert. It is rich in the antioxidants beta-carotene and selenium and supplies generous amounts of folic acid, calcium, iron, and magnesium—all nutrients that help to improve mood, memory, and general health.

CRUST

1 cup powdered pie crust mix (such as Krusteaz)

1 teaspoon orange or lemon zest

2 tablespoons water

flour

FILLING

1 (15-ounce) can pumpkin puree (not pumpkin pie filling)

½ cup brown sugar

¼ cup Splenda

⅔ cup fat-free half-and-half

⅔ cup fat-free evaporated milk

1 tablespoon cornstarch

½ teaspoon salt

¾ teaspoon ground cinnamon

½ teaspoon ground ginger

¼ teaspoon ground cloves

¼ teaspoon freshly ground nutmeg

¾ teaspoon rum extract

2 whole eggs

1 egg, separated into yolk and white

WHIPPED CREAM

½ pint carton of heavy whipping cream

2 tablespoons powdered sugar

¾ teaspoon rum extract

¼ teaspoon vanilla extract

Preheat oven to 425°.

1   In a medium bowl, place pie crust mix, zest, and water. Mix with a fork until dough is moistened. Pat together with hands to form a firm ball. Sprinkle a clean, flat surface with flour and roll dough into a circle, 2 inches larger than an inverted 9-inch pie pan. Fold dough in half, then into quarters. Place tip of folded sheet in center of pie pan and unfold. Press gently into pan and trim dough to 1 inch from edge of pie pan. Fold under and pinch to form fluted edges. Set aside. (This dough can be made ahead of time and refrigerated.)

2   In a large bowl, blend all filling ingredients from pumpkin puree through rum extract.

3   Place 2 whole eggs and 1 egg yolk in a small bowl and whip. Add to pumpkin mixture and blend thoroughly.

4   Whip remaining egg white with electric mixer until soft peaks form. Fold into pumpkin mixture until no white streaks remain.

5   Pour pumpkin filling into pie pan and bake at 425° for 15 minutes, reduce heat, and bake at 350° for 50 minutes or until a toothpick inserted into middle of pie comes out clean. Remove from oven and cool for at least 2 hours.

6   In a medium deep bowl, whip cream with a mixer on high speed. When cream begins to form peaks, add powdered sugar and extracts. Continue to whip until firm peaks form. Dollop 1 tablespoon of cream on top of each piece of pie.

MAKES 8 SERVINGS

NUTRITIONAL ANALYSIS PER SERVING OF PIE **208 calories** ▪ **33 percent fat (total fat 7.6 g, saturated fat 2 g)** ▪ **54 percent carbohydrate (2 g fiber)** ▪ **13 percent protein.**

NUTRITIONAL ANALYSIS PER TABLESPOON OF WHIPPED CREAM **26 calories** ▪ **89 percent fat (total fat 2.6 g, saturated fat 1.6 g)** ▪ **9 percent carbohydrate (0 g fiber)** ▪ **2 percent protein.**

Rum-Infused Tropical Fruit with Coconut

This refreshing, light dessert tastes sinfully delicious, yet is alcohol-free. Canned mandarin oranges can be used in place of the fresh orange.

FOOD TIP
Use a knife to cut the peel off the orange, so that all the pith is removed.

2 tablespoons sugar

2 tablespoons Splenda

¼ cup water

2 tablespoons fresh lime juice

¾ teaspoon rum extract

4 kiwi, peeled and quartered

1 mango, peeled and cubed

1 medium orange, peeled, quartered, and cubed

2 teaspoons sweetened coconut flakes

1   Place sugar, Splenda, and water in a small saucepan and warm over medium heat until sugar and Splenda dissolve, stirring occasionally. Remove from heat and allow to cool until warm. Add lime juice and extract.

2   Place fruit in a bowl and pour sugar mixture over fruit. Refrigerate for 30 minutes to 1 hour to allow rum flavors to blend with fruit.

3   Divide fruit mixture evenly between 2 glass serving bowls. Top each portion with 1 teaspoon of coconut and serve.

MAKES 2 SERVINGS

NUTRITIONAL ANALYSIS PER SERVING **258 calories** ▪ **6 percent fat (total fat 1.7 g, saturated fat < 1 g)** ▪ **90 percent carbohydrate (9.1 g fiber)** ▪ **4 percent protein.**

Q **S**

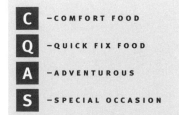

C –COMFORT FOOD
Q –QUICK FIX FOOD
A –ADVENTUROUS
S –SPECIAL OCCASION

Beverages

Boost Energy

IF THERE WAS an eternal fountain of vitality, it would flow with water. Next to oxygen, water is the most important nutrient for health and life. You can live without food for weeks, but most people can survive without water for only a few days. Water also reduces your risk for certain diseases, boosts energy, fights fatigue, and might even help with weight loss.

Why You Need Water

Your body is mostly water. Men are about 60 percent water (10 to 12 gallons), and women are about 55 percent water. (Water is more concentrated in muscle than in fat, and women have more body fat than men, in general.) For example, water makes up

- 83 percent of blood,

- 75 percent of brain,

- 70 percent of muscle,

- 20 to 30 percent of body fat, and

- 22 percent of bone.

Water fills every space inside and between cells. It is the body's universal solvent, coolant, lubricant, and transport agent, so it lubricates joints, maintains body temperature, hydrates the skin, transports toxins and waste out of the body, carries nutrients to tissues, and helps digest food.

Every system in your body—from reproduction and digestion to circulation, mood, and memory—depends on water. Consequently, it helps ward off fatigue, the number one health complaint in the United States, and might help boost alertness and feelings of vitality. It keeps tissues hydrated and wards off migraines, other headaches, kidney stones, and urinary tract infections. Water even might help lower cancer risk. In one study from the Harvard School of Public Health, men who drank 10 or more cups of water a day had half the risk of bladder cancer compared with men who drank 5 cups or less.

Even mild dehydration, such as losing 1 to 2 percent of body weight, results in a variety of problems, from headaches, fatigue, and weakness to light-headedness, poor stamina, reduced short-term memory, and poor concentration and reasoning ability. No wonder people often feel sluggish when they don't drink enough water!

What's Your Water Quota?

You can become dehydrated in one hot afternoon or slowly over days of drinking some, but not enough, fluids. Winter weather can dehydrate your body just as fast as a hot summer day; a household furnace dries the air inside, while winter winds outdoors also pull moisture from the body. You become dehydrated even faster if you exercise, travel by air, or work in hot climates. For example:

- A five-hour plane flight can cost the body 4 to 5 cups of water.

- Hiking for four hours in mild temperatures drains the body of 10 to 14 cups of water.

- Walking for one hour in 90° weather depletes the body of 4 cups of water.

- Watching a football game on TV results in a loss of 1 to 2 cups of water.

You lose about 64 to 80 ounces of fluid every day if you are sedentary. To replace this loss, many experts recommend that adults drink at least eight glasses (8 ounces each) of fluid daily, even more if they exercise, are pregnant or breast-feeding, or perspire heavily.

Many of us are walking around mildly dehydrated because thirst is a poor indicator of fluid needs, especially as we age. Mild dehydration can undermine energy level, mental function, and increase stress on the body. The three rules when it comes to fluids are:

1. Drink fluids frequently throughout the day to prevent dehydration.

2. Include lots of fluid-packed foods in the daily diet, such as fruits, vegetables, cooked cereals, pasta, yogurt, and soymilk.

3. Drink at least eight glasses of water daily or one cup of water for every 20 pounds of body weight. (A 150-pound person who does not exercise or work in hot climates needs seven and a half cups of water.)

Fruit and vegetable juices count as part of your quota, but not alcohol, since it has a diuretic, or dehydrating, effect. Drink one glass of water for every alcoholic beverage you consume to make up the difference. Despite arguments to the contrary, researchers at the University of Nebraska Medical Center in Omaha report that coffee and tea, while having a mild diuretic effect, also contribute to your water needs.

12 QUICK-FIX BEVERAGES

1. **PEACHY CREAMY SMOOTHIE:** Combine peach juice, peaches, strawberries, and orange sherbet in a blender and whip until smooth.

2. **SUNRISE SPECIAL:** Combine freshly squeezed orange juice, strawberries, 1 banana, and non-fat frozen yogurt in a blender and whip until smooth.

3. **MANGO WOW:** Combine freshly squeezed orange juice, 1 fresh peach (peeled and seeded), 1 mango (peeled and pitted), and 1 banana in a blender and whip until smooth.

4. **SOY BERRY SMOOTHIE:** Combine vanilla soymilk, strawberries, 2 tablespoons orange juice concentrate, and 1 banana in a blender and whip until smooth.

5. **MAPLE SYRUP SMOOTHIE:** Combine 1 cup vanilla soymilk, 6 graham cracker squares, 1/4 cup nonfat powdered milk, and 4 teaspoons maple syrup in a blender and whip until smooth.

6. **PB 'N' B SMOOTHIE:** Combine 1 cup vanilla soymilk, ½ cup fat-free cottage cheese, 2 tablespoons low-fat peanut butter, 1 banana, and 1 tablespoon honey in a blender and whip until smooth.

7. **HOMEMADE ORANGE JULIUS:** Blend ½ cup nonfat plain yogurt, half a (6-ounce) can of frozen orange juice concentrate, 1 cup nonfat milk, and a dash of vanilla until smooth.

8. **GRAPEFRUIT COOLER:** Fill a glass with ice and add ½ cup grapefruit juice and ⅔ cup sugar-free lemon-lime or Sprite soda.

9. **ICED HOT CHOCOLATE:** Make Frothy 'n' Rich Hot Chocolate (page 272) and refrigerate for 4 hours. Whip in blender and serve over ice.

10. **CAFÉ LATTE WITH ORANGE:** Mix strong coffee with fat-free half-and-half and ½ teaspoon finely grated orange rind. Sprinkle with nutmeg.

11. **CARROT-APPLE ZAPPER:** In a juicer, extract the juice from 1 apple, 2 carrots, and 1 thin slice fresh ginger.

12. **VEGETABLE COCKTAIL:** In a juicer, extract the juice from 1 medium tomato, 1 stalk celery, ½ red pepper, 1 carrot, and ½ cucumber.

How can you make sure you get enough fluids?

- Fill a pitcher with your daily allotment of water and keep it on your desk at work or the kitchen table at home.

- Fill eight glasses of water and place them in a convenient spot, such as the kitchen counter or dining room table.

- Take eight slurps of water every time you pass a water fountain (1 slurp = approximately 1 ounce).

- Need a little incentive to drink water? Try dressing it up with a twist of lemon, lime, or orange. Or mix a little fruit juice with sparkling water and ice.

- Drink your meals by fixing one or more of the yummy smoothies or fruit drinks in this chapter.

You'll know if you are getting enough fluid when your urine is pale yellow to clear and you urinate every two to four hours. Dark yellow urine is a sign your body is lacking in water and is trying to conserve. One exception to this rule is if you take large doses of vitamin B$_2$, since this vitamin colors the urine yellow even if you are well hydrated.

Drink to Lose Weight

Water might not directly cause weight loss, but including more water in your diet will help in a roundabout way to manage your appetite and waistline.

Your body doesn't register calories from clear liquids as well as it does from food, so the body doesn't compensate by cutting back on calories elsewhere. In one study, when people drank a sweetened beverage before or during lunch, they did not cut back on calories; consequently, the 166 calories in the drink were added to the total calories for the day. In another study, when people ate 450 calories of jelly beans, they cut back on calories later in the day, but they didn't cut back when they drank those calories as soda. "It doesn't matter if you drink soda pop with or before a meal, the calories are added to, they don't displace, the calories from food," says Barbara Rolls, Ph.D., at Pennsylvania State University. It also doesn't matter if the beverage is carbonated or not; nor does it matter what type of sugar is in the beverage. Water is a saving grace when it comes to weight management since it is a calorie-free beverage you can drink to your heart's content without worrying about your waistline.

GETTING YOUR WATER FROM FOOD

Water comes in more than a glass or bottle. You can also meet your daily quota from many water-packed foods. Here are four good sources and two not-so-good ones.

Food	Percent Water
Cucumbers	95
Milk	90
Oranges	85
Bananas	75
Pretzels	5
Nuts	2 to 5

Water versus Soda

Shouldn't a glass of water, soda, or lemonade fill us up? Apparently not, and the reason is found in our genes. For tens of thousands of years, our ancestors lived and evolved in a world where water was the only beverage. Food often was scarce, and our ancestors needed to pack in all the calories they could find, when they could find them. To "fill up" on water would mean they missed critical calories. For survival's sake, the human body learned to separate thirst from hunger.

Our modern thirst and appetite controls are identical to those of our ancestors, but we live in a toxic environment where soda, not calorie-free water, is the beverage of choice. Manufacturers pump out 15 billion gallons of soft drinks a year, or 54 gallons for every man, woman, and child. With soda at about 13 calories an ounce, it's not surprising that studies, such as one from the Harvard School of Public Health, report that people's weight problems are directly proportional to how many they drink. The Harvard study found that kids who drink soda consume about 200 extra calories a day, and a study from the University of Minnesota also found that children who drink daily as little as 9 ounces of soda consume 188 calories more every day than children who don't drink pop. At that excess calorie intake, you gain a pound in three weeks.

This is where water steps forward as the beverage of choice for weight management. It's fat-free, sugar-free, and calorie-free, and it works with, rather than against, our bodies' natural thirst and hunger systems. Replace the typical 19 ounces of soda guzzled every day with water, and you automatically quench your thirst and cut almost 250 calories from your daily diet!

Am I Thirsty or Hungry?

Some people mistake hunger for thirst, nibbling on ice cream rather than downing a glass of ice water. Granted, thirst is different from a hunger pang, but according to Debra Waterhouse, M.P.H., R.D., the author of *Outsmarting Female Fatigue*, "when people aren't connected with their bodies' hunger signals, they can't accurately distinguish one signal from another, including thirst and fatigue, so they eat in response to everything." Anne Fletcher, M.S., R.D., the author of *Eating Thin for Life*, a report on people who have lost weight and successfully maintained the weight loss, adds that she found two out of every three people interviewed made a concerted effort to drink water to help control their weight. So the next time you find yourself wanting to snack, but aren't really physically hungry, try drinking a glass of water and waiting 15 minutes; the urge to nibble might subside.

Have a Smoothie

To feel full and energized without gaining weight, you need to drink more water and add foods that have a high water content, such as fruits and vegetables, to your meals and snacks.

While soda adds unwanted calories, other beverages that have a thick consistency, such as vegetable juices and smoothies, fill you up and help cut back on calories later in the day. When Dr. Rolls and her colleagues asked people to drink tomato juice before lunch, they found that people consumed 136 fewer calories as a result. Smoothies, with their high water and fiber content, also help people feel full longer, so they eat less at the next meal.

In this section, you'll find 20 delicious beverages designed to boost energy. All are nutrient-packed and low-calorie. Many also have a high fiber content to keep you feeling satisfied longer. A few of the beverages are low-fat versions of high-calorie drinks served during holidays and on other special occasions. They allow you to have your celebration without jeopardizing your waistline or energy level.

Outrageous Fat-Free Eggnog

If you've had better eggnog than this, I'll eat my Christmas stocking! While traditional eggnogs pack in up to 19 grams of fat (that's almost 5 teaspoons of fat, and most of it is saturated), this recipe is fat- and cholesterol-free. It also has less than half the calories. Besides that—it is absolutely delicious! (You can make a nonalcoholic version using brandy or rum extract in place of the liquor.) Use the egg substitute listed, since this is the only egg substitute I found where the manufacturer guaranteed safety using its product uncooked.

FOOD TIP
Along with toasting to holiday cheer, eggnog can be used as a sauce for apple pie, fruit desserts, or baked apples. If you make nonalcoholic eggnog, add a little grated orange peel and pour the eggnog over oatmeal or other hot cereal or use it to make French toast.

1½ cups Papetti Foods Better'n Eggs substitute (1½ small cartons)

½ box powdered sugar

1 cup dark rum

4 cups fat-free half-and-half

5 large egg whites

freshly ground nutmeg

1   In a large bowl, whip egg substitute for 1 minute. Gradually add sugar. Gradually add rum.

2   Cover and refrigerate for 1 hour.

3   Add half-and-half, beating constantly with electric mixer. Cover and refrigerate for 3 hours.

4   In a medium bowl, whip egg whites until they form stiff peaks but are not dry. Gently fold egg whites into egg mixture.

5   Serve eggnog sprinkled with nutmeg.

MAKES 20 SERVINGS OF APPROXIMATELY 3 OUNCES EACH

NUTRITIONAL ANALYSIS PER SERVING **122 calories** ▪ **5 percent fat (total fat < 1 g, saturated fat 0 g)** ▪ **56 percent carbohydrate (0 g fiber)** ▪ **16 percent protein, 23 percent alcohol.**

S

Orange Frosty

This citrusy beverage is creamy and festive. It's partly sweetened with no-calorie Splenda, is cholesterol-free, and has the added benefit of soymilk, which lowers heart-disease risk. The mixture of soymilk and fruit juice helps knock out hunger because it provides a great balance of protein and carbohydrate.

FOOD TIP
Granted, juice does not have the fiber of the original fruit, but it has most of the fruit's original vitamins, minerals, and phytochemicals, which makes fruit juice far better than soft drinks or packaged fruit drinks made with sugar or concentrated pear, apple, or grape juice.

2 cups ice, crushed

1 cup 8th Continent vanilla soymilk

1 cup water

2 tablespoons Splenda

1 (6-ounce) can orange juice concentrate

5 teaspoons cranberry-orange relish

1   Place all ingredients except relish in a blender. Cover and blend on high speed 30 seconds or until smooth.

2   Pour into 5 (6-ounce) glasses and top with 1 teaspoon of relish per glass. Serve immediately.

MAKES 5 SERVINGS OF APPROXIMATELY 6 OUNCES EACH

Place fresh cranberries in ice cube trays, fill with water, and freeze. Once frozen, pop out the ice cubes and put two or three in glass before filling with Orange Frosty to make a pretty, festive drink.

NUTRITIONAL ANALYSIS PER SERVING **82 calories** ▪ **7 percent fat (total fat 0.6 g, saturated fat 0 g)** ▪ **83 percent carbohydrate (0.5 g fiber)** ▪ **10 percent protein.**

Banana-Pineapple Colada

This tropical smoothie is creamy and cool, just perfect for a quick breakfast or midafternoon refreshment. You also get a hefty dose of B vitamins, calcium, vitamin C, and magnesium in this delicious smoothie. And it's 57 percent water!

---

1 cup pineapple chunks, fresh or canned in juice

1 banana, peeled
½ cup low-fat vanilla soymilk

1 teaspoon coconut extract
crushed ice (optional)

1   Place all ingredients in a blender.
2   Blend on high speed until smooth.

MAKES 1 GENEROUS CUP

NUTRITIONAL ANALYSIS **225 calories** ▪ **10 percent fat (total fat 2.5 g, saturated fat 0 g)** ▪ **82 percent carbohydrate (4.3 g fiber)** ▪ **8 percent protein.**

Q

Mango-Lemon Daiquiri

Whipped mango is like silk in a glass. The rum extract adds a zing. At 82 percent water and packed with beta-carotene, vitamin C, B vitamins, calcium, and magnesium, this is the perfect way to start or end the day!

1 cup mango, peeled, pitted, and cubed (approximately 1 cup)

½ cup pineapple chunks, preferably fresh

1 (6-ounce) tub low-fat banana-flavored yogurt (such as "banana cream pie")

1 tablespoon fresh lemon juice

½ teaspoon vanilla extract

1 teaspoon rum extract

crushed ice (optional)

1   Place all ingredients in a blender.

2   Blend on high speed until smooth.

MAKES 1½ CUPS

NUTRITIONAL ANALYSIS **293 calories** ▪ **8 percent fat (total fat 2.6 g, saturated fat 1.5 g)** ▪ **79 percent carbohydrate (4.3 g fiber)** ▪ **13 percent protein.**

Apricot Cooler

This smoothie tastes so good it should be served in a champagne glass. The frozen yogurt gives it a creamy texture like a milk shake. Add Splenda if you want a sweet dessert drink.

---

1 can apricots canned in juice, drained (approximately 1 cup drained)

½ cup pineapple chunks

½ cup frozen vanilla nonfat yogurt

2 tablespoons fresh lemon juice

½ teaspoon rum extract

crushed ice (optional)

1   Place all ingredients in a blender.

2   Blend on high speed until smooth.

MAKES 1½ CUPS

NUTRITIONAL ANALYSIS **215 calories** ▪ **4 percent fat (total fat 1 g, saturated fat 0 g)** ▪ **83 percent carbohydrate (4 g fiber)** ▪ **13 percent protein.**

Q

Wake Up and Smell the Mocha Cooler

Need a little wake-up call in the morning? This morning brew is refreshing and packs a subtle jolt. It takes less than five minutes to make, so there's no excuse for not getting your soy and calcium today!

MOOD TIP

Adding soy-rich foods to the diet improved memory within 10 weeks in a group of men and women at King's College, London, while postmenopausal women who consumed the most soy-based phytoestrogens had the best memory in a study from University Medical Center, Utrecht, the Netherlands.

¾ cup 8th Continent vanilla soymilk (calcium and vitamin D–fortified)

¼ cup 8th Continent chocolate soymilk (calcium and vitamin D–fortified)

1 scoop or ¼ cup fat-free vanilla frozen yogurt

1 to 1½ teaspoons coffee crystals (or use decaffeinated coffee crystals)

1   Place all ingredients in blender.

2   Whip until smooth and crystals have dissolved, about 1 minute.

MAKES 1 SERVING OF 1 GENEROUS CUP

NUTRITIONAL ANALYSIS **142 calories** ▪ **18 percent fat (total fat 2.8 g, saturated fat < 1 g)** ▪ **56 percent carbohydrate (0.5 g fiber)** ▪ **26 percent protein** ▪ **38–57 mg caffeine if using caffeinated coffee.**

Q

Frothy 'n' Rich Hot Chocolate

You'll never go back to packaged mixes after making this ultra-rich, low-fat, homemade version. It's easy, too! Add an additional ½ ounce of chocolate if you're a real chocoholic.

FOOD TIP
While chocolate contains saturated fats, the predominant one is stearic acid, which does not harm your heart or arteries.

⅔ cup low-fat (1 percent) milk

⅓ cup fat-free half-and-half

1 tablespoon sugar

1 tablespoon Splenda

1 ounce bittersweet chocolate, chopped into small bits

¼ teaspoon vanilla extract

1 Bring milk and half-and-half just to a boil. Add sugar and Splenda, remove from heat, and stir until sugar dissolves.

2 Put chocolate into a blender and pour in hot milk mixture. Let stand for 5 minutes while chocolate melts.

3 Add vanilla, cover, and hold down lid while you blend the mixture for 30 seconds or until thoroughly mixed and frothy. Serve immediately. If desired, top with favorite low-fat topping, such as low-fat whipped cream, marshmallow, or chocolate whipped cream.

MAKES 1 SERVING OF 1 CUP

NUTRITIONAL ANALYSIS **303 calories** ▪ **36 percent fat** (total fat 12 g, saturated fat 7.4 g) ▪ **51 percent carbohydrate** (1 g fiber) ▪ **13 percent protein.**

C

Warm Milk with Honey and Orange

Time to sit back and relax. See who can get their pj's and socks on first. Then rendezvous for a warm, soothing mug of hot milk.

2 cups nonfat milk

2 cups fat-free half-and-half

2 tablespoons honey

1 teaspoon orange peel, grated

1 cinnamon stick

¼ teaspoon almond extract

pinch of ground nutmeg

orange peel (optional)

1 In a medium saucepan, place all ingredients, except almond extract and nutmeg. Bring to a simmer over medium heat. Whisk while warming to create a foam but do not boil. Once hot, remove from heat.

2 Whisk in almond extract. Discard cinnamon stick.

3 Pour into 4 mugs and sprinkle with nutmeg. Garnish with orange peel if desired.

MAKES 4 SERVINGS OF 1 CUP EACH

NUTRITIONAL ANALYSIS PER CUP **155 calories** ▪ **1 percent fat (total fat 0.5 g, saturated fat 0 g)** ▪ **75 percent carbohydrate (0 g fiber)** ▪ **24 percent protein.**

Chocolate Almond Joy-Soy Frappe

Craving chocolate and coconut? Look no farther! Take time to chill and enjoy this soy frappe.

---

3 cups chocolate nonfat frozen
yogurt

1 cup chocolate or vanilla soymilk

1 tablespoon shredded coconut

2 teaspoons coconut extract

½ teaspoon almond extract

fat-free chocolate syrup (optional)

1   Place all ingredients in a blender and puree until very smooth.

2   Serve in chilled glasses. Drizzle with fat-free chocolate syrup if desired.

MAKES 3 SERVINGS OF APPROXIMATELY 1 CUP EACH

NUTRITIONAL ANALYSIS PER SERVING **255 calories** ▪ **10 percent fat (total fat 3 g, saturated fat 1.5 g)**
▪ **70 percent carbohydrate (4.3 g fiber)** ▪ **20 percent protein.**

Strawberry-Banana Coconut Milk Smoothie

A rich and filling drink. The frozen strawberries add texture, flavor, and provide just the right amount of "chill."

MOOD TIP
Coconut is a good source of fiber and contains phytosterols, cholesterol-lowering compounds.

7 large frozen strawberries

½ cup light coconut milk

½ cup nonfat milk

1 banana, peeled and chopped

1 teaspoon Splenda

1 teaspoon vanilla extract

1 teaspoon shredded coconut (optional)

1   Place all ingredients in a blender and puree until smooth. (Add more milk if too thick.)

2   Serve in tall chilled glasses.

MAKES 2 SERVINGS

NUTRITIONAL ANALYSIS PER SERVING **148 calories** ▪ 21 percent fat (total fat 3.5 g, saturated fat 3 g) ▪ **68 percent carbohydrate (4 g fiber)** ▪ **11 percent protein.**

Q

Café Mocha Granita

A delicious alternative to a high-fat purchased iced mocha coffee, this drink is low in calories, fat, and sugar.

---

2 cups strong brewed coffee (regular or decaf), chilled

1½ cups chocolate soymilk

1 cup fat-free half-and-half

1 tablespoon Splenda

2 teaspoons vanilla extract

fat-free whipped cream

1   Pour chilled coffee into an ice cube tray and freeze overnight or up to several days.

2   When ready to use, place frozen coffee cubes in a Ziploc plastic bag and smash them with a rolling pin until coarsely crushed.

3   Place crushed cubes in a blender, add soymilk, half-and-half, Splenda, and vanilla. Blend until smooth.

4   Pour into 4 tall chilled glasses. Serve with a dollop of whipped cream and a straw.

MAKES 4 SERVINGS

NUTRITIONAL ANALYSIS PER SERVING **100 calories** ▪ **10 percent fat (total fat 1 g, saturated fat 0 g)** ▪ **69 percent carbohydrate (0 g fiber)** ▪ **21 percent protein.**

Q

Peach Blush Bellinis

Elegant and *refreshing* are words typically used to describe this traditional Italian beverage. The addition of raspberries provides our version with a hint of rosy color. For special occasions, return to tradition and substitute champagne for the apple juice.

---

1 cup fresh or thawed frozen peaches

⅔ cup peach nectar

2 tablespoons Splenda

½ cup frozen orange-peach-mango concentrate, thawed

1 tablespoon frozen or fresh raspberries

2 cups sparkling apple juice

1   Add peaches, peach nectar, Splenda, fruit concentrate, and raspberries to a blender and puree until smooth. (This puree can be made up to 24 hours ahead of time and refrigerated. Give it a quick turn in the blender just before serving.)

2   Pour equal portions of fruit puree into 4 wineglasses and top with ½ cup apple juice each. Serve immediately.

MAKES 4 SERVINGS OF APPROXIMATELY 1 CUP EACH

NUTRITIONAL ANALYSIS PER SERVING **151 calories** ▪ 1 percent fat (total fat < 0.5 g, saturated fat 0 g) ▪ **95 percent carbohydrate (1.4 g fiber)** ▪ 4 percent protein.

Classic Lemonade

We've found the perfect combination of Splenda and sugar so you can have your lemonade for half the calories. For an added treat, slice and seed a lemon and place a slice in each section of an ice cube tray, then fill the tray with water and freeze. The designer ice cubes add a nice touch to this old-fashioned refreshing drink.

FOOD TIP

Lemons give the most juice when they are at room temperature. Firmly roll lemons on the counter before slicing and squeezing to soften and release the most juice.

1 cup fresh lemon juice (approximately 10 small or 6 large lemons, juiced and seeded)

3 cups cold water

¼ cup Splenda

¼ cup plus 1 tablespoon sugar

4 lemon slices

ice cubes

1   Combine lemon juice, water, Splenda, and sugar in a large pitcher. Stir with a wire whisk until sugar is completely dissolved. Add lemon slices and refrigerate for 1 hour.

2   To serve, fill 4 glasses with ice and pour equal amounts of lemonade into each glass.

MAKES 4 SERVINGS OF APPROXIMATELY 1 CUP EACH

NUTRITIONAL ANALYSIS PER SERVING **76 calories** ▪ **1 percent fat (total fat < 0.5 g, saturated fat 0 g)** ▪ **98 percent carbohydrate (0 g fiber)** ▪ **1 percent protein.**

C

Hot Chai Tea

Look for chai tea bags in the tea section at your specialty food shop, health food store, or grocery. Relax and enjoy a cup at home.

MOOD TIP

Tea contains polyphenols— antioxidants that protect the brain from damage by free radicals.

4 cups water

6 chai tea bags

1/8 teaspoon ground cardamom

1/8 teaspoon ground cinnamon

3 tablespoons fat-free condensed milk (or 3 tablespoons fat-free half-and-half and 2 tablespoons honey)

1   In a medium saucepan, place water, tea bags (cut off strings), cardamom, and cinnamon. Over medium-high heat, bring mixture to a boil, reduce heat, and simmer for 1 to 2 minutes.

2   Remove from heat. Whisk in condensed milk. Stir well.

3   Pour into 4 coffee mugs or large teacups. Serve hot.

MAKES 4 CUPS

NUTRITIONAL ANALYSIS PER CUP 40 calories ▪ 0 percent fat (total fat 0 g, saturated fat 0 g) ▪ 96 percent carbohydrate (0 g fiber) ▪ 4 percent protein.

Raspberry Ice Tea

This is a refreshing iced tea beverage with a burst of raspberry flavor and a hint of lemon (or lime).

MOOD TIP

Drink tea between meals, rather than with meals, since compounds in tea called tannins block iron absorption by up to 80 percent, which contributes to iron deficiency and fatigue.

6 cups water

6 tea bags (Lipton, Red Rose, or other Darjeeling-like tea)

juice and zest of 1 lemon

¼ cup Splenda

¼ cup sugar

1 cup raspberries, frozen

sugar for rims of glasses (optional)

lemon or lime slices (optional)

1   In a medium saucepan, place water and tea bags (cut off strings). Over medium-high heat, bring mixture to a boil, reduce heat, and simmer for 2 minutes. Remove from heat and cool. Carefully press tea bags, then remove from pan. Add juice and zest of lemon, Splenda, and sugar. Mix well. Pour cool mixture into a large pitcher.

2   In a blender, combine 2 cups tea mixture and frozen raspberries. Blend until smooth.

3   Pour raspberry mixture into pitcher. Stir well to mix.

4   Fill 8 tall glasses with ice. Pour tea mixture over the ice. Garnish with a slice of lemon or lime or run a slice of lemon or lime around each glass rim and dip the rims in sugar. Serve immediately.

MAKES 8 SERVINGS

NUTRITIONAL ANALYSIS PER SERVING **34 calories** ▪ **3 percent fat (total fat ‹ 0.5 g, saturated fat 0 g)** ▪ **95 percent carbohydrate (1 g fiber)** ▪ **2 percent protein.**

Blueberry Limeade

It's surprising how well the flavors of sweet blueberries and tart lime work when combined for a refreshing, not-too-sweet beverage.

---

1 (12-ounce) can frozen limeade

3 cups cold water

1½ cups blueberries, frozen

zest of 1 lime

⅛ teaspoon ground cinnamon

1   In a large pitcher, whisk together limeade and water. Set aside.

2   In a blender, combine 1 cup limeade mixture, frozen blueberries, zest of lime, and cinnamon. Blend until smooth.

3   Pour mixture into pitcher of limeade. Stir well.

4   To serve, pour mixture over chilled glasses filled with ice. Short round glasses or tall slender ones work best.

MAKES 7 SERVINGS

NUTRITIONAL ANALYSIS PER SERVING **111 calories** ▪ **1 percent fat (total fat < 0.5 g, saturated fat 0 g)** ▪ **97 percent carbohydrate (1 g fiber)** ▪ **2 percent protein.**

Mango Maniac

Here is a cold, refreshing blend of raspberry tea, mango sorbet, strawberries, and fresh chopped mango. One taste will transform a mango lover into a mango maniac.

---

2 wild raspberry herbal tea bags

1 cup hot water

1 cup frozen mango sorbet

1 cup frozen or fresh strawberries, coarsely chopped

1 small mango, peeled, pitted, and coarsely chopped

1   Add tea bags to water, steep for 5 minutes. Remove tea bags and cool.

2   In a blender, combine sorbet, strawberries, and chilled raspberry tea. Blend until smooth. Add fresh mango, blend briefly to keep small pieces of mango intact. If too thick, add a little more tea or water.

3   Pour into festive glasses and add straws.

MAKES 3 SERVINGS

NUTRITIONAL ANALYSIS PER SERVING **125 calories** ▪ **2 percent fat (total fat < 0.5 g, saturated fat 0 g)** ▪ **96 percent carbohydrate (2.5 g fiber)** ▪ **2 percent protein.**

Sparkling Cider Mimosa with Raspberries

This traditional brunch drink gets an update! It usually contains fresh orange juice and champagne, which we have replaced with pureed raspberries, orange juice, and sparkling cider. Of course, you can switch back to champagne instead of apple cider for special occasions.

MOOD TIP

Most people recognize orange juice as a great source of vitamin C, but this refreshing juice is also one of the best dietary sources of folic acid, a B vitamin that helps curb depression.

⅓ cup frozen raspberries

juice and zest of 1 large orange

3 cups chilled orange juice

1 (25.4-ounce) bottle of nonalcoholic sparkling cider, well chilled

6 frozen raspberries

1   In a blender, combine frozen raspberries and juice and zest of orange. Blend until smooth. Pour into a small cup or bowl.

2   To each of 6 chilled wineglasses, add 2 tablespoons raspberry puree, ½ cup orange juice, and ½ cup sparkling cider. Stir to mix. Add 1 frozen raspberry to each glass and serve immediately. Pour any remaining juices or cider evenly into glasses.

MAKES 6 SERVINGS

NUTRITIONAL ANALYSIS PER SERVING 71 calories ▪ 2 percent fat (total fat < 0.5 g, saturated fat 0 g) ▪ **96 percent carbohydrate (1 g fiber)** ▪ **2 percent protein.**

Strawberry Lemonade

This drink is a kid pleaser and a great way to sneak fruit into the daily diet.

---

1 tub Crystal Light lemonade powder (comes in a 6-tub canister)   **6 cups cold water**   **1½ cups frozen strawberries**

1   In a large pitcher, combine Crystal Light powder and water, stirring well.

2   In a blender, pour 2 cups of Crystal Light lemonade and strawberries. Blend until smooth.

3   Add strawberry mixture to lemonade and mix well. Pour over tall glasses with ice.

MAKES 8 SERVINGS

NUTRITIONAL ANALYSIS PER SERVING **27 calories** ▪ **3 percent fat (total fat < 0.5 g, saturated fat 0 g)** ▪ **92 percent carbohydrate (0.7 g fiber)** ▪ **5 percent protein.**

Q

Instant Breakfast Fruit Smoothie

For those mornings when you don't have time to toast a waffle or scramble an egg, this smoothie packs a vitamin, mineral, and phytochemical punch and takes two minutes to prepare.

---

1 package vanilla Instant Breakfast flavor packet

1 cup nonfat milk or 1¼ cups fat-free half-and-half

½ cup ice cubes

1 cup strawberries, fresh or frozen

½ banana

1 tablespoon toasted wheat germ

1   In a blender, combine Instant Breakfast, milk, and ice cubes. Blend until smooth.

2   Add strawberries, blend until smooth.

3   Add banana and wheat germ, blend for about 10 seconds more. Serve immediately.

MAKES 2 GENEROUS SERVINGS

NUTRITIONAL ANALYSIS PER SERVING 227 calories = 4 percent fat (total fat 1 g, saturated fat 0 g) =
76 percent carbohydrate (3 g fiber) = 20 percent protein.

Q

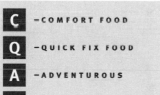

C —COMFORT FOOD

Q —QUICK FIX FOOD

A —ADVENTUROUS

S —SPECIAL OCCASION

· Selected References ·

Breakfasts and Breads: Fatigue Fighters

Bellisle F, Monneuse M, Steptoe A, et al: Weight concerns and eating patterns: A survey of university students in Europe. *Int J Obes* 1995;19:723–730.

Bertrais S, Luque M, Preziosi P, et al: Contribution of ready-to-eat cereals to nutrition intakes in French adults and relations with corpulence. *Ann Nutr M* 2000;44:249–255.

Gibson S, O'Sullivan K: Breakfast cereal consumption patterns and nutrient intakes of British schoolchildren. *J Roy S Hea* 1995;115:366–370.

Haines P, Guilkey D, Popkin B: Trends in breakfast consumption in U.S. adults between 1965 and 1991. *J Am Diet A* 1996;96:464–470.

Hill G: The impact of breakfast especially ready-to-eat cereals on nutrient intake and health of children. *Nutr Res* 1995;15:595–613.

Holt S, Delargy H, Lawton C, et al: The effects of high-carbohydrate vs high-fat breakfasts on feelings of fullness and alertness, and subsequent food intake. *Int J F S N* 1999;50:13–28.

Huang Y, Hoerr S, Song W: Breakfast is the lowest fat meal for young adult women. *J Nutr Educ* 1997;29:184–188.

Lloyd H, Rogers P, Hedderley D, et al: Acute effects of mood and cognitive performance of breakfasts differing in fat and carbohydrate content. *Appetite* 1996;27:151–164.

Moore R, Read N: The effects of breakfast skipping on physiological and psychological well-being. *P Nutr Soc* 2000;59:A127.

Nicklas T, Myers L, Reger C, et al: Impact of breakfast consumption on nutritional adequacy of the diets of young adults in Bogalusa, Louisiana: Ethnic and gender contrasts. *J Am Diet A* 1998;98:1432–1438.

Nicklas T, O'Neil C, Berenson G: Nutrient contribution of breakfast, secular trends, and the role of ready-to-eat cereals. *Am J Clin N* 1998;67:S757–S763.

Nicklas T, Reger C, Myers L, et al: Breakfast consumption with and without vitamin-mineral supplement use favorably impacts daily nutrient intake of ninth-grade students. *J Adoles H* 2000;27:314–321.

Ortega R, Requejo A, Lopez-Sobaler A, et al: The importance of breakfast in meeting daily recommended calcium intake in a group of schoolchildren. *J Am Col N* 1998;17:19–24.

Pollitt E: Does breakfast make a difference in school? *J Am Diet A* 1995;95:1134–1139.

Pollitt E, Lewis N, Garza C, et al: Fasting and cognitive function. *J Psych Res* 1982–83; 17:169–174.

Preziosi P, Galan P, Deheeger M, et al: Breakfast type, daily nutrient intakes and vitamin and mineral status of French children, adolescents, and adults. *J Am Col N* 1999; 18:171–178.

Richter L, Rose C, Griesel R: Cognitive and behavioral effects of a school breakfast. *S Afr Med J* 1997;87 (suppl):93–100.

Ruxton C, Kirk T: Breakfast: A review of association with measures of dietary intake, physiology, and biochemistry. *Br J Nutr* 1997;78:199–213.

Schlundt D, Hill J, Sbrocco T, et al: The role of breakfast in the treatment of obesity. A randomized clinical trial. *Am J Clin N* 1992;55:645–651.

Smith A: Breakfast consumption and intelligence in elderly persons. *Psychol Rep* 1998; 82:424–426.

Smith A, Bazzoni C, Beale J, et al: High fibre breakfast cereals reduce fatigue. *Appetite* 2001;37:249–250.

Smith A, Clark R, Gallagher J: Breakfast cereal and caffeinated coffee: Effects on working memory, attention, mood, and cardiovascular function. *Physl Behav* 1999;67:9–17.

Wyon D, Abrahamsson L, Jartelius M, et al: An experimental study of the effects of energy intake at breakfast on the test performance of 10-year-old children in school. *Int J F S N* 1997;48:5–12.

Appetizers, Snacks, and Quick Fixes: Eat to Relieve Stress and Improve Sleep

Askew E: Environmental and physical stress and nutrient requirements. *Am J Clin N* 1995;61:631S–637S.

Bjorntorp P: Do stress reactions cause abdominal obesity and comorbidities? *Obes Rev* 2001;2:73–86.

Brody S, Preut R, Schommer K: A randomized controlled trial of high dose ascorbic acid for reduction of blood pressure, cortisol, and subjective responses to psychological stress. *Psychophar* 2002;159:319–324.

Brody S, Preut R, Schommer K, et al: Ascorbic acid treatment decreases reactivity to stress: Randomized trial. *Psychophysl* 2001;38:S29 (meeting abstract).

Canetti L, Bachar E, Berry E: Food and emotion. *Behav Proc* 2002;60:157–164.

Carroll D, Ring C, Suter M, et al: The effects of an oral multivitamin combination with calcium, magnesium, and zinc on psychological well-being in healthy young male volunteers. *Psychophar* 2000;150:220–225.

Cernak I, Savic V, Kotur J, et al: Alterations in magnesium and oxidative status during chronic emotional stress. *Magnes Res* 2000;13:29–36.

Chollet D, Franken P, Raffin Y, et al: Magnesium involvement in sleep: Genetic and nutritional models. *Behav Genet* 2001;31:413–425.

Dietary stress may compromise bones. *Sci News* 2001;159:47.

Dixon J, Schachter L, O'Brien P: Sleep disturbance and obesity. *Arch in Med* 2001;161:102–106.

Duclos M, Corcuff J, Etcheverry N, et al: Abdominal obesity increases overnight cortisol excretion. *J Endoc Inv* 1999;22:465–471.

Greeno C, Wing R: Stress-induced eating. *Psychol B* 1994;115:444–464.

Huether G: The central adaptation syndrome: Psychosocial stress as a trigger for adaptive modifications of brain structure and brain function. *Prog Neurob* 1996. 48:569–612.

Kallner A: Influence of vitamin C status on the urinary excretion of catecholamines in stress. *Hum N Clin N* 1983;37:405–411.

Kansanen M, Vanninen E, Tyuunainen A, et al: The effect of a very low caloric diet-induced weight loss on the severity of obstructive sleep apnoea and autonomic nervous function in obese patients with obstructive sleep apnoea syndrome. *Clin Physl* 1999;18:377–385.

Kortella M, Kaprio J, Rissanen A, et al: Predictors of major weight gain in adult Finns: Stress, life satisfaction, and personality traits. *Int J Obes* 1998;22:949–957.

Laitinen J, Ek E, Sovio U: Stress-related eating and drinking behavior and body mass index and predictors of this behavior. *Prev Med* 2002;34:29–39.

Lopez J, Vazquez D, Chalmers D, et al: Regulation of 5-HT receptors and the hypothalamic-pituitary-adrenal axis. Implications for the neurobiology of suicide. *Ann NY Acad* 1997;836:106–134.

McClain C, McClain M, Boosalis M, et al: Zinc and the stress response. *Sc J Work E* 1993;19:132S–133S.

Mocci F, Canalis P, Tomasi P, et al: The effect of noise on serum and urinary magnesium and catecholamines in humans. *Occup Med* 2001;51:56–61.

Morgan C, Yanovski S, Nguyen T, et al: Loss of control over eating, adiposity, and the psychopathology in overweight children. *Int J Eat D* 2002;31:430–441.

Peters E, Anderson R, Nieman D, et al: Vitamin C supplementation attenuates the increases in circulating cortisol, adrenaline, and anti-inflammatory polypeptides following ultramarathon running. *Int J Sp M* 2001;22:537–543.

Peters E, Anderson R, Theron A: Attenuation of increase in circulating cortisol and enhancement of the acute phase protein response in vitamin C–supplemented ultramarathoners. *Int J Sp M* 2001;22:120–126.

Pizent A, Jurasovic J, Pavlovic M, et al: Serum copper, zinc, and selenium levels with regard to psychological stress in men. *J Tr Elem M* 1999;13:34–39.

Remer T, Pietrzik K, Manz F: Short-term impact of a lactovegetarian diet on adrenocortical activity and adrenal androgens. *J Clin End* 1998;83:2132–2137.

Roemmich J, Wright S, Epstein L: Dietary restraint and stress-induced snacking in youth. *Obes Res* 2002;10:1120–1126.

Rosch P: The stress-food-mood connection: Are there stress reducing foods and diets? *Stress Med* 1995;11:1–6.

Seelig M: Consequences of magnesium deficiency on the enhancement of stress reactions: Preventive and therapeutic implications. *J Am Col N* 1994;13:429–446.

Solomon M: Eating as both coping and stressor in overweight control. *J Adv Nurs* 2001;36:563–572.

Stone A, Bovbjerg D, Neale J, et al: Development of common cold symptoms following experimental rhinovirus infection is related to prior stressful life events. *Behav Med* 1992;18:115–120.

Stress and sleepless nights. *Sci News* 2000;158:40.

Tucker B, Tolbert B, Halver J, et al: Brain ascorbate depletion as a response to stress. *Int J Vit N* 1987;57:289–295.

Wardle J, Steptoe A, Oliver G, et al: Stress, dietary restraint, and food intake. *J Psychos Res* 2000;48:195–202.

Weinstein S, Shide D, Rolls B: Changes in food intake in response to stress in men and women: Psychological factors. *Appetite* 1997;28:7–18.

Lunchables and Sandwiches: Midday Energy Boosters

Crawley J: The role of galanin in feeding behavior. *Neuropeptid* 1999;33:369–375.

Glahn R, Wortley G, South P, et al: Inhibition of iron uptake by phytic acid, tannic acid, and ZnCl2: Studies using an in vitro digestion/Caco-2 cell model. *J Agr Food* 2002;50:390–395.

Jenkins D, Khan A, Jenkins A, et al: Effect of nibbling versus gorging on cardiovascular risk factors: Serum uric acid and blood lipids. *Metabolism* 1995; 44:549–555.

Jenkins D, Wolever T, Vuksan V, et al: Nibbling versus gorging: Metabolic advantages of increased meal frequency. *N Eng J Med* 1989;321:929–934.

Lawrence C, Baudoin F, Luckman S: Centrally administered galanin-like peptide modifies food intake in the rat: A comparison with galanin. *J Neuroendocr* 2002;14:853–860.

LeBlanc J, Mercier I: Components of postprandial thermogenesis in relation to meal frequency in humans. *Can J Physl* 1993;71:879–883.

Leibowitz S: Differential functions of hypothalamic galanin cell growth in the regulation of eating and body weight. *Ann NY Acad* 1998;863:206–220.

Leibowitz S, Akabayashi A, Wang J: Obesity on a high-fat diet: Role of hypothalamic galanin in neurons of the anterior paraventricular nucleus projecting to the median eminence. *J Neurosc* 1998;18:2709–2719.

Metzner H, Lamphiear D, Wheeler N, et al: Relationship between frequency of eating and adiposity in adult men and women in the Tecumseh Community Health Study. *Am J Clin N* 1977;30:712–715.

Patterson A, Brown W, Roberts D: Dietary and supplement treatment of iron deficiency results in improvements in general health and fatigue in Australian women of child-bearing age. *J Am Col N* 2001;20:337–342.

Ruidavets J, Bongard V, Bataille V, et al: Eating frequency and body fatness in middle-aged men. *Int J Obes* 2002;26:1476–1483.

Siega-Riz A, Bodnar L, Savitz D: What are pregnant women eating? Nutrient and food group differences by race. *Am J Obst G* 2002;186:480–486.

Speechly D, Buffenstein R: Greater appetite control associated with an increased frequency of eating in lean males. *Appetite* 1999;33:285–297.

Speechly D, Rogers G, Buffenstein R: Acute appetite reduction associated with an increased frequency of eating in obese males. *Int J Obes* 1999;23:1151–1159.

Tuntawiroon M, Sritongkul N, Brune M, et al: Dose-dependent inhibitory effect of phenolic compounds in foods on nonheme-iron absorption in men. *Am J Clin N* 1991;53:554–557.

Wang J, Akabayashi A, Yu H, et al: Hypothalamic galanin: Control by signals of fat metabolism. *Brain Res* 1998;804:7–20.

Westerterp-Plantenga M, Kovacs E, Melanson K: Habitual meal frequency and energy intake regulation in partially temporally isolated men. *Int J Obes* 2002;26:102–110.

Wilding J: Neuropeptides and appetite control. *Diabet Med* 2002;19:619–627.

Soups and Stews: Emotional Eating

Blair A, Lewis V, Booth D: Does emotional eating interfere with success in attempts at weight control? *Appetite* 1990;15:151–157.

Braet C, Van Strien T: Assessment of emotional, externally induced and restrained eating behaviors in nine- to twelve-year-old obese and non-obese children. *Behav Res* 1997;35:863–873.

Foreyt J, Brunner R, Goodrick G, et al: Psychological correlates of weight fluctuation. *Int J Eat D* 1995;17:263–275.

Greeno C, Wing R: Stress-induced eating. *Psychol B* 1994;115:444–464.

Himaya A, Louis-Sylvestre J: The effect of soup on satiation. *Appetite* 1998;30:199–210.

Holt S, Brand Miller J, Petocz P: Interrelationships among postprandial satiety, glucose and insulin responses, and changes in subsequent food intake. *Eur J Cl N* 1996;50:788–797.

Kent A, Waller G, Dagnan D: A greater role of emotional than physical or sexual abuse in predicting disordered eating attitudes: The role of mediating variables. *Int J Eat D* 1999;25:159–167.

Laitinen J, Ek E, Sovio U: Stress-related eating and drinking behavior and body mass index and predictors of this behavior. *Prev Med* 2002;34:29–39.

Lissau I, Sorensen T: Parental neglect during childhood and increased risk of obesity in young adulthood. *Lancet* 1994;343:324–327.

Lynch W, Everingham A, Dubitzky J, et al: Does binge eating play a role in the self-regulation of moods? *Integ Ph Be* 2000;35:298–313.

Macht M: Characteristics of eating in anger, fear, sadness and joy. *Appetite* 1999;33:129–139.

Macht M, Simons G: Emotions and eating in everyday life. *Appetite* 2000;35:65–71.

Meyer C, Waller G: The impact of emotion upon eating behavior: The role of subliminal visual processing of threat cues. *Int J Eat D* 1999;25:319–326.

Mueller W, Meininger J, Liehr P, et al: Adolescent blood pressure, anger expression, and hostility: Possible links to body fat. *Ann Hum Bio* 1998;25:295–307.

Oliver G, Wardle J, Gibson E: Stress and food choice: A laboratory study. *Psychos Med* 2000;62:853–865.

Patel K, Schlundt D: Impact of moods and social context on eating behavior. *Appetite* 2001;36:111–118.

Polivy J: Psychological consequences of food restriction. *J Am Diet A* 1996;96:589–592.

Rolls B, Bell E, Thorwart M: Water incorporated into a food but not served with a food decreases energy intake in lean women. *Am J Clin N* 1999;70:448–455.

Rolls B, Fedoroff I, Guthrie J, et al: Foods with different satiating effects in humans. *Appetite* 1990;15:115–126.

Solomon M: Eating as both coping and stressor in overweight control. *J Adv Nurs* 2001;36:563–572.

Timmerman G, Acton G: The relationship between basic need satisfaction and emotional eating. *Issues Ment He Nurs* 2001;22:691–701.

Uvnas-Moberg K: Endocrinologic control of food intake. *Nutr Rev* 1990;48:57–63.

Van Strien T: Ice cream consumption, tendency toward overeating, and personality. *Int J Eat D* 2000;28:460–464.

Williamson D, Thompson T, Anda R, et al: Body weight and obesity in adults and self-reported abuse in childhood. *Int J Obes* 2002;26:1075–1082.

Salads: Overcoming Overeating with Truly Tasty Foods

Alper C, Mattes R: Effects of chronic peanut consumption on energy balance and hedonics. *Int J Obes* 2002;26:1129–1132.

Clark J: Taste and flavour: Their importance in food choice and acceptance. *P Nutr Soc* 1998;57:639–643.

Drewnowski A: Taste preferences and food intake. *Ann R Nutr* 1997;17:237–253.

Glanz K, Basil M, Maibach E, et al: Why Americans eat what they do: Taste, nutrition, cost, convenience, and weight control concerns as influences on food consumption. *J Am Diet A* 1998;98:1118–1126.

Kaminski L, Henderson S, Drewnowski A: Young women's food preferences and taste responsiveness to 6-n-propylthiouracil (PROP). *Physl Behav* 2000;68:691–697.

Kurihara K, Kashiwayanagi M: Physiological studies on the umami taste. *J Nutr* 2000;130: S931–S934.

Porrini M, Crovetti R, Riso P, et al: Effects of physical and chemical characteristics of food on specific and general satiety. *Physl Behav* 1995;157:461–468.

Schiffman S: The use of flavor to enhance efficacy of reducing diets. *Hosp Pract* 1986; July:44H–44R.

Warwick Z, Hall W, Pappas T, et al: Taste and smell sensations enhance the satiating effect of both a high-carbohydrate and high-fat meal in humans. *Physl Behav* 1993;53:553–563.

Entrées: Taming Out-of-Control Appetites

Anderson K, Teuber S, Gobeille A, et al: Walnut polyphenolics inhibit in vitro human plasma and LDL oxidation. *J Nutr* 2001;131:2837–2842.

Barton C, Lin L, York D, et al: Differential effects of enterostatin, galanin, and opioids on high-fat diet consumption. *Brain Res* 1996;702:55–60.

Beebe D, Holmbeck G, Albright J, et al: Identification of "binge-prone" women: An experimentally and psychometrically validated cluster analysis in a college population. *Addict Beha* 1995;20:451–462.

Borah-Giddens J, Falciglia G: A meta-analysis of the relationship in food preferences between parents and children. *J Nutr Educ* 1993;25:102–107.

Brewerton T: Toward a unified theory of serotonin dysregulation in eating and related disorders. *Psychoneuro* 1995;20:561–590.

Caputo F, Mattes R: Human dietary responses to perceived manipulation of fat content in a midday meal. *Int J Obes* 1993;17:237–240.

deZwaan M, Mitchell J: Opiate antagonists and eating behavior in humans: A review. *J Clin Phar* 1992;32:1060–1072.

Dryden S, Frankish H, Wang Q, et al: Neuropeptide Y and energy balance: One way ahead for the treatment of obesity. *Eur J Cl In* 1994;24:293–308.

Feunekes G, deGraaf C, vanStaveren W: Social facilitation of food intake is mediated by meal duration. *Physl Beha* 1995;58:551–558.

Geiselman P: Control of food intake: A physiologically complex, motivated behavioral system. *End Metab C* 1996;25:815–829.

Green S, Burley V, Blundell J: Effect of fat- and sucrose-containing foods on the size of eating episodes and energy intake in lean males: Potential for causing overconsumption. *Eur J Cl N* 1994;48:547–555.

King N: The relationship between physical activity and food intake. *P Nutr Soc* 1998; 57:77–84.

Leibowitz S: Brain neuropeptide Y: An integrator of endocrine, metabolic, and behavioral processes. *Brain Res B* 1991;27:333–337.

Leibowitz S: Neurochemical-neuroendocrine systems in the brain controlling macronutrient intake and metabolism. *Trends Neur* 1992;15:491–497.

Mattes R: Fat preference and adherence to a reduced-fat diet. *Am J Clin N* 1993;57: 373–381.

Mattes R: Physiologic responses to sensory stimulation by food: Nutritional implications. *J Am Diet A* 1997;97:406–410,413.

Mercer M, Holder M: Food cravings, endogenous opioid peptides, and food intake: A review. *Appetite* 1997;29:325–352.

Mitchell S, Epstein L: Changes in taste and satiety in dietary-restrained women following stress. *Physl Behav* 1996;60:495–499.

Morley J: Appetite regulation by gut peptides. *Ann R Nutr* 1990;10:383–395.

Norton P, Falciglia G, Gist D: Physiologic control of food intake by neural and chemical mechanisms. *J Am Diet A* 1993;93:450–454,457.

Oygard L, Klepp K: Influences of social groups on eating patterns: A study among young adults. *J Behav Med* 1996;19:1.

Peters G, Rappoport L, Huff-Corzine L, et al: Food preferences in daily life: Cognitive, affective and social predictors. *Ecol Food N* 1995;33:215–228.

Pijl H, Koppeschaar P, Cohen A, et al: Evidence for brain serotonin-mediated control of carbohydrate consumption in normal weight and obese humans. *Int J Obes* 1993;17:513–520.

Putnam J, Allshouse J, Kantor L: U.S. per capita food supply trends: More calories, refined carbohydrates, and fats. *Food Rev* 2002;25:2–15.

Reidelberger R: Cholecystokinin and control of food intake. *J Nutr* 1994;124:1327S–1333S.

Severus W, Littman A, Stoll A: Omega-3 fatty acids, homocysteine, and the increased risk of cardiovascular mortality in major depressive disorder. *Harv R Psyc* 2001; 9:280–293.

Staten M: The effect of exercise on food intake in men and women. *Am J Clin N* 1991;53:27–31.

Teff K, Englelman K: Palatability and dietary restraint: Effect on cephalic phase insulin release in women. *Physl Behav* 1996;60:567–573.

Uvnas-Moberg K: Endocrinologic control of food intake. *Nutr Rev* 1990;48:57–63.

Woods S, Strubbe J: The psychobiology of meals. *Psychon B R* 1994;1:141–155.

Wurtman J: The involvement of brain serotonin in excessive carbohydrate snacking by obese carbohydrate cravers. *J Am Diet A* 1984;84:1004–1007.

Pasta, Rice, and Potato Dishes: Carbs for PMS, SAD, and Depression

Bendich A: The potential for dietary supplements to reduce premenstrual syndrome (PMS) symptoms. *J Am Col N* 2000;19:3–12.

Cross G, Marley J, Miles H, et al: Changes in nutrient intake during the menstrual cycle of overweight women with premenstrual syndrome. *Br J Nutr* 2001;85:475–482.

Dye L, Warner P, Bancroft J: Food craving during the menstrual cycle and its relationship to stress, happiness of relationship, and depression: A preliminary enquiry. *J Affect D* 1995;34:157–164.

Johnson R: Diagnosing and managing seasonal affective disorder. *Nurse Pract* 2000;25:56, 59–62,68–70.

McKeown N, Meigs J, Liu S, et al: Whole-grain intake is favorably associated with metabolic risk factors for type 2 diabetes and cardiovascular disease in the Framingham Offspring Study. *Am J Clin N* 2002;76:390–398.

Penaskovic K, Baker P, Bamman M, et al: Depressive symptoms and physical activity in older adults. *J Am Ger So* 2002;50:P233.

Pinchasov B, Shurgaja A, Grischin O, et al: Mood and energy regulation in seasonal and non-seasonal depression before and after midday treatment with physical exercise or bright light. *Psychi Res* 2000;94:29–42.

Pins J, Geleva D, Keenan J, et al: Do whole-grain oat cereals reduce the need for antihypertensive medications and improve blood pressure control? *J Fam Pract* 2002;51: 353–359.

Truswell A: Cereal grains and coronary heart disease. *Eur J Cl N* 2002;56:1–14.

Wurtman J: Depression and weight gain: The serotonin connection. *J Affect D* 1993; 29:183–192.

Vegetables: Antiaging Mind Boosters

Berr C, Balansard B, Arnaud J, et al: Cognitive decline is associated with systemic oxidative stress: The EVA study. *J Am Ger So* 2000;48:1285–1291.

Bryan J, Calvaresi E, Hughes D: Foods for thinking and memory. *Food Aust* 2001; 53:477–479.

Bryan J, Calvaresi E, Hughes D: Short-term folate, vitamin B_{12}, or vitamin B_6 supplementation slightly affects memory performance but not mood in women of various ages. *J Nutr* 2002;132:1345–1356.

Duthie S, Whalley L, Collins A, et al: Homocysteine, B vitamin status, and cognitive function in the elderly. *Am J Clin N* 2002;75:908–913.

Fabre C, Chamari K, Mucci P, et al: Improvement of cognitive function by mental and/or individualized aerobic training in healthy elderly subjects. *Int J Spt Med* 2002;23:415–421.

Flabby minds: A fatty diet can clog your brain as well as your arteries. *New Scientist* 2001;March 3:10.

Joseph J, Shukitt-Hale B, Denisova N, et al: Reversals of age-related declines in neuronal signal transduction, cognitive, and motor behavioral deficits with blueberry, spinach, or strawberry dietary supplementation. *J Neurosc* 1999;19:8114–8121.

Kalmijn S, Feskens E, Launer L, et al: Polyunsaturated fatty acids, antioxidants, and cognitive function in very old men. *Am J Epidem* 1997;145:33–41.

Kim H, Xia H, Li L, et al: Attenuation of neurodegeneration-relevant modifications of brain proteins by dietary soy. *Biofactors* 2000;12:243–250.

Kreijkamp-Kaspers S, Kok L, Grobbee D, et al: Phytoestrogen intake in the Western diet and memory function in postmenopausal women. *J Nutr* 2002;132:S612–S613.

Laurin D, Verreault R, Lindsay J, et al: Physical activity and risk of cognitive impairment and dementia in elderly persons. *Arch Neurol* 2001;58:498–504.

Lee L, Kang S, Lee H, et al: Relationships between dietary intake and cognitive function level in Korean elderly people. *Publ Heal* 2001;115:133–138.

McBride J: Can foods forestall aging: Some with high antioxidant activity appear to aid memory. *Agri Res* 1999;February:14–17.

Molteni R, Barnard R, Ying Z, et al: A high-fat, refined sugar diet reduces hippocampal brain-derived neurotrophic factor, neuronal plasticity, and learning. *Neuroscienc* 2002;112:803–814.

Ortega R, Requejo A, Andres P, et al: Dietary intake and cognitive function in a group of elderly people. *Am J Clin N* 1997;66:803–809.

Paleologos M, Cumming R, Lazarus R: Cohort study of vitamin C intake and cognitive impairment. *Am J Epidem* 1998;148:45–50.

Prins N, den Heijer T, Hofman A, et al: Homocysteine and cognitive function in the elderly: The Rotterdam Scan Study. *Neurology* 2002;59:1375–1380.

Rogers P: A healthy body, a healthy mind: Long-term impact of diet on mood and cognitive function. *P Nutr Soc* 2001;60:135–143.

Solfrizzi V, Panza F, Torres F, et al: High monounsaturated fatty acids intake protects against age-related cognitive decline. *Neurology* 1999;52:1563–1569.

Stevens L, Zentall S, Abate M, et al: Omega-3 fatty acids in boys with behavior, learning, and health problems. *Physl Behav* 1996;59:915–920.

Wells A, Read N, Craig A: Influences of dietary and intraduodenal lipid on alertness, mood, and sustained concentration. *Br J Nutr* 1995;74:115–123.

Youdim K, Martin A, Joseph J: Essential fatty acids and the brain: Possible health implications. *Int J Dev N* 2000;18:383–399.

Desserts, Chocolate, and Other Sweets: Curbing Sweet Cravings

Avena N, Hoebel B: Amphetamine-sensitized rats show sugar-induced hyperactivity (cross-sensitization) and sugar hyperphagia. *Pharm Bio B* 2003;74:635–639.

Barkeling B, Linne Y, Lindross A, et al: Intake of sweet foods and counts of cariogenic microorganisms in relation to body mass index and psychometric variables in women. *Int J Obes* 2002;26:1239–1244.

Christensen L, Pettijohn L: Mood and carbohydrate craving. *Appetite* 2001;36:137–145.

Colantuoni C, Rada P, McCarthy J, et al: Evidence that intermittent, excessive sugar intake causes endogenous opioid dependence. *Obes Res* 2002;10:478–488.

Colantuoni C, Schwenker J, McCarthy J, et al: Excessive sugar intake alters binding to dopamine and muopiod receptors in the brain. *Neuroreport* 2001;12:3549–3552.

Drewnowski A, Massien C, Louis-Sylvestre J, et al: Comparing the effects of aspartame and sucrose on motivational ratings, taste preferences, and energy intakes in humans. *Am J Clin N* 1994;59:338–345.

Hao S, Avraham Y, Mechoulam R, et al: Low dose anandamide affects food intake, cognitive function, neurotransmitter and corticosterone levels in diet-restricted mice. *Eur J Pharm* 2000;392:147–156.

Helm K, Rada P, Hoebel B: Cholecystokinin combined with serotonin in the hypothalamus limits accumbens dopamine release while increasing acetylcholine: A possible satiation mechanism. *Brain Res* 2003;963:290–297.

Hoebel B, Colantuoni C, Schwenker J, et al: Sugar dependence: Neural and behavioral signs of sensitization and withdrawal. *Am J Clin N* 2002;75:241.

Ludwig D, Peterson K, Gortmaker S: Relation between consumption of sugar-sweetened drinks and childhood obesity: A prospective, observational analysis. *Lancet* 2001;357: 505–508.

Meguid M, Fetissov S, Varma M, et al: Hypothalamic dopamine and serotonin in the regulation of food intake. *Nutrition* 2000;16:843–857.

Michener W, Rozin P: Pharmacological versus sensory factors in the satiation of chocolate cravings. *Physl Behav* 1994;56:419–422.

Pelchat M: Food cravings in young and elderly adults. *Appetite* 1997;28:103–113.

Pelchat M: Of human bondage: Food craving, obsession, compulsion, and addiction. *Physl Behav* 2002;76:347–352.

Pelchat M, Schaefer S: Dietary monotony and food cravings in young and elderly adults. *Physl Behav* 2000;68:353–359.

Putnam J, Allshouse J, Kantor L: U.S. per capita food supply trends: More calories, refined carbohydrates, and fats. *Food Rev* 2002;25:2–15.

Rogers P, Smit H: Food craving and food "addiction": A critical review of the evidence from a biopsychosocial perspective. *Pharm Bio B* 2000;66:3–14.

Schlundt D, Virts K, Sbrocco T, et al: A sequential behavioral analysis of craving sweets in obese women. *Addict Beha* 1993;18:67–80.

Somer E: *The Origin Diet*. New York, Owl Books, 2000.

White M, Whisenhunt B, Williamson D, et al: Development and validation of the food-craving inventory. *Obes Res* 2002;10:107–114.

Willner P, Benton D, Brown E, et al: Depression increases craving for sweet rewards in animal and human models of depression and craving. *Psychopharm* 1998;136:272–283.

Zador D, Wall P, Webster I: High sugar intake in a group of women on methadone maintenance in South Western Sydney, Australia. *Addiction* 1996;91:1053–1061.

Beverages: Boost Energy

Ainslie P, Campbell I, Frayn K, et al: Energy balance, metabolism, hydration, and performance during strenuous hill walking: The effect of age. *J App Physl* 2002;93:714–723.

DiMeglio D, Mattes R: Liquid versus solid carbohydrate: Effects on food intake and body weight. *Int J Obes* 2000;24:794–800.

Duffy R, Jarrett N, Fluck E, et al: Dietary soy improves memory in humans. *J Nutr* 2002;132:S587.

Grandjean A, Reimers K, Bannick K, et al: The effect of caffeinated and non-caffeinated, caloric and non-caloric beverages on hydration. *J Am Col N* 2000;19:591–600 (meeting abstract).

Kleiner S: Water: An essential but overlooked nutrient. *J Am Diet A* 1999;99:200–206.

Kreijkamp-Kaspers S, Kok L, Grobbee D, et al: Phytoestrogen intake in the Western diet and memory function in postmenopausal women. *J Nutr* 2002;132:S612–S613 (meeting abstract).

Rogers P, Kainth A, Smit H: A drink of water can improve or impair mental performance depending on small differences in thirst. *Appetite* 2001;36:57–58.

Rolls B, Bell E, Thorwart M: Water incorporated into a food but not served with a food decreases energy intake in lean women. *Am J Clin N* 1999;70:448–455.

Rolls B, Castellanos V, Halford J, et al: Volume of food consumed affects satiety in men. *Am J Clin N* 1998;67:1170–1177.

Rolls B, Roe L: Effect of the volume of liquid food infused intragastrically on satiety in women. *Physl Behav* 2002;76:623–631.

Stookey J: The diuretic effects of alcohol and caffeine and total water intake misclassification. *Eur J Epid* 1999;15:181–188.

Stricker E, Sved A: Thirst. *Nutrition* 2000;16:821–826.

Thys-Jacobs S, Starkey P, Bernstein D, et al: Calcium carbonate and the premenstrual syndrome: Effects on premenstrual and menstrual symptoms. *Am J Obstet Gyn* 1998; 179:444–452.

Tordoff M, Alleva A: Effects of drinking soda sweetened with aspartame or high-fructose corn syrup on food intake and body weight. *Am J Clin N* 1990;51:963–969.

▪ Acknowledgments ▪

WE ARE SO grateful to all the special people in our lives who have made this cookbook possible. A special thank-you to Jeanette's daughter Alex for typing and retyping the endless recipes without rolling her eyes. To Jeanette's daughter Amy for not offering to type the recipes; she's too much like her mother! To Gary, Jeanette's wonderful, dutiful husband, who often drove to the store for another ingredient at 10 P.M. To Patrick, Lauren, and Will, who tried every recipe and gave such honest critiques. And to Walloby and Meg, the family dogs, who mostly ate burned food.

Our literary agent, David Hale Smith, is the best agent in the world, and our editor, Deborah Brody, is the best editor (along with a great bike buddy!). Sweet Leah Kaufman's help in the kitchen, analyzing the recipes and preparing the references was invaluable. Just having her precious spirit around was a joy! Thanks to Victoria Dolby-Toews, for yet again traipsing to the medical library week after week to retrieve the research; to Miriam at Salem Public Library, for locating hundreds of hard-to-find research articles; and to Jodi Schwindt, for making copies of studies and attempting to keep Elizabeth's office in working order. What would Elizabeth do without Mark, the computer wizard recently promoted to computer saint, who miraculously kept the equipment running, right up to the deadline? Thank you to Roth's Supermarkets, especially to the employees at Vista and Sunnyslope, for having all the ingredients we needed and always being so willing to search for them on the shelves.

We acknowledge our friends who enthusiastically volunteered to help with taste-testing duties. One of the greatest joys in creating this book has been the time we shared with them. They make us laugh and dance in the kitchen. With thanks to Kim and Cort Garrison; Deb, Sid, Eric, and Alex Green; Gloria Hettle; Joanna and Christopher Kaufman; Janice and Justine Keudell; Joan Roberts; Sherry West; and Rollie and Dolores Wisbrock.

Much gratitude to all the wonderful cooks in our lives. Their influence remains one of our most prized possessions. What we remember most is how they all danced and celebrated in and around the kitchen. Our love affair with food has never stopped. Thanks to Jeanette's dearest Auntie Mim; to Jeanette's six siblings, who made it impossible to sit at the Sunday dinner table with a straight face; to Elizabeth's sisters, Gayle and Lovey, who are still shocked that she wrote a cookbook; and to Jeanette's brother, Paul ("Rocky"), for his inspiring New American Cuisine creations at his successful restaurant in Steamboat Springs, Colorado.

Finally, a heartfelt thank-you to all the researchers and clinicians whose work forms the foundation of this book, especially to those who took time out of their day to answer Elizabeth's questions. These include: Dr. Bruce Arnow at Stanford University Medical Center, Dr. Kelly Brownell at Yale University, Dr. C. Wayne Callaway at George Washington University, Dr. Larry Christensen at the University of South Alabama, Sharon Edelstein, Sc.M., at George Washington University, Anne Fletcher, M.S., R.D., Rosanne Gold, and Dr. David Jenkins at St. Michael's Hospital, Dr. Jan Johnson-Shane at Illinois State University, Dr. Sarah Leibowitz at Rockefeller University, Dr. Barry Popkin at the University of North Carolina, Dr. Barbara Rolls at Pennsylvania State University, Dr. David Schlundt at Vanderbilt University, Dr. Gayle Timmerman at the University of Texas, and Dr. Zoe Warwick at the University of Maryland.

· Index ·

Italic page numbers indicate recipes; boldface page numbers indicate box text.

age/aging, 5, 30, 201, 202, 204
alcohol, 31, 32, 146, 261
Almonds, Toasted Slivered, Green Beans and, 216
anandamide, 230
ancestors, ancient, 59, 232; appetite control systems, 116, 230; thirst control, 264
animals: under stress, 31
anthocyanins, 206
antioxidant-rich foods, **207**
antioxidants, 5, 12, 31, 33, 150, 204–5, 206, 214, 220
appetite, 3, 113, 171; versus hunger, 144; taming out-of-control, 143–70
appetite-control systems, 116, 147, 230, 264
appetizers, 29–55; recipes, 35–55
apples:
    Apple 'n' Nut Tossed Salad, **115**
    Apple Snacks, **34**
    Baked Apple-Cinnamon Pancake, 13

Baked Stuffed Apples with Toasted Walnuts, Currants, and Maple Syrup, 251
Baked Sweet Potatoes Topped with Apples, Cranberries, and Nuts, 220
Caramelized Leek Tart with Apples and Blue Cheese, 48
Tart Apple, Pecan, and Dried Cherry Salad, 123
Apricot Cooler, 270
aroma, 113–14, 117, 118, 119, 120
artichokes:
    Artichoke Dip, 37
    Creamy Artichoke Soup with Roasted Hazelnuts, 101
Arugula and Garlic Balsamic Vinaigrette, Roasted Veggie Focaccia Layered with Eggplant, Roasted Peppers, Portabello Mushrooms, Feta Cheese and, 79
Asian Cucumber Salad, 140
Asian-Style Noodles, **175**

asparagus:
    Cream of Asparagus Soup, **91**
    Pan-Seared Asparagus with Gingered Onions, 208
    Prawn and Asparagus Lettuce Wraps with Hoisin Sauce, 69
Avocado-Lime Salsa, 36

B vitamins, 3, 10, 12, 31, 39, 70, 94, 130, 131, 132, 184, 203, 268, 269
Baby Greens and Orange Salad with Pecans and Celery Seed Dressing, 133
bagels, 120:
    Toasted Whole Wheat Bagels with Brie and Strawberries, 71
    Veggie Bagel Bites, 68
Baked Apple-Cinnamon Pancake, 13
Baked Lima and Butter Beans in a Thick BBQ Sauce, 223
Baked Pork Florentine with Wild Rice, 168

Baked Stuffed Apples with Toasted
  Walnuts, Currants, and Maple
  Syrup, *251*
Baked Sweet Potatoes Topped with
  Apples, Cranberries, and Nuts,
  220
Balsamic Vinaigrette, Grilled
  Vegetables with Garlic and,
  227
Balsamic Vinegar, Quick-Baked
  Cherry Tomatoes with Olive
  Oil, and Basil, *222*
bananas:
  Banana-Pineapple Colada, *268*
  Quick Oatmeal with Bananas and
    Maple Syrup, *20*
  Rice Cakes Layered with Low-Fat
    Peanut Butter, Toasted Wheat
    Germ, Bananas, and Honey,
    49
  Whole Wheat Banana French
    Toast, *16*
Barbecued Chicken, **145**
barley:
  Barley, Red Pepper, and Green
    Onion Pilaf, *199*
  Hearty Lamb and Barley Stew,
    102
basil:
  Creamy Hummus Dip with Fresh
    Tomatoes and Basil, *39*
  Fresh Sliced Tomatoes with Basil,
    115
  Garden Tomato Soup with Fresh
    Basil, *93*
  Halibut with Tomatoes, Basil,
    and Capers, *157*
  Linguine and Pesto, **175**
  Linguine with Tomatoes and
    Fresh Basil, *190*
  Quick-Baked Cherry Tomatoes
    with Olive Oil, Balsamic
    Vinegar, and Basil, *222*
  Slow-Roasted Tomatoes and
    Pesto on Polenta Pizzas, *51*
  Sunshine Rice with Basil and
    Parmesan, *179*
  Thai Curry Pasta with Fresh Crab
    and Basil, *195*
  Toasted Tomato and Fresh Basil
    on Sourdough, *81*

Bay Shrimp Omelet with Sautéed
  Spinach and Gruyère Cheese,
  28
beans:
  Baked Lima and Butter Beans in a
    Thick BBQ Sauce, *223*
  Bean 'n' Vegetable Burrito, **60**
  Beans, Greens, and Roasted
    Garlic Soup, *110*
  Black Bean Burritos, *64*
  Black Bean Chili with Chicken,
    95
  Black Bean Dip with Pita
    Wedges, *38*
  Black Beans with Cumin and
    Chipotle Peppers, *154*
  Curried Couscous with Garbanzo
    Beans and Mandarin Oranges,
    136
  Red Rice and Kidney Bean Salad,
    134
  Veggie Stir-Fry with Ginger and
    Black Bean Sauce, *212*
beef:
  Grilled Asian Flank Steak with
    Wasabi Cream Sauce, *165*
  Old-Fashioned Country
    Vegetable-Beef Stew, *97*
beets, *131*:
  Beet Salad, **115**
  Roasted Beet Salad with Orange
    Vinaigrette, *131*
Bellini Peach Blush, *277*
berries, *5*:
  Berry Parfait, **231**
  Mixed Berries with Custard
    Sauce, *248*
beta-carotene, *94, 182, 203, 214,*
  218, 220, 269; sources of, *206*
beverages, *259–85;* quick-fix,
  261–62; recipes, *266–85*
binge(ing), *3, 33, 60, 87, 176;*
  sugar, *232–33*
Bite-Size Lettuce Wraps, *54*
bitter (taste), *113, 117*
Black Bean Burritos, *64*
Black Bean Chili with Chicken, *95*
Black Bean Dip with Pita Wedges,
  38
Black Bean Sauce, Veggie Stir-Fry
  with Ginger and, *212*

Black Beans with Cumin and
  Chipotle Peppers, *154*
blood sugar, *5, 29, 32, 173, 174,*
  176
BLT, **61**
Blue Cheese, Caramelized Leek Tart
  with Apples and, *48*
blueberries:
  Blueberry Frozen Yogurt, **231**
  Blueberry Limeade, *281*
  Blueberry Waffles, **4**
  Lemon Cheesecake Piled High
    with Blueberries, *236–37*
  Peach 'n' Blueberry Crisp with a
    Hint of Orange, *255*
  Strawberry-Blueberry Cobbler,
    252
  Very Berry Lemon Pancakes with
    Blueberry Sauce, *10–11*
brain, *1–2, 5, 201;* control center
  for cravings in, *230;* needs
  antioxidants, *204–5*
brain cells, *203, 204–5*
brain chemistry, *58, 144, 176, 230,*
  233
brain food, *202–3*
Braised Chicken Parmesan, *166*
breads, quick-fix, **4;** recipes, *8–28:*
  Cranberry-Orange Bread, *9*
  Crusty French Bread, *18*
  Individual Bread Puddings with
    Brandy White Sauce, *239*
breakfast eaters/skippers, *2–3*
Breakfast Oat Scone Cake, *19*
Breakfast Parfait, **4**
breakfast rules, *6–7*
breakfasts, *1–28, 33, 176;* and
  mental health, *202;* quick-fix,
  4; recipes, *8–28;* superstars,
  5–6; what you eat, *3–5*
Brie, Spicy Shrimp, and Peach
  Chutney, Toasted Crostini
  with, *43*
Brie and Strawberries, Toasted
  Whole Wheat Bagels with, *71*
British McMuffin, **4**
broccoli, **205:**
  Quick Steamed Broccoli with
    Parmesan Cheese, *228*
Broiled Tomatoes, **205**
Brownie, Raspberry, Sundae, **231**

Brownies, Busy-Day, *249*
Bruschetta with Baked
    Mediterranean Marinara and
    Goat Cheese, *47*
Brussels Sprouts, **205**:
    Maple-Glazed Brussels Sprouts
    with Portabello Mushrooms
    and Walnuts, *213*
Build-Your-Own Fish Tacos, *78*
burritos:
    Bean 'n' Vegetable Burrito, **60**
    Black Bean Burritos, *64*
    California-Style Roasted Veggie
    Burrito, *76*
Busy-Day Brownies, *249*
Butternut Squash Soup with
    Cranberry Chutney and
    Roasted Pecans, *100*

Caesar Salad, Low-Fat, *142*
Café Latte with Orange, **262**
Café Mocha Granita, *276*
caffeine, 32, 62–63, 174, 230
Cajun Sweet Potatoes, **205**
cakes:
    Carrot Cake with Coconut Cream
    Frosting, *246*
    Lemon Bundt Cake with
    Raspberry Filling, *247*
calcium, 3, 12, 31, 94, 244, 268,
    269
California-Style Roasted Veggie
    Burrito, *76*
caloric density, 89–91; lowdown on,
    89
calories, 5, 57, 60, 120, 233;
    concentrated, 230; consumed,
    144, 146; and liquids, 263;
    storing, 31, 59
cancer, 59, 174, 204, 225, 260
cannabinoids, 230
Cantaloupe Cups, **4**
Capers, Halibut with Tomatoes,
    Basil, and, *157*
Caramel Flan, Citrus-Scented, *238*
Caramelized Leek Tart with Apples
    and Blue Cheese, *48*
carb dishes, quick-fix, **174–75**
carbohydrates, 6, 57–58, 230; for
    PMS, SAD, depression,
    171–77; quality, 173–77

Cardamon, Coconut Rice with
    Ginger and, *194*
Caribbean Chicken, **145**
CaribBean One-Pot Stew, *111*
carrots, **205**:
    Carrot Cake with Coconut Cream
    Frosting, *246*
    Carrot-Apple Zapper, **262**
    Creamy Mashed Potatoes,
    Parsnips, and Carrots, *182*
    Glazed Carrots, *215*
casseroles:
    Chilies Rellenos Casserole with
    Red Sauce, *160–61*
    Southwest Fiesta Casserole with
    Corn Bread Topping, *167*
cataracts, 204
Cauliflower Puree, Creamy, *225*
Celery Logs, **34**
Celery Seed Dressing, Baby Greens
    and Orange Salad with Pecans
    and, *133*
Cereal Twist, **4**
cereals, 2, 5–6
cheese:
    Fresh Green Beans with Shallots,
    Red Onion, and Feta Cheese,
    219
    Grilled Cheese, Tomato, and
    Roasted Yellow Pepper
    Sandwich, *67*
    Ham, Cheese, and Spinach
    Frittata, *17*
    intensely flavored cheese, **117**
    Old-Fashioned (Low-Fat)
    Macaroni and Cheese, *197*
    Parmesan Cheese, *119*
    Potato Gratin with Light Boursin
    Cheese, *200*
    Quick Steamed Broccoli with
    Parmesan Cheese, *228*
    Roasted Veggie Focaccia Layered
    with Eggplant, Roasted
    Peppers, Portabello
    Mushrooms, Feta Cheese,
    Arugula, and Garlic Balsamic
    Vinaigrette, *79*
Cheesecake, Lemon, Piled High
    with Blueberries, *236–37*
Cherry, Dried, Pecan, Tart Apple
    and, Salad, *123*

Cherry Tomatoes, Quick-Baked,
    with Olive Oil, Balsamic
    Vinegar, and Basil, *222*
chicken, 149, 185, 221:
    Barbecued Chicken, **145**
    Black Bean Chili with Chicken,
    95
    Braised Chicken Parmesan, *166*
    Caribbean Chicken, **145**
    Chicken and Peanut Wraps, *83*
    Chicken Mango Sandwich, **60**
    Chicken 'n' Mushrooms in Sherry
    Cream Gravy, *156*
    chicken salad, 152
    Chicken Salad Pitas with Red
    Pepper and Dill, *65*
    Chicken Salad with Chutney and
    Toasted Coconut, *130*
    Chicken Satay Chop Salad in
    Lettuce Parcels with Peanut
    Sauce, *139*
    Chicken with Mushrooms in
    Creamy Garlic-Pecan Sauce,
    151
    Chunky Chicken Noodle Soup,
    108
    Classic Chicken Pot Pie, *164*
    Grandma's Homemade Chicken
    'n' Noodles, *180–81*
    Herb-Roasted Chicken, *152*
    Stir-Fried Mu-Shu Chicken, *153*
    Tandoori Chicken Made Simple,
    170
    Thai Fettuccine with Chicken,
    184
Chickpeas, Spicy Couscous and, *185*
Chili, Black Bean, with Chicken, *95*
Chilies Rellenos Casserole with
    Red Sauce, *160–61*
Chili-Spiced Shrimp Salad with
    Mango-Pineapple Salsa, *129*
Chili-Spiced Shrimp Spring Rolls,
    52
Chilled Fruit Soup, **91**
chipotle peppers, **118**, 167, 169:
    Black Beans with Cumin and
    Chipotle Peppers, *154*
    Creamy Sweet Potatoes and Yams
    with Chipotle Peppers, *217*
    Fish Fajitas with Creamy
    Chipotle Coleslaw, *169*

chocolate, 173, 229–58; recipes, 235–58:
    Chocolate Almond Joy-Soy Frappe, *274*
    Chocolate Chip Frozen Yogurt, **231**
    Chocolate Chip Granola Cookies, **234**, *254*
    Chocolate Fondue, **231**
    Chocolate-Orange Sauce, Poached Pears with, *250*
    The Ultimate Bittersweet Chocolate Pudding, **233**, *242*
cholesterol, 3, 4, 59
Chowder, Old-Fashioned New England Seafood, *105*
Chunky Chicken Noodle Soup, *108*
Chunky Tomato Soup, **91**
chutney:
    Butternut Squash Soup with Cranberry Chutney and Roasted Pecans, *100*
    Chicken Salad with Chutney and Toasted Coconut, *130*
    Cranberry Chutney, *53*
    Grilled Halibut with Ginger-Mango Chutney, *149*
    Sweet Potato Chutney Salad, *122*
    Toasted Crostini with Brie, Spicy Shrimp, and Peach Chutney, *43*
    Tomato Chutney with Ginger, *46*
Cioppino in a Robust Tomato Base, Infused with Fresh Fennel and Orange, *99*
Citrus Rice, **175**
Citrus-Scented Caramel Flan, *238*
Clafouti, Pear, Rum-Scented, *253*
clams:
    Instant Clam Chowder, **91**
    Linguine with Clams, **145**
    Spicy Linguine with Red Clam Sauce, *189*
Classic Chicken Pot Pie, 62, *164*
Classic Lemonade, 78, *278*
Cobbler, Strawberry-Blueberry, *252*
coconut:
    Carrot Cake with Coconut Cream Frosting, *246*
    Chicken Salad with Chutney and Toasted Coconut, *130*

Coconut Rice with Ginger and Cardamon, *194*
    Rum-Infused Tropical Fruit with Coconut, *258*
    Strawberry Yogurt Pancakes with Coconut, *15*
    Strawberry-Banana Coconut Milk Smoothie, *275*
    Thai-Grilled Prawns with Coconut Dipping Sauce, *44–45*
coffee, 62–63, **234**, 261
Colada, Banana-Pineapple, *268*
coleslaw:
    Fish Fajitas with Creamy Chipotle Coleslaw, *169*
    Pineapple Coleslaw, **115**
    Sesame-Ginger Coleslaw, *121*
Comfort Breakfast, The, **4**
comfort foods, 88, 180, 200:
    Classic Chicken Pot Pie, *164*
    Creamy Comfort-Food Mashed Potatoes, *186*
    Creamy Mashed Potatoes, Parsnips, and Carrots, *182*
    meat loaf, 162
    Old-Fashioned (Low-Fat) Macaroni and Cheese, *197*
    personalized list of, 114
concentration, 62, 203
condiments, salty, **117**
cookies:
    Chocolate Chip Granola Cookies, *254*
    Ice Cream Cookies, **231**
Cooler, Apricot, *270*
Cooler, Grapefruit, **262**
Cooler, Mocha, the, Wake Up and Smell, 26, *271*
copper, 132
corn:
    Dilled Corn, **174**
    Smoky Sweet Potato 'n', Corn Chowder, *92*
    Southwest Corn-Potato Cakes, *183*
    Southwest Fiesta Casserole with Corn Bread Topping, *167*
cortisol, 30–31, 33, 204–5
Coulis, Strawberry, Fresh Fruit Parfaits with, *24*

Coulis, Strawberry, Ricotta Tart with, *243*
couscous, **174**:
    Curried Couscous with Garbanzo Beans and Mandarin Oranges, *136*
    Spicy Couscous and Chickpeas, *185*
    Spicy Shrimp Gumbo over Couscous, *107*
Crab, Fresh, and Basil, Thai Curry Pasta with, *195*
Crab and Veggie Cakes with Garlic-Chili Cream, *150*
crabmeat, 28
cranberries:
    Baked Sweet Potatoes Topped with Apples, Cranberries, and Nuts, *220*
    Butternut Squash Soup with Cranberry Chutney and Roasted Pecans, *100*
    Cranberry Chutney, *53*
    Cranberry-Orange Bread, *9*
    Crusty Cranberry Salmon, *155*
cravings, 58, 86, 88, 171–72, 173, 176; control center for, 230; giving in to, 229; gone bad, 172; identifying, 176; sugar, 230–31, 232; for sweets, 31, 86, 172, 229–34; 12-Step Program for, **233**; working with, 176
Cream Cheese, Toast and, **4**
Cream of Asparagus Soup, **91**
Creamed Tuna, **145**
Creamy, Low-Fat Fudge, *235*
Creamy Artichoke Soup with Roasted Hazelnuts, *101*
Creamy Cauliflower Puree, *225*
Creamy Comfort-Food Mashed Potatoes, *186*
Creamy Hummus Dip with Fresh Tomatoes and Basil, *39*
Creamy Mashed Potatoes, Parsnips, and Carrots, *182*
Creamy Risotto with Wild Mushrooms and Fresh Thyme, *196*
Creamy Sweet Potatoes and Yams with Chipotle Peppers, *217*

Crunchy Cucumbers, **115**
Crusty Cranberry Salmon, *155*
Crusty French Bread, *18*
cucumber:
    Asian Cucumber Salad, *140*
    Crunchy Cucumber, **115**
    Shrimp on Cucumber Rounds, **34**
Cumin and Chipotle Peppers, Black Beans with, *154*
Currants, and Maple Syrup, Baked Stuffed Apples with Toasted Walnuts and, *251*
curry:
    Curried Chicken Sandwich, **61**
    Curried Couscous with Garbanzo Beans and Mandarin Oranges, *136*
    Curried Rice, **175**
    Shrimp Curry in a Hurry, *163*
Custard Sauce, Mixed Berries with, *248*

Daiquiri, Mango-Lemon, *269*
dehydration, 32, 260, 261
Denver Egg 'n' Cheese Muffins, *21*
depression, 6, 31, 33, 63, 202, 203; carbohydrates for, 171–77; common thread with PMS and SAD, 172–73
desserts, 229–58; best, **234**; quick-fix, **231**; recipes, 235–58; skip or split, **234**
diabetes, 30, 58, 59, 174
diet, 29, 30, 146, 203
dieting, 86, 144
dill:
    Chicken Salad Pitas with Red Pepper and Dill, *65*
    Dilled Corn, **174**
    Salmon Hash with Dill Cream, *22*
dips, 33:
    Artichoke Dip, *37*
    Black Bean Dip with Pita Wedges, *38*
    Creamy Hummus Dip with Fresh Tomatoes and Basil, *39*
    Veggie Dip, **34**
disease(s), 30; water and, 259, 260
dopamine, 58, 232

East Coast Goulash, *198*
eating: mindfully, 146; out of habit, 177; regularly, 33, **234**; stress and, 32–33
eating habits/patterns, 3, 29, 30, 58–59, 144, 176
egg(s):
    Bay Shrimp Omelet with Sautéed Spinach and Gruyère Cheese, *28*
    Denver Egg 'n' Cheese Muffins, *21*
    Egg and Sausage Enchiladas, *26*
    egg substitute, 254, 266
    Ham, Cheese, and Spinach Frittata, *17*
    Low-Fat Eggs Benedict Florentine, *27*
    Spinach and Ham Quiche Cups, *8*
Eggnog, Outrageous Fat-Free, *266*
eggplant:
    Polenta-Crusted Eggplant Parmesan, *224*
    Roasted Veggie Focaccia Layered with Eggplant, Roasted Peppers, Portabello Mushrooms, Feta Cheese, Arugula, and Garlic Balsamic Vinaigrette, *79*
ellagic acid, 206
emotional eating/emotions, 85–91, 144; taste and, 114
Enchiladas, Egg and Sausage, *26*
endorphins, 33, 230, 232
energy, 2, 5, 148, 176; boosting, with beverages, 259–65; sugar and, 63
entrées, 143–70; planning, 147, quick-fix, **145**; recipes, 149–70
European Snack, The, **34**
exercise, 33, 147, 176, 202, 261
extracts, **118**

Fall Fruit Salad, **115**
fat (body), 30, 59
fats:
    fat (dietary), 60, 146; and brain, 203; in breakfast, 3, 4, 5, 6, 7; and flavor, 116; at lunch, 57, 58; in salad dressing, 119, 120

fat busters, **117**
fat metabolism, 59
fat substitutes, **234**, 235
fat-free half-and-half, 146, 151
fatigue, 33, 58, 61–62, 63; and memory, 202; water and, 259, 260
fatigue fighters, 1–7
feast-or-fast scenario, 59
feeling full, 90, 148, 265
fettuccine:
    Fettuccine Alfredo, **175**
    Sautéed Scallops with a Creamy Pink Sauce over Fettuccine, *191*
    Thai Fettuccine with Chicken, *184*
fiber, 3, 6, 90, 218, 233, 265; focus on, 32, 60
fish, 35, 146, 149, 203, 221:
    Build-Your-Own Fish Tacos, *78*
    Fish Fajitas with Creamy Chipotle Coleslaw, *169*
    fish oils, 203
    fish soup, 99
Flan, Citrus-Scented Caramel, *238*
flavonoids, 206
flavor(s), 113–14, 117, 119, 120; fat and, 116; in salad dressing, 120; in salads, 120; smoking and, **117**
flavor boosters, **117**
flavorings: as salt substitutes, **118**
Fluffy Mashed Potatoes with Horseradish, 158, *187*
fluids, 261, 262–63
Focaccia, Roasted Veggie, Layered with Eggplant, Roasted Peppers, Portabello Mushrooms, Feta Cheese, Arugula, and Garlic Balsamic Vinaigrette, *79*
folic acid, 3, 39, 121, 131, 149, 172, 203, 208, 218
food(s), 144; emotions and, 86, 87, 88; focus on real, 148; getting water from, **263**; mood and, **234**; soothing, 117–18
food choices, 57, 230, 232; serotonin levels and, 172; of stressed people, 30

Frappe, Chocolate Almond Joy-Soy,
    274
free radicals, 31, 204
French Bread, Crusty, 18
French toast:
    Overnight Crunchy French Toast,
        25
    Whole Wheat Banana French
        Toast, 16
Fresh Fruit Parfaits with Strawberry
    Coulis, 24
Fresh Fruit Salad with Yogurt
    Dressing, 137
Fresh Green Beans with Shallots,
    Red Onion, and Feta Cheese,
    219
Fresh Sliced Tomatoes with Basil,
    115
Frittata, Ham, Cheese, and Spinach,
    17
Frothy 'n' Rich Hot Chocolate, 272
Frozen Yogurt Pie, 231
fruits, 1, 33, 119, 206, 265:
    Chilled Fruit Soup, 91
    Fall Fruit Salad, 115
    Fruit Dunk, 231
    Fresh Fruit Parfaits with
        Strawberry Coulis, 24
    Fresh Fruit Salad with Yogurt
        Dressing, 137
    fruit juices, 261
    Fruit Sandwich, 60
    Fruit Tortilla, 34
    Instant Breakfast Fruit Smoothie,
        285
    Rum-Infused Tropical Fruit with
        Coconut, 258
Fudge, Creamy, Low-Fat, 235

galanin, 58, 230
Garbanzo Toss with Sun-Dried
    Tomatoes, Red Pepper, and
    Fresh Parsley, 128
Garden Tomato Soup with Fresh
    Basil, 93
garlic, 118:
    Beans, Greens, and Roasted
        Garlic Soup, 110
    Chicken with Mushrooms in
        Creamy Garlic-Pecan Sauce,
        151

Crab and Veggie Cakes with
    Garlic-Chili Cream, 150
Gourmet Pizza with White Clam
    Sauce, Spinach, Garlic, and
    Fresh Tomatoes, 72
Grilled Vegetables with Garlic and
    Balsamic Vinaigrette, 227
Roasted Veggie Focaccia Layered
    with Eggplant, Roasted
    Peppers, Portabello
    Mushrooms, Feta Cheese,
    Arugula, and Garlic Balsamic
    Vinaigrette, 79
Slow-Roasted Tomatoes with
    Garlic and Herbs, 221
Swiss Chard with Garlic and
    Oregano, 218
ginger:
    Coconut Rice with Ginger and
        Cardamon, 194
    Ginger Squash, 209
    Ginger-Pumpkin Muffins, 14
    Ginger-Teriyaki Rice Bowls, 192
    Grilled Halibut with
        Ginger-Mango Chutney, 149
    Pan-Seared Asparagus with
        Gingered Onions, 208
    Tofu Cakes in Sweet Ginger
        Sauce, 75
    Tomato Chutney with Ginger,
        46
    Veggie Stir-Fry with Ginger and
        Black Bean Sauce, 212
Glazed Carrots, 215
glucose, 1–2, 233
Goat Cheese, Bruschetta with
    Baked Mediterranean Marinara
    and, 47
Goulash, East Coast, 198
Gourmet Pizza with White Clam
    Sauce, Spinach, Garlic, and
    Fresh Tomatoes, 72
grains, 1, 2, 174, 176; serving size,
    146; see also whole grains
Grandma's Homemade Chicken 'n'
    Noodles, 180–81
Granola Cookies, Chocolate Chip,
    254
Grapefruit Cooler, 262
Greek Pasta Salad with Red Wine
    Vinaigrette, 132

Green and Red Chunky Salad with
    Oregano, 93, 125
green beans, 205:
    Fresh Green Beans with Shallots,
        Red Onion, and Feta Cheese,
        219
    Green Beans and Toasted Slivered
        Almonds, 216
    Green Onion Pilaf, Barley, Red
        Pepper, and, 199
    Green Pepper Seviche, Shrimp and
        Roasted, 55
greens, 117, 119:
    Baby Greens and Orange Salad
        with Pecans and Celery Seed
        Dressing, 133
    Beans, Greens, and Roasted
        Garlic Soup, 110
Grilled Asian Flank Steak with
    Wasabi Cream Sauce, 165
Grilled Cheese, Tomato, and
    Roasted Yellow Pepper
    Sandwich, 67
Grilled Halibut with
    Ginger-Mango Chutney, 149
Grilled Polenta Rounds with
    Tomato Caponata, 41
Grilled Pork Tenderloin with
    Rosemary-Orange Sauce,
    158–59
Grilled Salmon, 145
Grilled Turkey Reuben on Dark Rye,
    77
Grilled Vegetables with Garlic and
    Balsamic Vinaigrette, 227
Gruyère Cheese, Bay Shrimp Omelet
    with Sautéed Shrimp and, 28
Guacamole, Low-Fat Chunky, 40
Gumbo, Spicy Shrimp, over
    Couscous, 107

halibut:
    Grilled Halibut with
        Ginger-Mango Chutney, 149
    Halibut Vera Cruz, 145
    Halibut with Tomatoes, Basil,
        and Capers, 157
ham:
    Ham, Cheese, and Spinach
        Frittata, 17
    Spinach and Ham Quiche Cups, 8

Hash, Salmon, with Dill Cream, 22
hazelnuts:
    Creamy Artichoke Soup with
      Roasted Hazelnuts, *101*
    Wilted Spinach Salad with Warm
      Raspberry Vinaigrette and
      Toasted Hazelnuts, *141*
heart disease, 6, 58, 204; risk for, 5,
    30, 59, 121, 174
Heartwarming Winter Vegetable
    Soup, *98*
Hearty Lamb and Barley Stew, *102*
Herbed Baked Potato, **175**
Herbed Rice, **175**
Herb-Roasted Chicken, *152*
herbs:
    fresh herbs, **117**
    Slow-Roasted Tomatoes with
      Garlic and Herbs, *221*
    Wild Rice and Mushroom Soup
      with Fresh Herbs, *104*
hippocampus, 201
Hoisin Sauce, Prawn and Asparagus
    Lettuce Wraps with, *69*
Homemade Orange Julius, **262**
homocysteine, 203
honey:
    Hot Polenta Cereal with Honey,
      23
    Minted Lamb Pockets with
      Honey Yogurt Dressing, *66*
    Rice Cakes Layered with Low-Fat
      Peanut Butter, Toasted Wheat
      Germ, and Honey, *49*
    Warm Milk with Honey and
      Orange, *273*
hormones, 30–31
Horseradish, Fluffy Mashed
    Potatoes with, *187*
Hot Chai Tea, *279*
hot chocolate:
    Frothy 'n' Rich Hot Chocolate,
      272
    Iced Hot Chocolate, **262**
Hot Dog, **61**
Hot Polenta Cereal with Honey, *23*
Hummus Dip, Creamy, with Fresh
    Tomatoes and Basil, *39*
hunger: appetite versus, 144;
    managing, 59, 60; thirst or,
    264

hunger response, 86, 144
hypertension, 58, 174
hypothalamus, 58

Ice Cream Cookies, **231**
Ice Tea, Raspberry, *280*
Iced Hot Chocolate, **262**
Individual Bread Puddings with
    Brandy White Sauce, *239*
Individual Meat Loaves with Fresh
    Thyme, *162*
indole, 225
Indonesian Rice Salad Medley, *138*
Instant Breakfast Fruit Smoothie,
    285
Instant Clam Chowder, **91**
Instant Creamed Soups, **91**
Instant Stir Fry, **145**
insulin, 31, 59
iron, 3, 12, 39, 63, 94, 118, 121,
    130, 132, 149, 203, 208, 218;
    in beets, 131; and fatigue,
    61–62; heme/nonheme, 62;
    need for, 31
irritability, 6, 31, 58
isoflavones, 5
Italian Sausage, Hot, Lentil Soup
    with, *103*

junk food, 3, 172

Kidney Bean, Red Rice and, Salad,
    134

labels, reading, 174, **234**, 243
lamb:
    Hearty Lamb and Barley Stew,
      102
    Minted Lamb Pockets with
      Honey Yogurt Dressing, *66*
Lasagna, Zucchini-Tomato, with
    Fresh Thyme and Caramelized
    Onions, *210–11*
Leek Tart, Caramelized, with
    Apples and Blue Cheese, *48*
leftovers, 8, 149, 152, 160, 183,
    190, 207:
    Classic Chicken Pot Pie, *164*
    Crusty French Bread, *18*
    meat loaf, 162
    Salmon Hash with Dill Cream, 22

Slow-Roasted Tomatoes with
    Garlic and Herbs, *221*
Swiss Chard with Garlic and
    Oregano, *218*
Lemon Bundt Cake with Raspberry
    Filling, *247*
Lemon Cheesecake Piled High with
    Blueberries, *236–37*
lemon peel, **118**
lemonade:
    Classic Lemonade, *278*
    Strawberry Lemonade, *284*
Lentil Soup with Hot Italian
    Sausage, *103*
lettuce, 119:
    Bite-Size Lettuce Wraps, *54*
    Chicken Satay Chop Salad in
      Lettuce Parcels with Peanut
      Sauce, *139*
    Prawn and Asparagus Lettuce
      Wraps with Hoisin Sauce, *69*
light therapy, 176
lima beans:
    Baked Lima and Butter Beans in a
      Thick BBQ Sauce, *223*
Limeade, Blueberry, *281*
linguine:
    Linguine and Pesto, **175**
    Linguine with Clams, **145**
    Linguine with Tomatoes and
      Fresh Basil, *190*
    Spicy Linguine with Red Clam
      Sauce, *189*
low-carbohydrate diet, 144, 203
Low-Fat Caesar Salad, *142*
Low-Fat Chunky Guacamole, *40*
Low-Fat Eggs Benedict Florentine,
    27
Low-Fat Panna Cotta with Fresh
    Raspberry Sauce, *240–41*
Low-Fat Potato Latkes, *178*
lunchables, 57–83; recipes, 64–83
lunches: quick-fix, **60–61**; healthy,
    63; power, 57–58
lutein, 206
lycopene, 206

Macaroni and Cheese,
    Old-Fashioned (Low-Fat), *197*
magnesium, 12, 31, 39, 94, 133,
    268, 269

Mandarin Toss with Mint-Lemon Dressing, *135*

manganese, 132, 182

mango:
Chili-Spiced Shrimp Salad with Mango-Pineapple Salsa, *129*
Mango Maniac, *282*
Mango Wow, **261**
Mango-Lemon Daiquiri, *269*
Mango-Pineapple Salsa, *35*

maple:
maple flavoring, **118**
Baked Stuffed Apples with Toasted Walnuts, Currants, and Maple Syrup, *251*
Maple Syrup Smoothie, **261**
Maple-Glazed Brussels Sprouts with Portabello Mushrooms and Walnuts, *213*
Quick Oatmeal with Bananas and Maple Syrup, *20*
Sweet Potatoes with Maple Syrup, **206**

marinade, *165*; as salt substitute, **118**

Marinated Veggies, **115**

meals: regular, 58–60, 87; small, frequent, 33

meat:
Individual Meat Loaves with Fresh Thyme, *162*
limiting, 62; serving size, 146

medication(s): and taste, **117**

Mediterranean Marinara and Goat Cheese, Bruschetta with Baked, *47*

memory, 2, 113, 121, 171, 203, 206; short-term, 202, 205; taste and, 114

memory loss, 5, 6, 201, 202, 203, 204

mental function, 5, 171

mental health, 202–3

Mexican Five-Layered Spread, *50*

midday energy boosters, 57–63

midday quick fix, 62–63

Milk, Warm, with Honey and Orange, *273*

Mimosa, Sparkling Cider, with Raspberries, *283*

mind, exercising, 202

mind boosters, antiaging, 201–7

minerals, 3, 5, 70, 203, 233

Minestrone with Spinach and Orzo Pasta, *106*

mini-meals, 58–59, 60

Mini-Tomato Bowls, **34**

mint:
Mandarin Toss with Mint-Lemon Dressing, *135*
Minted Lamb Pockets with Honey Yogurt Dressing, *66*
Quinoa Tabbouleh with Fresh Mint, *73*

Mixed Berries with Custard Sauce, *248*

Mixed Berry Trifle, *244–45*

Mocha Cooler, the, Wake Up and Smell, *271*

Mock Taco Salad, **115**

Mock Waldorf Salad, **115**

monosodium glutamate (MSG), 32, 114

monounsaturated fats, 203

mood, 5, 6, 62, 113, 148; eating and, 58, 85–86, 87; and food, **234**; quality carbohydrates and, 173–77; nerve chemicals and, 171–72, 176

Mu-Shu, Stir-Fried Chicken, *153*

muffins, 120:
Denver Egg 'n' Cheese Muffins, *21*
Ginger-Pumpkin Muffins, *14*
Oat 'n' Dried Plum Muffins, *12*

mushrooms:
Chicken 'n' Mushrooms in Sherry Cream Gravy, *156*
Chicken with Mushrooms in Creamy Garlic-Pecan Sauce, *151*
Creamy Risotto with Wild Mushrooms and Fresh Thyme, *196*
Petite Peas with Shiitake Mushrooms, *226*
Quick Cream of Mushroom Soup, **91**
Portabello Mushrooms and Walnuts with Maple-Glazed Brussels Sprouts, *213*

Roasted Veggie Focaccia Layered with Eggplant, Roasted Peppers, and Portabello Mushrooms, Feta Cheese, Arugula, and Garlic Balsamic Vinaigrette, *79*
Wild Rice and Mushroom Soup with Fresh Herbs, *104*

Nachos, **145**

National Weight Control Registry, 2

nerve chemicals, 171–72, 176, 203

nervous system, 62, 113, 171

neuropeptide Y (NPY), 1–2, 3, 58, 144, 230

neurotransmitters, 171, 172, 176

nibbling, 31, 59, 60

noodles:
Asian-Style Noodles, **175**
Grandma's Homemade Chicken 'n' Noodles, *180–81*
Soba Noodles with Spicy Peanut Sauce, *193*
see also pasta

norepinephrine, 58

Northwest Sushi Roll-Ups with Smoked Salmon, *80*

nuts, **118**:
Baked Sweet Potatoes Topped with Apples, Cranberries, and Nuts, *220*
Nut Bread Spread, **61**
nut butters, 49
nut milk, 151

nutrients, 60, 174, 203; from breakfast, 5; fatigue-fighting, 3; mood boosting, 118; stress and need for, 31–33

Oat 'n' Dried Plum Muffins, *12*

oatmeal, 2, 5:
Quick Oatmeal with Bananas and Maple Syrup, *20*

obesity, 31

oils, **117**, 119; flavored, **118**

Old-Fashioned Country Vegetable-Beef Stew, *97*

Old-Fashioned (Low-Fat) Macaroni and Cheese, *197*

Old-Fashioned New England Seafood Chowder, *105*

olive oil, **117**

Olive Oil, Balsamic Vinegar, and Basil, Quick-Baked Cherry Tomatoes with, 222

omega-3 fats, 5, 6, 22, 70, 155, 172, 203

Omelet, Bay Shrimp, with Sautéed Spinach and Gruyère Cheese, 28

One-Dish Tacos, **145**

One-Minute Pancake, The, **4**

1-Minute Snack, **34**

1-2-3 Sloppy Joes, 82

onions:

  Pan-Seared Asparagus with Gingered Onions, 208

  Turkey Burgers with Caramelized Onions, 74

  Zucchini-Tomato Lasagna with Fresh Thyme and Caramelized Onions, 210–11

oranges:

  Baby Greens and Orange Salad with Pecans and Celery Seed Dressing, 133

  Café Latte with Orange, **262**

  Cioppino in a Robust Tomato Base, Infused with French Fennel and Orange, 99

  Curried Couscous with Garbanzo Beans and Mandarin Oranges, 136

  Homemade Orange Julius, **262**

  Orange Frosty, 267

  orange peel, 110

  Oranges with a Zing, **231**

  Peach 'n' Blueberry Crisp with a Hint of Orange, 255

  Roasted Beet Salad with Orange Vinaigrette, 131

  Spinach Orange Salad, **115**

  Warm Milk with Honey and Orange, 273

oregano:

  Green and Red Chunky Salad with Oregano, 125

  Swiss Chard with Garlic and Oregano, 218

Orzo Pasta, Minestrone with Spinach and, 106

osteoporosis, 204

Outrageous Fat-Free Eggnog, 266

Oven-Fried Potato Wedges, **175**

overeating, 86, 144, 148; overcoming, with tasty foods, 113–20; reasons for, 143

Overnight Crunchy French Toast, 25

oxidants/oxidation, 204, 205

oxytocin, 86

Paella, Quick, **145**

pancakes, 2, 58; potato, 183:

  Baked Apple–Cinnamon Pancake, 13

  Pancake Wrap, 6

  Strawberry Yogurt Pancakes with Coconut, 15

  The One-Minute Pancake, **4**

  Very Berry Lemon Pancakes with Blueberry Sauce, 10–11

Panna Cotta, Low-Fat, with Fresh Raspberry Sauce, 240–41

Pan-Seared Asparagus with Gingered Onions, 208

parfait:

  Berry Parfait, **231**

  Fresh Fruit Parfaits with Strawberry Coulis, 24

Parmesan, Sunshine Rice with Basil and, 179

Parsley, Fresh, Garbanzo Toss with Sun-Dried Tomatoes, Red Pepper, and, 128

Parsnips, and Carrots, Creamy Mashed Potatoes, 182

pasta dishes, 171–200, **175**; recipes, 178–200:

  Greek Pasta Salad with Red Wine Vinaigrette, 132

  Minestrone with Spinach and Orzo Pasta, 106

  Pasta Fagioli, 109

  Pasta Pronto, **145**

  Thai Curry Pasta with Fresh Crab and Basil, 195

  Tomato 'n' Herb Pasta, **175**

  see also noodles

PB 'n' B Smoothie, **262**

peaches:

  Peach Blush Bellinis, 277

  Peach 'n' Blueberry Crisp with a Hint of Orange, 255

Peachy Creamy Smoothie, **261**

Toasted Crostini with Brie, Spicy Shrimp, and Peach Chutney, 43

peanut butter:

  Chicken and Peanut Wraps, 83

  Peanut Butter Candy Sandwich, **60**

  Peanut Butter Krispies, **4**

  Peanut Butter Wraps, **4**

  Rice Cakes Layered with Low-Fat Peanut Butter, Toasted Wheat Germ, Bananas, and Honey, 49

Peanut Sauce, Chicken Satay Chop Salad in Lettuce Parcels with, 139

Peanut Sauce, Spicy, Soba Noodles with, 193

pears:

  Pear and Pomegranate Toss, **115**

  Poached Pears with Chocolate-Orange Sauce, 250

  Rum-Scented Pear Clafouti, 253

Peas, Petite, with Shiitake Mushrooms, 226

pecans:

  Baby Greens and Orange Salad with Pecans and Celery Seed Dressing, 133

  Butternut Squash Soup with Cranberry Chutney and Roasted Pecans, 100

  Chicken with Mushrooms in Creamy Garlic-Pecan Sauce, 151

  Tart Apple, Pecan, and Dried Cherry Salad, 123

Peppers, Roasted, Portabello Mushrooms, Feta Cheese, Arugula, and Garlic Balsamic Vinaigrette, Roasted Veggie Focaccia Layered with Eggplant and, 79

pesto:

  Linguine and Pesto, **175**

  Slow-Roasted Tomatoes and Pesto on Polenta Pizzas, 51

Petite Peas with Shiitake Mushrooms, 226

phenylethylamine (PEA), 230

phytochemicals, 206, 233
pies:
   Pumpkin Pie with Rum Whipped
     Cream, 256–57
Pilaf, Barley, Red Pepper, and Green
   Onion, *199*
Pineapple Coleslaw, **115**
Pita Wedges, Black Bean Dip with,
   38
Pitas, Chicken Salad, with Red
   Pepper and Dill, *65*
pizza:
   Gourmet Pizza with White Clam
     Sauce, Spinach, Garlic, and
     Fresh Tomatoes, *72*
   Slow-Roasted Tomatoes and
     Pesto on Polenta Pizzas, *51*
   Veggie Pizza, **60**
plums, dried, 5
PMS Soup, **91**
Poached Pears with
     Chocolate-Orange Sauce, *250*
Pocket Breakfast, **4**, 6
polenta:
   Grilled Polenta Rounds with
     Tomato Caponata, *41*
   Hot Polenta Cereal with Honey, *23*
   Plenty of Polenta,**175**
   Polenta-Crusted Eggplant
     Parmesan, *224*
   Slow-Roasted Tomatoes and
     Pesto on Polenta Pizzas, *51*
polyphenols, 5
Pomegranate, Pear and, Toss, **115**
pork:
   Baked Pork Florentine with Wild
     Rice, *168*
   Grilled Pork Tenderloin with
     Rosemary-Orange Sauce,
     158–59
portions, 6, 146, **147**, 233
Posole Soup, *96*
Pot Pie, Classic Chicken, *164*
potassium, 130, 131, 182
potatoes, 171–200; recipes, *178–200*:
   Creamy Comfort-Food Mashed
     Potatoes, *186*
   Creamy Mashed Potatoes,
     Parsnips, and Carrots, *182*
   Fluffy Mashed Potatoes with
     Horseradish, *187*

Herbed Baked Potato, **175**
Low-Fat Potato Latkes, *178*
Oven-Fried Potato Wedges, **175**
Potato Gratin with Light Boursin
   Cheese, *200*
potato pancakes, *183*
Southwest Corn-Potato Cakes, *183*
Prawn and Asparagus Lettuce
   Wraps with Hoisin Sauce, *69*
Prawns, Thai-Grilled, with Coconut
   Dipping Sauce, *44–45*
premenstrual syndrome (PMS):
   carbohydrates for, 171–77;
   common thread with SAD and
   depression, 172–73
processed foods, 172, 174, 203,
   206; sugar in, 233
protein, 6, 57–58, 119
Pumpkin, Ginger-, Muffins, *14*
Pumpkin Pie with Rum Whipped
   Cream, *256–57*
Pumpkin-Corn Soup with Creamy
   Lime-Ginger Sauce, *94*

Quesadillas, **60**
Quiche Cups, Spinach and Ham, *8*
Quick Cream of Mushroom Soup, **91**
quick fixes, 29–55; beverages,
   261–62; breakfasts and breads,
   4; carb dishes, **174–75**;
   desserts, **231**; entrées, **145**;
   lunches, **60–61**; midday,
   62–63; recipes, *35–55*; salads,
   115; snacks, **34**; soups, **91**;
   vegetables, **205–6**
Quick Oatmeal with Bananas and
   Maple Syrup, *20*
Quick Paella, **145**
Quick Steamed Broccoli with
   Parmesan Cheese, *228*
Quick-Baked Cherry Tomatoes with
   Olive Oil, Balsamic Vinegar,
   and Basil, *222*
Quinoa Tabbouleh with Fresh Mint,
   73

raspberries:
   Lemon Bundt Cake with
     Raspberry Filling, *247*
   Low-Fat Panna Cotta with Fresh
     Raspberry Sauce, *240–41*

Raspberry Brownie Sundae, **231**
Raspberry Ice Tea, *280*
Sparkling Cider Mimosa with
   Raspberries, *283*
red bell peppers:
   Barley, Red Pepper, and Green
     Onion Pilaf, *199*
   Chicken Salad Pitas with Red
     Pepper and Dill, *65*
   Garbanzo Toss with Sun-Dried
     Tomatoes, Red Pepper, and
     Fresh Parsley, *128*
   Stuffed Red Bell Peppers, **206**
Red Onion and Feta Cheese, Fresh
   Green Beans with Shallots and,
   219
Red Rice and Kidney Bean Salad,
   134
Red Sauce, Chilies Rellenos
   Casserole with, *160–61*, 188
REM (Rapid Eye Movement) sleep,
   32
rice dishes, 171–200, **175**; recipes,
   178–200:
   Citrus Rice, **175**
   Coconut Rice with Ginger and
     Cardamon, *194*
   Curried Rice, **175**
   Ginger-Teriyaki Rice Bowls, *192*
   Herbed Rice, **175**
   Indonesian Rice Salad Medley,
     138
   Red Rice and Kidney Bean Salad,
     134
   Rice Cakes Layered with
     Low-Fat Peanut Butter,
     Toasted Wheat Germ,
     Bananas, and Honey, *49*
   South-of-the-Border Rice, *188*
   Sunshine Rice with Basil and
     Parmesan, *179*
Ricotta Tart with Strawberry
   Coulis, *243*
Risotto, Creamy, with Wild
   Mushrooms and Fresh Thyme,
   196
Roasted Beet Salad with Orange
   Vinaigrette, *131*
Roasted Corn Salsa, *42*
Roasted Gingered Vegetables, *214*
Roasted Vegetables, **205**

Roasted Veggie Focaccia Layered
with Eggplant, Roasted
Peppers, Portabello
Mushrooms, Feta Cheese,
Arugula, and Garlic Balsamic
Vinaigrette, 79
Rum-Infused Tropical Fruit with
Coconut, 258
Rum-Scented Pear Clafouti, 253

salad dressing, 120; Celery Seed,
72, 133; fat in, 119; low-fat,
120; for Low-Fat Caesar Salad,
142; Mint-Lemon, 135; as salt
substitute, **118**
salads, 113–42; accompaniments,
120; golden rules of, 119–20;
quick-fix, **115**; recipes, 121–42:
Apple 'n' Nut Tossed Salad,
115
Asian Cucumber Salad, 140
Baby Greens and Orange Salad
with Pecans and Celery Seed
Dressing, 133
Beet Salad, **115**
chicken salad, 152
Chicken Salad with Chutney and
Toasted Coconut, 130
Chili-Spiced Shrimp Salad with
Mango-Pineapple Salsa, 129
Curried Couscous with Garbanzo
Beans and Mandarin Oranges,
136
Fish Fajitas with Creamy
Chipotle Coleslaw, 169
Greek Pasta Salad with Red Wine
Vinaigrette, 132
Green and Red Chunky Salad
with Oregano, 125
Low Fat Caesar Salad, 142
Mandarin Toss with Mint-Lemon
Dressing, 135
Pineapple Coleslaw, **115**
Mock Taco Salad, **115**
Mock Waldorf Salad, **115**
Red Rice and Kidney Bean Salad,
134
Roasted Beet Salad with Orange
Vinaigrette, 131
Sesame Salmon and Spinach Salad
with Asian Vinaigrette, 124

Sesame-Ginger Coleslaw, 121
Shrimp Louis, **115**
Spinach Orange Salad, **115**
Sweet Potato Chutney Salad, 122
Tart Apple, Pecan, and Dried
Cherry Salad, 123
Wild Rice and Roasted
Vegetables with Thyme
Vinaigrette, 126–27
Wilted Spinach Salad with Warm
Raspberry Vinaigrette and
Toasted Hazelnuts, 141
salmon, 5:
Salmon, Crusty Cranberry, 155
Salmon, Grilled, **145**
Salmon, Sesame, and Spinach
Salad with Asian Vinaigrette,
124
Salmon, Sesame, Sandwich, 70
Salmon, Smoked, Northwest
Sushi Roll-Ups with, 80
Salmon Hash with Dill Cream,
22
salsa:
Salsa, Avocado-Lime, 36
Salsa, Mango-Pineapple, 35
Salsa, Mango-Pineapple,
Chili-Spiced Shrimp Salad
with, 129
Salsa, Roasted Corn, 42
sandwiches, 57–83; quick-fix
lunches, 60–61; recipes,
64–83:
Chicken and Peanut Wraps, 83
Chicken Mango Sandwich, 60
Chicken Salad Pitas with Red
Pepper and Dill, 65
Curried Chicken Sandwich, **61**
Fruit Sandwich, **60**
Grilled Cheese, Tomato, and
Roasted Yellow Pepper
Sandwich, 67
Grilled Turkey Reuben on Dark
Rye, 77
Minted Lamb Pockets with
Honey Yogurt Dressing, 66
Peanut Butter Candy Sandwich,
60
Sesame Salmon Sandwich, 70
Sloppy Joes, 1-2-3, 82
Veggie Sandwich, 61

"Satiety Index," 90
saturated fat, 3, 203, 206
sauce(s):
Black Bean Sauce, 212
Blueberry Sauce, 10
Brandy White Sauce, 239
Chocolate-Orange Sauce, 250
Coconut Dipping Sauce, 44–45
Creamy Garlic-Pecan Sauce, 151
Creamy Lime-Ginger Sauce, 94
Creamy Pink Sauce, 191
Custard Sauce, 248
fish, 52
Fresh Raspberry Sauce, 240
Hoisin Sauce, 69
for Low-Fat Eggs Benedict
Florentine, 27
Peanut Sauce, 139
Red Clam Sauce, 189
Red Sauce, 160–61
Rosemary-Orange Sauce,
158–59
Spicy Peanut Sauce, 193
Sweet Ginger Sauce, 75
Thai peanut sauce, 52
Thick BBQ Sauce, 233
tomato sauce, 47
Wasabi Cream Sauce, 165
White Clam Sauce, 72
Sausage, Egg and, Enchiladas, 26
Sautéed Scallops with a Creamy
Pink Sauce over Fettuccine,
191
Scone Cake, Breakfast Oat, 19
Scotch broth, 102
Seafood Chowder, Old-Fashioned
New England, 105
seasonal affective disorder (SAD):
carbohydrates for, 171–77;
common thread with PMS and
depression, 172–73
selenium, 31, 94, 130, 184, 208
serotonin, 3, 31, 33, 58, 144, 171,
230; and food choices, 172;
and mood, 86; and PMS, SAD,
depression, 173; raising,
176
Sesame Salmon and Spinach Salad
with Asian Vinaigrette, 124
Sesame Salmon Sandwich, 62, 70
Sesame-Ginger Coleslaw, 121

Shallots, Red Onion, and Feta
Cheese, Fresh Green Beans
with, 165, *219*
Sherry Cream Gravy, Chicken 'n'
Mushrooms in, *156*
shrimp:
Bay Shrimp Omelet with Sautéed
Spinach and Gruyère Cheese,
28
Prawn and Asparagus Lettuce
Wraps with Hoisin Sauce, *69*
Shrimp and Roasted Green
Pepper Seviche, *55*
Shrimp Cocktail, **145**
Shrimp Curry in a Hurry, *163*
Shrimp Louis, **115**
Shrimp on Cucumber Rounds,
34
Shrimp Salad, Chili-Spiced, with
Mango-Pineapple Salsa, *129*
Shrimp Spring Rolls,
Chili-Spiced, *52*
Spicy Shrimp Gumbo over
Couscous, *107*
Toasted Crostini with Brie, Spicy
Shrimp, and Peach Chutney, *43*
skipping meals, 2–3, 33, 171, 176,
202–3
sleep: eating to improve, 29–55; lack
of, and memory, 202;
magnesium and, 31; serotonin
and, 171; snacks and, 33; and
stress and diet, 29–30
sleep problems, 30; depression and,
173; eliminating caffeine for,
32
Sloppy Joes, 1–2–3, *82*
Slow-Roasted Tomatoes and Pesto
on Polenta Pizzas, *51*
Slow-Roasted Tomatoes with Garlic
and Herbs, *221*
smoking, 31, **117**, 202
Smoky Sweet Potato 'n' Corn
Chowder, *92*, 118
smoky "umami" taste, **117**
smoothies, 265:
Apricot Cooler, *270*
Banana-Pineapple Colada, *268*
Instant Breakfast Fruit Smoothie,
285
Maple Syrup Smoothie, **261**

PB 'n' B Smoothie, **262**
Peachy Creamy Smoothie, **261**
Soy Berry Smoothie, **261**
Strawberry-Banana Coconut Milk
Smoothie, *275*
snacks, 29–55, 58, 59;
carbohydrate-rich, 176; as
habit, 177; low-fat, 31;
quick-fix, **34**; recipes, *35–55*;
and stress, 33
Snow Peas, **205**
Soba Noodles with Spicy Peanut
Sauce, *193*
soda, 174, 263, 265; water versus,
264
soft drinks, 233, **234**
soups, 85–111; case for, 89–91; as
comfort food, 88, 89; quick-fix,
91; with salad, 120; recipes,
92–111:
Beans, Greens, and Roasted
Garlic Soup, *110*
Butternut Squash Soup with
Cranberry Chutney and
Roasted Pecans, *100*
Chilled Fruit Soup, **91**
Chunky Chicken Noodle Soup,
108
Chunky Tomato Soup, **91**
Cioppino in a Robust Tomato
Base, Infused with Fresh
Fennel and Orange, *99*
Instant Clam Chowder, **91**
Cream of Asparagus Soup, **91**
Creamy Artichoke Soup with
Roasted Hazelnuts, *101*
Garden Tomato Soup with Fresh
Basil, *93*
Heartwarming Winter Vegetable
Soup, *98*
Instant Clam Chowder, **91**
Instant Creamed Soups, **91**
Minestrone with Spinach and
Orzo Pasta, *106*
Old-Fashioned New England
Seafood, Chowder, *105*
PMS Soup, **91**
Pumpkin-Corn Soup with
Creamy Lime-Ginger Sauce, *94*
Quick Cream of Mushroom
Soup, **91**

Smoky Sweet Potato 'n' Corn
Chowder, *92*
Wild Rice and Mushroom Soup
with Fresh Herbs, *104*
sour (taste), 113, 117, 120
Sourdough, Toasted Tomato and
Fresh Basil on, *81*
South-of-the-Border Rice, *188*
Southwest Corn-Potato Cakes, *183*
Southwest Fiesta Casserole with
Corn Bread Topping, *167*
soy, 5
Soy Berry Smoothie, **261**
soymilk, 5, 267
Sparkling Cider Mimosa with
Raspberries, *283*
Spiced-Up Tuna, **61**
spicy (taste), 120
Spicy Couscous and Chickpeas,
185
Spicy Linguine with Red Clam
Sauce, *189*
Spicy Shrimp Gumbo over
Couscous, *107*
spinach, 119:
Bay Shrimp Omelet with Sautéed
Spinach and Gruyère Cheese,
28
Gourmet Pizza with White Clam
Sauce, Spinach, Garlic, and
Fresh Tomatoes, *72*
Ham, Cheese, and Spinach
Frittata, *17*
Minestrone with Spinach and
Orzo Pasta, *106*
Sesame Salmon and Spinach
Salad with Asian Vinaigrette,
124
Spinach and Ham Quiche Cups, *8*
Spinach Orange Salad, **115**
Wilted Spinach Salad with Warm
Raspberry Vinaigrette and
Toasted Hazelnuts, *141*
Splenda, 10, **234**, 235, 254, 267,
270, 278
spreads:
Cranberry Chutney, 53
Mexican Five-Layered Spread, *50*
Nut Bread, **61**
Spring Rolls, Chili-Spiced Shrimp,
52

Squash, Ginger, *209*
Steak, Grilled Asian Flank, with
    Wasabi Cream Sauce, *165*
stews, 85–111; case for, 89–91; as
    comfort food, 89; recipes,
    92–111:
    Caribbean One-Pot Stew, *111*
    Hearty Lamb and Barley Stew,
        102
    Old-Fashioned Country
        Vegetable-Beef Stew, *97*
stir fries:
    Instant Stir Fry, **145**
    Stir-Fried Chicken Mu-Shu, *153*
strawberries:
    Fresh Fruit Parfaits with
        Strawberry Coulis, *24*
    Ricotta Tart with Strawberry
        Coulis, *243*
    Strawberry Custard Sundae, **231**
    Strawberry Lemonade, *284*
    Strawberry Shortcake, **231**
    Strawberry Yogurt Pancakes with
        Coconut, *15*
    Strawberry-Banana Coconut Milk
        Smoothie, *275*
    Strawberry-Blueberry Cobbler,
        252
    Toasted Whole Wheat Bagels with
        Brie and Strawberries, *71*
stress: and brain cells, 204–5;
    chronic, 30–31; eating to
    relieve, 29–55; and hormones
    and weight gain, 30–31; and
    memory, 202; nutrition
    meltdown, 31–33; and sleep
    and diet, 29–30; snacks and,
    33
stress cycle, breaking, 32–33
stress hormones, 29, 30, 33
Stuffed Red Bell Peppers, **205**
sugar, 60, 62; addiction, 230–32; in
    breakfasts, 5, 7; and energy
    level, 63; and flavor, 116; on
    labels, **234**; limiting, 174, 206;
    and mental health, 203; natural,
    233; saying "no" to, 32;
    temporary fix, 173
sugar binge, 232–33
sugar substitutes, 10, **234**, 235
sulfur compounds, 206

sulphorophane, 206
Sunrise Special, **261**
Sunshine Rice with Basil and
    Parmesan, *179*
Super-Simple Breakfast, 7
Sushi Roll-Ups, Northwest, with
    Smoked Salmon, *80*
sweet (taste), 113, 117, 120
sweet potato:
    Baked Sweet Potatoes Topped
        with Apples, Cranberries, and
        Nuts, *220*
    Cajun Sweet Potatoes, **205**
    Creamy Sweet Potatoes and
        Yams with Chipotle Peppers,
        217
    Smoky Sweet Potato 'n' Corn
        Chowder, *92*
    Sweet Potato Chutney Salad, *122*
    Sweet Potato with Maple Syrup,
        205
sweets, 171, 173, 229–58; cravings,
    31, 86, 172, 229–34; recipes,
    235–58
Swiss Chard with Garlic and
    Oregano, *218*

Tabbouleh, Quinoa, with Fresh
    Mint, *73*
tacos:
    Build-Your-Own Fish Tacos, *78*
    Mock Taco Salad, **115**
    One-Dish Tacos, **145**
Tandoori Chicken Made Simple,
    170
tannins, 63
tarts:
    Caramelized Leek Tart with
        Apples and Blue Cheese, *48*
    Ricotta Tart with Strawberry
        Coulis, *243*
taste, 113, 117, 118; and health,
    116; and memories/emotions,
    114; qualities in, 113–14
tea, 5, 62–63, 261:
    Hot Chai Tea, *279*
    Raspberry Ice Tea, *280*
Teriyaki, Ginger-, Rice Bowls, *192*
Thai Curry Pasta with Fresh Crab
    and Basil, *195*
Thai Fettuccine with Chicken, *184*

Thai-Grilled Prawns with Coconut
    Dipping Sauce, *44–45*
theobromine, 230
thermogenesis, 59
thirst, 264
thyme:
    Creamy Risotto with Wild
        Mushrooms and Fresh Thyme,
        196
    Individual Meat Loaves with
        Fresh Thyme, *162*
    Zucchini-Tomato Lasagna with
        Fresh Thyme and Caramelized
        Onions, *210–11*
Toast and Cream Cheese, **4**
Toasted Crostini with Brie, Spicy
    Shrimp, and Peach Chutney,
    43
Toasted Tomato and Fresh Basil on
    Sourdough, *81*
Toasted Whole Wheat Bagels with
    Brie and Strawberries, *71*
Tofu Cakes in Sweet Ginger Sauce,
    75
tomatoes:
    Broiled Tomatoes, **205**
    Cioppino in a Robust Tomato
        Base, Infused with Fresh
        Fennel and Orange, *99*
    Creamy Hummus Dip with
        Fresh Tomatoes and Basil,
        39
    Fresh Sliced Tomatoes with Basil,
        115
    Garbanzo Toss with Sun-Dried
        Tomatoes, Red Pepper, and
        Fresh Parsley, *128*
    Garden Tomato Soup with Fresh
        Basil, *93*
    Gourmet Pizza with White Clam
        Sauce, Spinach, Garlic, and
        Fresh Tomatoes, *72*
    Grilled Cheese, Tomato, and
        Roasted Yellow Pepper
        Sandwich, *67*
    Grilled Polenta Rounds with
        Tomato Caponata, *41*
    Halibut with Tomatoes, Basil,
        and Capers, *157*
    Linguine with Tomatoes and
        Fresh Basil, *190*

tomatoes (*cont'd*)
Slow-Roasted Tomatoes and
Pesto on Polenta Pizzas, *51*
Slow-Roasted Tomatoes with
Garlic and Herbs, *221*
sun-dried tomatoes **118**
Toasted Tomato and Fresh Basil
on Sourdough, *81*
Tomato Chutney with Ginger,
46
Tomato 'n' Herb Pasta, **175**
tomato sauce, 47
Zucchini-Tomato Lasagna with
Fresh Thyme and Caramelized
Onions, *210–11*
toxic environment, 116, 264
trace minerals, 132, 184
trans fatty acids, 6, 203
Trifle, Mixed Berry, *224–45*
tryptophan, 33, 172
tuna:
Creamed Tuna, **145**
Spiced-Up Tuna, **61**
turkey:
Grilled Turkey Reuben on Dark
Rye, *77*
Turkey Burgers with Caramelized
Onions, *74*
12-Step Program, **233–34**

Ultimate Bittersweet Chocolate
Pudding, The, *242*
umami, 113–14

vegetables, 33, 201–28; bitter, **117**;
crunchy, 33; and fruits, 119,
206; quantity of, 206–7;
quick-fix, **205–6**; recipes,
208–28; sugar solution for,
117; water content, 265:
California-Style Roasted Veggie
Burrito, *76*
Crab and Veggie Cakes with
Garlic-Chili Cream, *150*
Grilled Vegetables with Garlic
and Balsamic Vinaigrette, *227*
Heartwarming Winter Vegetable
Soup, *98*
Marinated Veggies, **115**
Old-Fashioned Country
Vegetable-Beef Stew, *97*

Roasted Gingered Vegetables,
214
Roasted Veggie Focaccia Layered
with Eggplant, Roasted
Peppers, Portabello
Mushrooms, Feta Cheese,
Arugula, and Garlic Balsamic
Vinaigrette, *79*
Vegetable Cocktail, **262**
vegetable juices, 261
Veggie Bagel Bites, *68*
Veggie Dip, **34**
Veggie Pizza, **60**
Veggie Sandwich, **61**
Veggie Stir-Fry with Ginger and
Black Bean Sauce, *212*
Veggies à la Campbells, **91**
Wild Rice and Roasted
Vegetables with Thyme
Vinaigrette, *126–27*
Very Berry Lemon Pancakes with
Blueberry Sauce, *10–11*
vicious cycle(s): galanin/fatty
foods, 58; sleep/stress/eating
habits/weight problems, **30**;
sugar/energy levels, 63; sugar
fix, 173
Vinaigrette, Asian, Sesame
Salmon and Spinach Salad
with, *124*
Vinaigrette, Garlic Balsamic,
Roasted Veggie Focaccia
Layered with Eggplant,
Roasted Peppers, Portabello
Mushrooms, Feta Cheese,
Arugula, and, *79*
Vinaigrette, Orange, Roasted Beet
Salad with, *131*
Vinaigrette, Red Wine, Greek Pasta
Salad with, *132*
Vinaigrette, Thyme, Wild Rice and
Roasted Vegetables with,
126–27
Vinaigrette, Warm Raspberry, and
Toasted Hazelnuts, Wilted
Spinach Salad with, *141*
vinegars, flavored, **118**
vitamin A, 3, 70, 149
vitamin B$_2$, 244, 263
vitamin B$_6$, 172, 203
vitamin B$_{12}$, 172, 203

vitamin C, 3, 31, 62, 70, 131, 132,
149, 182, 184, 203, 208, 214,
218, 220, 244, 268, 269;
sources of, 206
vitamin E, 3, 10, 31, 70, 94, 131,
220
vitamins, 3, 5, 203, 233

waffles, 2, 58:
Blueberry Waffles, **4**
Wake Up and Smell the Mocha
Cooler, 26, *271*
Waldorf Salad, Mock, **115**
Warm Milk with Honey and
Orange, *273*
water, 32, 90, 203, 233, 265;
getting from food, **263**; need
for, 259–60; versus soda, 264;
and weight control, 263,
264
weight gain, 86, 146, 174;
depression and, 173; in
emotional eating, 87; and
stress and hormones, 30–31
weight loss: breakfast and, 2–3;
drinking and, 263; eating style
and, 58–59; in emotional
eating, 87; water and, 259
weight management, 146, 174;
water in, 264
weight problems: dieting and, 144;
soda in, 264
wheat germ, 10, 20
Wheat Germ, Toasted, Bananas,
and Honey, Rice Cakes Layered
with Low-Fat Peanut Butter
and, *49*
Whipped Cream, Rum, Pumpkin
Pie with, *256*
White Clam Sauce, Spinach, Garlic,
and Fresh Tomatoes, Gourmet
Pizza with, *72*
whole grains, 5–6, 173, 174
Whole Wheat Banana French Toast,
16
Wild Rice, Baked Pork Florentine
with, *168*
Wild Rice and Mushroom Soup
with Fresh Herbs, *104*
Wild Rice and Roasted Vegetables
with Thyme Vinaigrette, *126–27*

Wilted Spinach Salad with Warm
  Raspberry Vinaigrette and
  Toasted Hazelnuts, *141*
wraps:
  Bite-Size Lettuce Wraps, *54*
  Chicken and Peanut Wraps, *83*
  Mexican wraps, 188
  Peanut Butter Wraps, **4**
  Prawn and Asparagus Lettuce
    Wraps with Hoisin Sauce, *69*

Yams, Creamy Sweet Potatoes
  and, with Chipotle Peppers,
  217
Yellow Pepper, Roasted, Grilled
  Cheese, Tomato and,
  Sandwich, *67*
Yogurt, Blueberry Frozen,
  231
Yogurt, Chocolate Chip Frozen,
  231

Yogurt Dressing, Fresh Fruit Salad
  with, *137*
Yogurt Pie, Frozen, **231**

zest **118**
zinc, 10, 31, 130, 132, 203
Zucchini, **205**
Zucchini-Tomato Lasagna with
  Fresh Thyme and Caramelized
  Onions, *210–11*

ABOUT THE AUTHORS

ELIZABETH SOMER, M.A., R.D., is the author of several books, including *The Origin Diet, Food & Mood, Age-Proof Your Body,* and *Nutrition for Women.* She is the editor in chief of *Nutrition Alert,* a newsletter that summarizes current research from more than 6,000 journals, and serves on the advisory board of *Shape* magazine. Elizabeth has appeared frequently as a nutrition correspondent on *Today, Good Morning America,* and *AMNorthWest,* in Portland, Oregon. Her hour-long special, *Age-Proof Your Body,* aired on national public television in 2001.

JEANETTE WILLIAMS is a registered nurse who attributes her culinary passion to the "melting pot" of her hometown, Newton, Massachusetts. In this densely populated city with many small ethnic neighborhoods, her family, friends, and neighbors shared gardens, recipes, stories, and traditions. Jeanette put herself through nursing school waiting tables at a local restaurant, where she also spent time in the kitchen learning the chefs' secrets. She has worked with Elizabeth for years developing recipes for numerous projects, including such books as *Food & Mood, The Origin Diet,* and *Nutrition for a Healthy Pregnancy,* and is a consultant and recipe developer for numerous companies, including the California Fruit and Tomato Kitchens. She lives in Salem, Oregon, with her husband and two daughters.